Autism Spectrum Disorders

D1519946

AUTISM SPECTRUM DISORDERS: APPLIED BEHAVIOR ANALYSIS, EVIDENCE, AND PRACTICE

Edited by
Peter Sturmey
Adrienne Fitzer

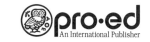
An International Publisher

8700 Shoal Creek Boulevard
Austin, Texas 78757-6897
800/897-3202 Fax 800/397-7633
www.proedinc.com

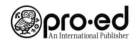
An International Publisher

© 2007 by PRO-ED, Inc.
8700 Shoal Creek Boulevard
Austin, Texas 78757-6897
800/897-3202   Fax 800/397-7633
www.proedinc.com

Library of Congress Cataloging-in-Publication Data

    Autism spectrum disorders : applied behavior analysis, evidence,
and practice / edited by Peter Sturmey and Adrienne Fitzer.
       p. ; cm.
    Includes bibliographical references and index.
    ISBN-13: 978-1-4164-0209-1
    ISBN-10: 1-4164-0209-8
    1. Autism in children.   2. Autistic children—Rehabilitation.
3. Behavioral assessment.   4. Education.   I. Sturmey, Peter.   II. Fitzer,
Adrienne.
    [DNLM: 1. Autistic Disorder—therapy.   2. Behavioral Medicine—
methods.   WM 203.5 A93845 2007]
RJ506.A9A98   2007
618.92'85882—dc22

                                  2006012485

Art Director: Jason Crosier
Designer: Nancy McKinney
This book is designed in Goudy.

Printed in the United States of America

1 2 3 4 5 6 7 8 9 10   11 10 09 08 07

Dedicated

to

William Jack Palmore

and

Adam Jay Fitzer

CONTENTS

PREFACE

The last 20 years have seen an increasing interest in applied behavior analysis (ABA) and Autism Spectrum Disorders (ASDs). This reflects the increasing prevalence of ASD, the potential for ABA to provide significant habilitation or even perhaps recovery from autism, recognition of milder forms of the disorder such as Pervasive Developmental Disorder–Not Otherwise Specified and Asperger syndrome, earlier detection, considerable parental and legal advocacy for early interventions and other services, and greater public awareness of these issues in the media.

Treatment of ASD remains controversial. It has continued to attract treatments that are unsubstantiated and even harmful; some have even referred to autism as a "fad magnet." There has been extensive biological research, including fairly robust evidence of a significant genetic contribution to the cause of autism. However, although this research has described some of the biological features of autism more clearly than hitherto had been known, it has not yet led to highly specified models of the causes of autism that have translated into effective treatments. Although various biological treatments have been heralded as effective, these hopes have not been substantiated by research. For example, the use of secretin has been repeatedly shown to be ineffective, and the evidence for the effectiveness of popular psychotropic medications such as risperidone has also been questioned. In addition, many popular nonbiological-based treatments have also been shown to be ineffective or have not been evaluated in controlled studies. Thus, we have the problem of more and more children being identified with ASD, a need for rapid expansion of services for these children, and a plethora of unevaluated or ineffective treatments.

In contrast with other approaches, ABA has extensive empirical support for use with people with ASD dating back to the early 1960s. It is not the work or opinion of one researcher, school, or center that defines ABA but the collective work of many over a period of 50 years or more. ABA is a strong and coherent science that is the basis for the technologies and procedures supported by research that are typically used in practice with learners with ASD. This research is on public record, has been conducted by many researchers, and has been independently replicated many times.

ABA is not synonymous with discrete trial teaching (DTT), nor is it a different science from applied verbal behavior (AVB). DTT and AVB are examples of procedures that were developed from the science of applied behavior analysis, yet many who claim to be trained in ABA are not aware of these distinctions or the other myths and misconceptions about ABA.

With the increased demand for applied behavior analytic services, the number of practitioners has expanded in such a way that many practitioners have limited or no professional training in ABA or may have received training that was explicitly hostile to ABA. Even worse, many who have little or no effective professional supervision are put in charge of running home-based and school-based ABA programs.

Autism Spectrum Disorders: Applied Behavior Analysis, Evidence, and Practice is not a replacement for formal training in ABA, but we believe that this single volume concisely summarizes the science of behavior analysis and its application to people with autism. This book was written for those familiar with the elementary concepts of ABA such as are provided in an undergraduate course in learning theory or gained through a few months of experience working with learners in ABA-based programs. Readers from different backgrounds will be exposed to the breadth of areas that are researched within the field of ABA and the technologies and procedures that are used in the most well-known and well-developed programs for learners with ASD. Masters- and doctoral-level psychologists, speech pathologists, occupational and physical therapists, psychiatrists, pediatricians' supervisors, behavior analysts, educational administrators, special education and mainstream teachers, classroom assistants, and primary caregivers working and living with children and adults with autism spectrum disorders will find the information in this volume helpful when developing and providing services. In addition, researchers and professors teaching undergraduate and graduate students will find this book well suited for use as a reference or class text.

Organization of the Book

The book is organized into eight chapters. The chapters are written by authors who are currently active researchers and practitioners and leaders in the field of autism spectrum disorders. Hence, each chapter contains up-to-date summaries of the research literature and explicit practitioner recommendations based on this literature. These recommendations, found at the end of each chapter, provide the reader with a practical summary of what research has identified as the most effective practices.

In Chapter 1 Tristram Smith, David McAdam, and Deborah Napolitano describe the defining features of ASD and describe the wide range of skills and abilities of people with ASD. The authors take a historical perspective as they show how behavior analysis began with laboratory demonstrations of operant conditioning in children with ASD and then moved to applications to individual behavior, such as training specific skills and reducing specific maladaptive behaviors. In the final section of the chapter, the authors note that although there is extensive research on ABA and ASD, further research is still needed in many areas.

In Chapter 2 William H. Ahearn, Rebecca MacDonald, Richard B. Graff, and William V. Dube consider the nature of behaviorism and identify and address some of the misconceptions regarding behaviorism. They then provide a detailed account of ABA and ASD that systematically bridges basic and applied behavioral research. They describe the basic processes of learning, including operant conditioning, response differentiation, operant extinction, stimulus control, discrimination, and generalization. They then discuss the application of these basic concepts to teach people with ASD by distinguishing between simple and conditional discriminations, identity and arbitrary matching to sample procedures, equivalence class formation and stimulus overselectivity and its remediation in people with ASD. They describe the variety of prompting procedures and discuss the technology of transfer of stimulus control. In the section on consequence operations, they provide a concise account of the limits of informal methods of reinforcer assessment and describe the varieties of stimulus preference assessment methods that have been developed. This chapter is conceptually sophisticated and contains a concise account of all the basic learning processes that practitioners and parents should be familiar with when using ABA with people with ASD.

In Chapter 3 Ruth Anne Rehfeldt and Rocio Rosales review the research on readiness skills and lay out how to teach such skills as sitting, eye contact, joint attention, attention to materials, and generalized imitation. They also review reinforcement control and methods for establishing compliance. If readiness skills are not successfully taught to children with ASD, their lives will be greatly restricted. It is urgent that these skills be effectively taught within the first few years of life if children are to learn.

Chapter 4, also by Rehfeldt and Rosales, addresses self-help skills, which are essential for effective functioning. People who are not toilet trained, do not dress or feed themselves, and so on are significantly disabled, may be viewed negatively by others, and consume expensive public services because they require additional staff or parent time to perform these basic functions for them. Rehfeldt and Rosales summarize the wide range of approaches to teaching these skills that are so vital to effective daily functioning. The authors review commonly used behavioral technologies, including task analysis and response chaining, programming generalization through multiple exemplar training and general case training, activity schedules and other visually based methods of teaching, various forms of modeling, and self-management. The final part of this chapter reviews interventions to teach more sophisticated community skills.

In Chapter 5 Dorothea C. Lerman, Valerie M. Volkert, and Linda LeBlanc review some of the common deficits and excesses in social behavior in people with ASD and outline beginning, intermediate, and advanced social skills. They distinguish interventions that are mediated through the behavior of adults and those mediated through peers. Finally, they note the importance of analyzing and planning generalization of social behavior in any program.

Children and adults with ASD demonstrate a wide range of communication disorders ranging from complete lack of spoken or any other functional communicative behavior through subtle deficits in content, grammar, or nonverbal aspects of communication. In Chapter 6 Jeff Sigafoos, Mark F. O'Reilly, Ralf W. Schlosser, and Giulio E. Lancioni review this full range of behavioral deficits and excesses and provide an analysis of these problems by referencing Skinner's *Verbal Behavior*. The authors review Skinner's approach to language and the distinctions between different classes of verbal behavior. Mutism, echolalia, and lack of spontaneity are all examples of common communication problems in ASD. The authors present an analysis and review of interventions for each of these problems and address the issues of generalization and environmental modification to promote appropriate verbal behavior.

Maladaptive behaviors such as aggression, self-injury, and tantrums are some of the most restricting and dangerous that people with ASD display. Rigidity in routines, food selectivity and refusal, and extreme fearful behavior can also restrict their lives a great deal. In Chapter 7 Richard G. Smith, Timothy R. Vollmer, and Claire St. Peter Pipkin provide a comprehensive and conceptually coherent account of behavioral explanations and treatments for these severely challenging problems. The authors begin by reviewing the evidence that problem behavior is maintained by one of four types of contingencies: positive social, negative social, automatic positive, and automatic negative reinforcement. They describe experimental analysis, descriptive analysis, and anecdotal assessment, the three kinds of technologies used to identify the contingencies maintaining problem behavior. The authors then describe function-based treatments such as extinction, differential reinforcement, interventions based on establishing operations, and skills training. They also review other behavioral interventions that are not clearly function based, such as response blocking and punishment, as well as a variety of antecedent-based interventions. Knowing the function of the problem behavior and developing a treatment based on that function is not enough to implement an effective behavioral treatment. Smith and his colleagues describe staff and training methods, considerations relating to the ecology of intervention, and how to address maintenance and prevent relapse.

Teaching skills and treatment of individual problem behavior does not take place in a vacuum. These interventions take place in the context of busy and sometimes stressed families and in classrooms and residential services with multiple demands on staff. In Chapter 8 Sandra L. Harris, Robert H. LaRue, and Mary Jane Weiss review these issues, drawing from their own extensive work teaching ABA and other skills to family members as well as providing support to family members, such as support groups for siblings. They discuss the importance of using behavioral skills training—combinations of instruction, rehearsal, and feedback—as an essential and effective method of teaching skills to family members and staff. In the second and third parts of the chapter, the authors address special issues concerning parents and siblings and professionals providing services to people with autism spectrum disorders, including stress management and the dissemination of services to learners of different social and economic backgrounds.

Acknowledgments

Several colleagues and friends have assisted us in this project. Professor Susan Croll, Dr. Daphna El-Roy, John Ward-Horner, Ron Lee, and Robin M. Havens all read early versions of portions of the book. We are grateful to them for their feedback. We would also like to acknowledge the faculty of the Learning Processes Doctoral Program, The Graduate Center, City University of New York, Professors Alvero, Brown, Fields, Hemmes, Lanson, Poulson, and Ranaldi, whose teaching and collegial input over the last 5 years has been instrumental in sharpening our thinking. We also thank the numerous graduate students at Queens College whose research has provoked, stimulated, and provided us with further education. Finally, we thank those people with autism spectrum disorders, their families, and the staff who work with them who have inspired us to research, write, and teach and to give more of ourselves for the improvement of services for people with ASD.

Thanks to the Authors

We would like to thank our chapter authors. We selected them because of their active contributions to research and practice in this area. We hoped for high-quality, research-based chapters and practical recommendations that readers of this volume could act upon; we were not disappointed. We thank them for the excellent quality and timeliness of their contributions and their responsiveness to our feedback. They fulfilled our high expectations and were fun to work with. We could ask for nothing more.

CHAPTER

AUTISM AND
APPLIED BEHAVIOR ANALYSIS

Tristram Smith, David McAdam, and Deborah Napolitano
University of Rochester Medical School

Singing "Twinkle, Twinkle Little Star" as he plays, 3-year-old Jason skillfully assembles jigsaw puzzles, puts objects through a shape sorter, and writes letters with a marker. Apart from singing, however, he seldom speaks, and during most activities he flicks his fingers in front of his eyes. He does not seem to notice other people coming and going in the room, and he screams when they ask to play with him. Over time, it becomes evident that he is repeating the same song, activities, and movements again and again.

Ryan, who is 10 years old, is an "A" student in his fifth-grade class. He enjoys schoolwork, and he likes talking to his teachers. However, he talks only about different kinds of trains, avoids eye contact, and ignores attempts to change the topic. He spends most of his free time reading about trains and organizing his train collection. He tries to interact with his classmates. However, he has no friends, and some children rebuff him because of his eccentricities. Changes in routine such as field trips are a source of great distress to him.

F or parents, teachers, and other caregivers, children like Jason and Ryan raise many questions and concerns. The two children, whose names have been changed to protect their confidentiality, are very different from each other, yet each has a diagnosis of autism. Both struggle to cope with everyday situations, yet they also display remarkable abilities, notably Jason's proficiency with puzzles, letters, and shapes and Ryan's excellent academic achievement. What, then, is autism, and why did both children receive this diagnosis? Why do they struggle, and will they continue to do so all their lives, or are their abilities a sign that it is possible to help them?

Fortunately, research has answered some of these questions, though much remains to be learned. We now have reliable descriptions of the types of behavior that are associated with autism. These descriptions make it possible to identify autism in children like Jason and Ryan at various ages and levels of functioning. Identification of children with autism is important because effective interventions have been found to address their skill deficits and problem behavior. Despite substantial gaps in our understanding of autism, and despite the limitations of available interventions, enough is known that when caregivers are well informed they and their children can benefit. Accordingly, this chapter gives an overview of what we know about autism and interventions for children with this diagnosis.

Autism

There is no biological marker or simple laboratory test on which clinicians can rely to diagnose autism. Rather, the diagnosis is based on behavior that children display. Diagnosticians conduct careful observations and interviews to identify such behavior, and they refer to standard criteria for determining whether these forms of behavior meet requirements for a classification of autism. The most widely accepted criteria are presented in the *Diagnostic and Statistical Manual of Mental Disorders—Fourth Edition Text Revision* (DSM–IV–TR; American Psychiatric Association [APA], 2000) and the *International Classification of Diseases—10th Edition* (World Health Organization, 1994). In these diagnostic systems, autism has three defining characteristics:

1. qualitative impairment in reciprocal social interaction,

2. qualitative impairment in verbal and nonverbal communication and in imaginative activity, and

3. markedly restricted and repetitive repertoire of behavior, activities, and interests.

The severity of these difficulties varies greatly across children, as illustrated by Jason and Ryan. Like Jason, some children with autism are so socially impaired that they appear almost completely unaware of others. However, many display attachments to caregivers and a desire to interact with peers, although they may have poor eye contact and lack important conversational and social skills. Similarly, some children with autism have essentially no verbal or nonverbal language. Jason will echo words, songs, or scripts that he has heard, and some, like Ryan, have communicative speech, although it may be limited to stating requests or delivering monologues on topics that preoccupy them. The restricted activities of children with autism may comprise stereotypies, such as rocking their bodies back and forth or flapping their hands in front of their eyes as Jason does. Some may engage in actions with objects, such as arranging toys into neat rows, making wheels spin, turning light switches on and off, or pouring water over and over again. In other cases, restricted activities may follow a complex pattern, such as insisting on adhering to a routine or developing a fascination with a highly specific topic; Ryan's perseveration with trains is a typical example.

In addition to the defining features of autism, many other characteristics are common but not universal. About 75% of children with autism have delays in development such as slow acquisition of language skills or performance in the range of mental retardation on standardized tests (APA, 2000). Like Jason, many show uneven development, often with more advanced visual–spatial than verbal skills. Approximately 10% may show skills that are far more advanced than their overall developmental level (Treffert, 1988); these savant or splinter skills may include precocious reading, rapid mathematical calculations, or strong memory for particular facts. Behavioral difficulties are frequent, with more than 90% of children diagnosed with autism having tantrums of some form and perhaps 10% to 20% engaging in either self-injurious or aggressive behavior (Lovaas, 1987). Many children with autism also display unusually picky eating habits, problems initiating and maintaining sleep, and sensory anomalies, such as apparent lack of response to sounds or physical pain (APA, 2000).

Other Pervasive Developmental Disorders and the Autism Spectrum

In the *DSM–IV–TR* (APA, 2000), autism is classified as one of five pervasive developmental disorders (PDDs), along with Rett's Disorder, Childhood

Disintegrative Disorder, Asperger's Disorder, and Pervasive Developmental Disorder–Not Otherwise Specified (PDD-NOS). Rett's Disorder is a degenerative disorder that occurs almost exclusively in girls. Although it may resemble autism during the preschool years, its etiology, presentation, course, and response to treatment are distinct from autism (Kerr & Ravine, 2003); for this reason, it should be classified separately in future editions of diagnostic manuals. Childhood Disintegrative Disorder is diagnosed when signs of autism emerge between the ages of 3 and 5 years, following a history of typical development. This diagnosis is rare and poorly understood (Mouridsen, 2003) and therefore will not be considered further here.

Current criteria for Asperger's Disorder emphasize impairments in social interaction and nonverbal communication similar to those found in autism but without delays in development of cognitive or language skills (APA, 2000). Children with Asperger's Disorder have pedantic and poorly modulated speech, poor conversational skills, literal use of language, and intense preoccupation with circumscribed topics, such as train timetables or power pylons. They are usually unable to form friends because of their naive, inappropriate, and one-sided social interactions. However, many individuals with Asperger's Disorder reportedly desire successful interpersonal relationships and are puzzled when they do not achieve them. Diagnostic manuals such as the *DSM–IV–TR* (APA, 2000) also note that individuals with Asperger's Disorder commonly have deficits in motor skills and may appear to be clumsy.

Children who display features of autism but do not meet criteria for Autistic Disorder might be classified as having PDD-NOS. Thus, the criteria for this diagnosis substantially overlap with those for Autistic and Asperger's Disorders. Because of the many similarities among Autistic Disorder, Asperger's Disorder, and PDD-NOS, much debate has taken place over whether these three classifications are really separate disorders or are simply variations of the same condition. In support of the latter view, Wing (1988) introduced the concept of a spectrum or continuum to capture the idea that the same disorder may vary in severity of presentation. From this perspective, the problems seen in Autistic Disorder, Asperger's Disorder, and PDD-NOS may reflect different degrees of impaired social understanding, with the mildest impairments "shad[ing] into the eccentric end of the wide range of normal behavior" (Wing, 1992, p. 138). Proponents of the "continuum" perspective commonly refer to autism, Asperger's Disorder, and PDD-NOS collectively as Autism Spectrum Disorders (ASD).

Other investigators favor the current *DSM* classification scheme. They distinguish Asperger's Disorder from autism by citing evidence that children with Asperger's Disorder tend to have higher verbal than visual–motor skills, whereas the reverse tends to be true for children with autism (Ghaziuddin & Mountain-Kimchi, 2004). Also, children with Asperger's Disorder are described as making awkward social approaches and having intellectual preoccupations, whereas children with Autistic Disorder may tend to avoid all social contact and focus on repetitive motor activities (Szatmari, Archer, Fisman, Streiner, & Wilson, 1995). However, many studies have failed to detect two distinct groups (Manjiviona & Prior, 1999; Miller & Ozonoff, 2000; Prior et al., 1998). Reliable criteria for differentiating between groups are not currently available. For example, some clinicians might diagnose a child like Ryan with Asperger's Disorder, whereas others might consider him to be a high-functioning child with autism. At present, there are no standard methods for deciding which diagnosis is correct. Also, the important issue of whether the diagnosis makes a meaningful difference for planning and implementing treatment has yet to be answered; there are no known implications for behavioral, psychopharmacological, or other intervention.

An additional argument for the spectrum view is that the behavior in which children with autism, Asperger's Disorder, and PDD-NOS may engage is not unique to children with these diagnoses. For example, many children with mental retardation display high rates of repetitive behavior and intense preoccupations, and many preschoolers show behavior that is associated with autism, such as tantrums, picky eating, and poor sleeping. Indeed, research indicates that everyone occasionally displays autistic traits such as difficulty maintaining a back-and-forth conversation, repetitive behavior, or insistence on a routine (Constantino & Todd, 2003; Rafaeli-Mor, Foster, & Berkson, 1999).

Although research continues on whether the spectrum or discrete disorder view is more accurate, the absence of a clear demarcation between autism and other PDDs, or even between autism and typical behavior, has led most clinicians and researchers to favor the spectrum view. In keeping with this preference, the term *ASD* rather than *PDD* will be used hereafter.

Etiology and Epidemiology

ASDs appear to have a strong genetic basis, and many individuals with ASD show signs of atypical neurobiological development. Evidence for the role of genetics comes from studies showing that ASD clusters in families and that the risk for a particular family member is linked to the genetic similarity of the affected individual. Identical twins share 100% of their genes with each other. When one identical twin has autism, the risk for the other is approximately 60%, rising as high as 93% if milder variants such as Asperger's Disorder are included (Bailey et al., 1995). Fraternal twins and other siblings share 50% of their genes. When one sibling has autism, the risk for the other is about 3% to 7% (Simonoff, 1998). Recently, investigators have identified several specific genes that may confer vulnerability to autism, although more studies of these genes are needed (Nicolson & Szatmari, 2003).

Studies consistently show that children with autism have an enlarged head circumference (Courchesne, Carper, & Akshoomoff, 2003). Brain imaging studies allow investigators to explore this finding by looking inside the head to examine brain structure and activity. Although studies to date have not yet given clear answers as to why the enlarged head circumference occurs, some noteworthy findings have emerged. For example, most but not all studies show abnormalities in the cerebellum (Courchesne, Yeung-Courchesne, Press, Hesselink, & Jernigan, 1988), which may be involved in sequencing movements in order to perform a complex activity (e.g., grooming and hygiene tasks, sports). Most also show abnormalities in the amygdala, which may contribute to recognizing faces and decoding emotional expressions (Baron-Cohen et al., 2000). Several additional studies indicate abnormalities in the posterior hippocampus (Saitoh, Courschesne, Egaas, Lincoln, & Schreibman, 1995), which may be associated with complex (nonrote) learning. Several structures in the brain stem associated with attention also have been implicated (Rodier, 2000). Finally, individuals with autism appear to show unusual patterns of activation in the cortex when shown faces (Schultz et al., 2000); these patterns may be linked to their difficulties in identifying faces and facial expressions. However, much remains unknown about how these abnormalities give rise to the types of behavior that people with autism exhibit.

In the past, autism was considered rare. Since the late 1980s, however, reported prevalence rates have risen. For example, in the California Regional Centers, which coordinate services for individuals with developmental disabilities who reside in the state, the number of individuals who were diagnosed with autism grew by about 250% from 1987 to 1998 (Department of Developmental Services, 1999). In public schools, the number of children who were classified as having autism more than doubled during the 1990s (U.S. Department of Education, 2002). In the 1980s, it was estimated that autism occurred in 1 of every 2,500 children, but the current estimate is that it occurs in 1 of 750 to 1,000 children (Fombonne, 2003). For all ASDs, the prevalence may be about 1 in 200 (Chakrabarti & Fombonne, 2001).

Importantly, these numbers may reflect changes in diagnostic practice, rather than a real increase in the prevalence of autism. For example, the 1987 revision of the *DSM* significantly expanded the number of children who met criteria for a diagnosis of autism (Volkmar, Cicchetti, Bregman, & Cohen, 1992). In 1990, federal law changed to include autism as a classification that qualified students for special education services (Individuals with Disabilities Education Act of 1990 [IDEA]). In the 1990s, the concept of the autism spectrum gained widespread acceptance, and Asperger's Disorder was included for the first time in standard diagnostic systems such as *DSM–IV*. In 2000, the American Association of Neurology and the American Academy of Pediatrics began recommending that physicians screen all young children for autism (American

Academy of Pediatrics, 2000). Recent studies of the prevalence of autism have used broader criteria for diagnosing autism and ASD than did earlier studies (Fombonne, 2003).

The Centers for Disease Control have initiated long-term investigations to monitor the rate of autism using the same diagnostic criteria from year to year (Yeargin-Allsopp et al., 2003). These investigations will answer definitively whether the rate of autism is increasing or remaining the same. Certainly, however, criteria for diagnosing autism have evolved, and children who would not have qualified for a diagnosis of autism or ASD a few years ago do qualify now.

A few investigators believe the rise in prevalence estimates reflects an actual increase in the disorder, and they implicate vaccines (Wakefield et al., 1998), toxicity from metals such as mercury (Geier & Geier, 2003), pollutants (Kreiling, Stephens, & Reinisch, 2005), and toxins in foods (Reichelt, Knivsberg, Lind, & Nodland, 1991). However, at the time of printing, no conclusive evidence has demonstrated a causal relationship between vaccines and the onset of autism (Institute of Medicine, 2004), and no relationship has been found between autism and metal toxicity, pollutants, or foods (Volkmar & Pauls, 2003).

Interventions for Children with ASD

Because ASDs are associated with problems in learning, a logical intervention approach is to provide specialized instruction to teach skills that children with ASD have been otherwise unable to learn. Indeed, research indicates that such instruction is currently the most effective intervention for these children (New York State Department of Health, 2001). Most studies on specialized instruction focus on teaching approaches derived from applied behavior analysis (ABA). These approaches are described later in this chapter and elaborated in subsequent chapters.

Two other teaching approaches that have generated some research are the Project for the Treatment and Education of Autistic and Related Communication Handicapped Children (TEACCH) and the Denver Model. Project TEACCH emphasizes relationship development between professionals and parents; the teaching of vocational, social, and independent living skills; and the use of visual supports to promote self-management of one's own behavior (Marcus, Schopler, & Lord, 2001). In the Denver Model, teachers aim to establish "warm, affectionate, playful relationships" and encourage individuals with autism to exercise control in these relationships by choosing activities, asking to finish activities, and taking turns in songs and games (Rogers, Hall, Osaki, Reaven, & Herbison, 2001). These interventions have not yet been evaluated in well-designed studies, but preliminary evidence suggests that the TEACCH and Denver models might be beneficial for some persons with ASD (Marcus et al., 2001; Rogers et al., 2001).

Another influential intervention approach, the Developmental Individual-difference Relationship-based (DIR) model, involves a combination of specialized instruction and "Floor Time" (Greenspan, 2000). The goal of Floor Time is to follow the child's lead and invite interactions in order to foster social and emotional development. DIR has many proponents, but systematic evaluations are needed to determine whether or not it is effective.

Although specialized instruction is the primary intervention for individuals with ASD, psychoactive medications (i.e., medications that alter brain function) also are a logical approach. Research confirms that they may augment specialized instruction in treating problem behavior displayed by some individuals with ASD, such as self-injury, aggression toward others, repetitive behavior, or overactivity (Volkmar & Weisner, 2004). For example, risperidone (Risperdal), which is an atypical antipsychotic medication, often reduces self-injury and aggression (McCracken et al., 2002); recently, it was approved as a treatment for children with ASD who display high levels of these types of behavior. Selective Serotonin Reuptake Inhibitors (SSRIs) such as Prozac, which are commonly used to treat anxiety and depression, also may reduce repetitive behavior or perseveration exhibited by some children with ASD, such as Jason's hand-flapping and Ryan's preoccupation with trains. A network of research centers has now undertaken a large study to evaluate the effects of an SSRI on repetitive and perseverative behavior (Vitiello & Wagner, 2004).

Although specialized instruction and in some cases medication are effective interventions, they are not cures for ASD. Thus, practitioners and families are eager to implement other treatments that would improve outcomes. Unfortunately, this eagerness has led to a proliferation of unproven or fad treatments, many of which attract a great deal of publicity (Jacobson, Foxx, & Mulick, 2004). For example, Facilitated Communication is an intervention in which a trained instructor holds the hand of an individual with autism and guides the person to type messages on a keyboard. A film that touted this intervention was nominated for an Academy Award in 2005, many years after research had exposed the intervention as having no value (Jacobson, Mulick, & Schwartz, 1995). In 1998, news stories on television and in other media reported dramatic success from prescribing the pancreatic hormone secretin; however, these stories were based on results obtained with only one individual with autism, and numerous well-designed investigations subsequently failed to show any benefit for other individuals (Sturmey, 2004). Complementary and alternative medicines such as high doses of vitamins or diets that restrict consumption of certain foods also are commonly used (Smith & Antolovich, 2000); however, these interventions are unsupported by research and are viewed skeptically by many researchers and data-based practitioners. This skepticism is based on the lack of a logical theoretical link between how a particular intervention works and what is known about biology and behavior in children with ASD.

Behaviorism

As noted, teaching approaches derived from ABA are the most extensively studied interventions for teaching new skills to individuals with ASD: hundreds of empirical studies have now been published in professional peer-reviewed journals.

ABA grew out of the work of B. F. Skinner and other scientists who described their philosophy of science as behaviorism. According to behaviorists, three factors determine the types of behavior that persons acquire during their lifetime: (a) their biological makeup, (b) the culture in which they live, and (c) their individual learning history. The interaction among these factors creates each person's unique characteristics and explains the differences among humans (Chiesa, 1994).

While recognizing that biology and culture are crucial to human development, behavior analysts are especially interested in learning. For this reason, behavior analysts who work with children with ASD focus mainly on what behavior the child has learned and how to help him or her learn new skills. To behavior analysts, biological studies such as the ones previously discussed are likely to be helpful in understanding ASD and may one day lead to effective treatments. Cultural factors also are relevant; for example, culture may influence what behavior families and practitioners want the children to learn and which methods of instruction are acceptable. Nevertheless, behavior analysts consider learning to be important and worthy of study in its own right.

Skinner advocated a science of learning and behavior that emphasizes identifying functional relationships between behavior and environmental events (Bijou, 1993; Skinner, 1938, 1953). He distinguished this approach from the practice of attempting to explain behavior in terms of hypothesized internal states such as anxiety. For example, to understand the behavior of children with disabilities such as ASD, Skinner and his colleagues emphasized observing how their behavior was influenced by environmental events such as children's physical surroundings or the reactions they received from others (e.g., parental attention).

Skinner did not deny that internal states or events exist. Rather, he argued that internal (or private) events are unique to each individual and difficult to objectively measure and study (Skinner, 1950, 1953). For example, Jason might experience what is commonly called "anxiety" when other people ask him to play. Because of his limited communication skills, however, he cannot report feeling anxious. Even if he were able to do so, listeners would not know whether his report truly reflected his internal state or was a response to social contingencies. The only evidence of anxiety that observers may have is that he clenches his fists, tenses and raises his shoulder muscles, and screams when approached by other people. Therefore, the most promising way to find an effective intervention may be to examine the relationship between the behavior and the environment. Given that the antecedent is the approach of others, parents and practitioners might give him the opportunity to earn access to favorite toys or activities if he keeps his hands open, shoulders down, and voice quiet after being in close proximity to others for a short time. Then they could gradually increase the amount of time he spends in close proximity to others. Evidence that this intervention is successful might be a decrease or absence of screaming and an increase in peer interaction. Thus, in this example, it was beneficial to identify the behavior that Jason was displaying and its antecedent in order to change aspects of the environment. Because a functional relationship between the behavior of screaming and the antecedent of proximity to others was evident, it does not appear to have been necessary to label the behavior as anxiety or to say that anxiety caused Jason to scream (Friman, Hayes, & Wilson, 1998).

In addition to emphasizing functional relationships between behavior and environmental events, Skinner set the occasion for the development of behavior analysis by distinguishing between respondent conditioning and operant learning. Respondent behavior is elicited by antecedent stimuli. For example, a young boy who is bitten by a vicious dog might, in the future, display a conditioned physiological arousal, including increased heart rate and sweating, whenever he sees a dog, no matter how docile it appears. Thus, dogs have become antecedent stimuli for physiological arousal.

In contrast, operant learning occurs because of the relationship between particular classes of behavior and the consequences that follow them. It requires that three conditions are met: (a) a behavior must be emitted in the presence of an antecedent stimulus, (b) the behavior is followed by a consequent event (called a reinforcer or punisher), and (c) future likelihood of the behavior increases or decreases). Behavior analysts use the term "three-term contingency" to describe this relationship among the antecedent, behavior, and consequence.

An example of operant learning is reading sight words. A girl may respond to the antecedent stimulus of a written word by emitting the behavior of correctly reading it. If she receives the consequence of verbal praise and social attention from her mother contingent on this behavior, and if that attention increases her future rate of correct reading, operant learning has occurred. Experiences such as these make up a person's individualized learning history (see Chapter 2 for more on operant learning).

In humans, operant conditioning is usually combined with other behavioral processes. These processes include rule-governed behavior (i.e., behavior shaped by either the verbal behavior of another person or the combination of the verbal behavior of another person in direct contact with contingencies), imitation (i.e., repeating actions performed by another individual), and shaping (i.e., the differential reinforcement of approximations to a targeted behavior). For example, typically developing young children learning to hit a baseball might be initially told by their parents to place their hands on the bat, to position their feet in a particular way, and to swing at the ball only if it crosses home plate. The parents might also demonstrate these actions. When playing in a baseball game with their friends, correct hitting then might be further shaped by the nonverbal contingencies between hitting form and correctly hitting the baseball. Many cultural practices in which we participate, such as playing baseball, are shaped and reinforced by the culture in which we live because members of our culture have determined them to be socially important practices to continue.

Another important behavioral process is the "establishing operation" (EO). This term describes events that influence whether or not a person is motivated to behave in a particular way (Keller & Schoenfeld, 1950). According to Michael (1993), an EO can be defined as

> an environmental event, operation, or stimulus condition that affects an organism by momentarily altering (a) the reinforcing effectiveness of other events and (b) the frequency of occurrence of that part of the organism's repertoire relevant to those events as consequences. (p. 192)

In this definition, an EO has two main effects, which Michael (1982) called *reinforcer establishing* and *evocative*. For example, briefly depriving a child with autism of liquids such as fruit juice or water is an EO that establishes these liquids as having reinforcement value for the child. It also may have the evocative effect of increasing behavior that the child has previously used to obtain a drink (e.g., verbally requesting a drink).

ABA for Children with Autism

Origins

ABA, like all other natural sciences, has been developed step-by-step, with new studies building on earlier ones (Lovaas & Smith, 1989). Thus, these interventions are not the same now as they were in the past, and they are not the product of any one investigator or any single research report. Rather, they have evolved gradually and continually over time, with contributions from many investigators.

Applications of behavior analysis to children with autism began in the early 1960s. At that time, most investigators hypothesized that autistic behavior resulted from trauma in infancy and did not expect that behavioral intervention strategies could change the behavior of persons with autism. In the initial behavior analytic study, Ferster and DeMeyer (1962) used operant conditioning to teach behavior such as pulling levers to three children with autism. Although teaching these responses did not help the children function more effectively in everyday situations, the potential usefulness of behavioral education strategies was clear, and investigators soon extended these findings to important clinical problems such as the ones that challenge Jason and Ryan. In the first of these investigations, Wolf, Risley, and Mees (1964) successfully increased cooperation and language skills in one boy with autism. Shortly thereafter, Lovaas, Freitag, Gold, and Kassorla (1965) found that self-injurious behavior of a child with autism was reinforced by social attention from other people, and they reduced the self-injury by withholding attention. This study provided one of the first examples of how problem behavior of persons with ASD may have a specific environmental function (i.e., may serve to obtain a particular consequence that is reinforcing to the individual, such as attention from others). As such, the study confirmed behaviorists' belief that environmental events, such as the actions of other people, influence the problem behavior of persons with ASD. The work of Lovaas and colleagues was a forerunner of what is now called the functional analysis of problem behavior (Iwata, Vollmer, & Zarcone, 1990).

During this period, investigators also reported that behavior analysis could be effective for many other groups of children and adults. These studies produced considerable excitement and led to the recognition of ABA as a science and burgeoning profession. Baer, Wolf, and Risley (1968) outlined the key elements of this new profession: *applied* means that the focus is on socially important issues; *behavioral* indicates that it emphasizes measurable outcomes; and *analytic* refers to the use of a well-controlled experimental design to document whether an intervention works and, if so, why. Baer and colleagues (1968) noted that other essential aspects of ABA are that it is technological (describing interventions operationally), conceptually systematic (relying on established behavioral principles such as reinforcement), effective (aiming to produce large, socially significant behavior changes), and general (intended to yield changes that are durable across time and environments).

Development

Behavior analysts work continually to expand their understanding of human behavior and to improve interventions for socially important problems. Consistent with this approach, investigators in the late 1960s and early 1970s expanded on early studies of ABA for children with autism by documenting procedures for enhancing individual skills (e.g., expressive language, toileting) and reducing problem behavior (e.g., flapping hands, hitting others). By this time, researchers and clinicians recognized that children with autism did not learn in the same manner as typically developing children (Lovaas, Schreibman, Koegel, & Rehm, 1971). To increase the likelihood that a child would acquire skills necessary to be successful in coping with everyday situations, specific instructional formats such as discrete trial teaching were developed. Discrete trial teaching is a highly structured teaching procedure characterized by (a) one-to-one interaction between the practitioner and the child in a distraction-free environment, (b) clear and concise instructions from the practitioner, (c) highly specific procedures for prompting and fading, and (d) immediate reinforcement such as praise or a preferred toy for correct responses (Leaf & McEachin, 1999).

Despite many successes, however, data on long-term outcomes of behavioral interventions were disappointing (e.g., Lovaas, Koegel, Simmons, & Long, 1973). It appeared that the gains children made when they received an ABA intervention did not transfer to environments outside the treatment setting or maintain over time. As a result, many professionals and parents lost interest in ABA, though others continued to work on increasing its effectiveness.

Observing that poor generalization and maintenance of skills was a problem not only for children with autism but also for many other persons who received ABA interventions, Stokes and Baer (1977) recommended developing a technology of generalization. They suggested several generalization strategies that might be effective, such as teaching communication skills across environments (e.g., home and school), presenting common stimuli across environments (e.g., having parents participate in both teaching the skill to their son or daughter in the treatment setting and then promoting the use of the skill in their home), and using "loose" teaching methods, rather than relying exclusively on approaches such as discrete trial teaching. Investigators put these strategies into practice. For example, they increasingly emphasized implementing interventions in the child's everyday environments instead of in clinical settings (e.g., Lovaas et al., 1981), involving parents and peers as change agents in the natural environment (Strain, Shores, & Timm, 1977), and identifying alternate teaching methods (Koegel, O'Dell, & Koegel, 1987).

By the late 1980s, investigators were reporting favorable long-term outcomes with ABA intervention. In an influential study, Lovaas (1987) compared three groups of children who began intervention when they were younger than 4 years old. One group received intensive ABA intervention (40 hours per week for 2 or more years.) The other two groups of children received either a less intensive behavioral intervention or no intervention. At follow-up evaluations conducted at the ages of 7 and 13 years, the group that received intensive intervention showed significant improvement, relative to the two other groups, in educational placement and IQ. Almost half of the children in the intensive group achieved unassisted placements in regular education classes and IQs in the average range.

Several researchers have built upon Lovaas's (1987) findings by demonstrating that participation in intensive behavioral intervention at a very early age resulted in some children with autism making significant improvements (Green, Brennan, & Fein, 2002). In addition to these encouraging findings on intensive early intervention, other developments in ABA have occurred. An example is the increased use of incidental teaching methods (Matson, Benavidez, Compton, Paclawskyj, & Baglio, 1996). These methods involve teaching during the course of naturally occurring activities, as opposed to setting aside a time and place to provide instruction. Incidental teaching situations arise from a child's motivation or desire for something (an EO). For example, snack time may present an opportunity to teach requesting or to require increasingly elaborate requests. A teacher can require a child to ask for a cookie before receiving it. To help the child with this request, the teacher can use a cue (e.g., asking, "What do you want?"), decide what form of communication will be expected (e.g., spoken words, manual sign language, or presentation of a picture corresponding to the desired object), and prompt a more elaborate language form, such as saying, "I want a cookie" instead of simply "cookie" (Hart & Risley, 1975, 1980). If the child communicates accurately, the consequence is that the child receives the desired cookie (see Chapter 6 for more on communication and verbal behavior). In most contemporary ABA programs, a combination of discrete trial, incidental, and other teaching methods are used to increase the likelihood that the skills acquired will maintain across time and generalize across people and settings (Smith, 2001).

Other developments have enhanced the ability of practitioners to individualize ABA interventions to match the needs of a particular child with ASD. Procedures have been refined for identifying high-preference stimuli that may act as reinforcers for a child. A multitude of preference assessment procedures now exist, including surveys and methods for directly testing children's preferences (e.g., Fisher et al., 1992; Hagopian, Rush, Lewin, & Long, 2001; Matson et al., 1999). Advances also have occurred in procedures for evaluating the functions that problem behavior may serve for a particular child and designing an individualized intervention plan based on this information. Iwata, Dorsey, Slifer, Bauman, and Richman (1982/1994) described a standardized procedure for systematically varying events in the environment and ascertaining the effects that these changes had on the frequency or severity of problem behavior. This assessment tool has been widely used to prescribe treatments based on the function of problem behavior displayed by persons with various developmental disabilities including autism. (See Chapter 7 for more on assessment of problem behavior.) Other assessment tools also are available, including surveys and observations of the behavior as it occurs in everyday situations. Because many children with autism have idiosyncratic preferences and functions of problem behavior (Carr, Yarbrough, & Langdon, 1997), preference assessments and functional analyses have a substantial role in treatment planning.

Most autism research in ABA has been directed toward helping individual children with ASD. A recent area of interest, however, has been a systems level approach to behavior change. In this approach, the unit of analysis is a social system such as an entire school or state. One service delivery model that focuses on systems is Positive Behavior Support (PBS; Wacker & Berg, 2002). As an illustration of PBS, Luiselli, Putnam, and Sunderland (2002) collaborated with personnel in a middle school to implement a schoolwide plan for reinforcing outstanding student behavior and academic achievement (e.g., "caught being good" cards were distributed and subsequently entered into a lottery). Through the successful application of this plan, the authors reduced the number of student detentions from 1,326 in the first year to 599 by the fourth year. In another study, Reid et al. (2003) reported on disseminating a PBS staff training model throughout the state of South Carolina.

Current Status

Since the early 1960s, ABA interventions for children with autism have generated a large body of research. As the field has matured, a variety of well-established techniques for teaching new skills and promoting generalization and maintenance of these skills have been identified, and research continues to add to this technology. Moreover, studies have generally confirmed Lovaas's (1987) finding that, when implemented intensively (up to 40 hours per week) and early (beginning prior to 4 years of age), ABA may produce major gains such as increases in IQ and other standardized test scores, along with a reduction in need for services such as special education (Smith, 1999). Thus, a child like 3-year-old Jason has the potential to benefit substantially. However, additional studies of long-term outcomes from early intensive intervention are still needed because previous studies have had limitations such as examining outcomes for only a small number of children.

Older children also benefit from teaching procedures derived from ABA. Although gains may be more circumscribed than those made by young children, such teaching procedures are successful in teaching most older children to learn important new skills and decrease problem behavior (Newsom, 1998).

Techniques developed within the field of ABA could be used to teach 9-year-old Ryan how to interact with peers and how to behave when there are changes in his routine.

Research indicates that some children benefit much more than others from behavior analytic–based teaching procedures, and reliable predictors of how much a particular child will benefit are not yet available. For this reason, practitioners are not able to tell Jason's or Ryan's families exactly what outcomes they could expect from ABA, though they could say, in general, that most children are likely to make some improvements.

ABA for Difficult Problems

Despite the extensive research on ABA, questions linger regarding its appropriateness as an intervention for children with autism. Notably, because ABA is based on operant learning and other behavioral processes that occur in both humans and nonhuman species, some have doubted how well it can address the defining features of ASD, which involve difficulties with skills that are unique to humans, such as reciprocal communication and social interaction (Greenspan, 2000). However, ABA has focused extensively on these difficulties.

Verbal Behavior

Language, as a probably uniquely human form of behavior, was one apparent difficulty for behaviorism (Skinner, 1957, pp. 456–460). Yet, Skinner viewed communication as just a particular variant of operant behavior and referred to it as *verbal behavior*. According to Skinner's analysis, verbal behavior can take vocal, gestural, or textual forms. For example, both Jason's screaming when others approach and Ryan's talking about trains are types of verbal behavior, though they have different forms.

Influenced by Skinner's analysis, a model of ABA intervention was developed called verbal behavior (Sundberg & Partington, 2001). Other ABA models have different names but are also strongly influenced by Skinner's (1957) analysis of verbal behavior (e.g., Bondy, Tincani, & Frost, 2004). Research has demonstrated that teaching procedures based on engaging in appropriate verbal behavior enables children with ASD to improve their social connections. Chapter 6 by Sigafoos, O'Reilly, Schlosser, and Lancioni provides an extensive review of Skinner's analysis of verbal behavior and the assessment and teaching procedures developed based on his analysis.

Related to their difficulties in communication, a defining feature of ASD is limited creativity and imagination. Behavior analysts define creativity in terms of fluency (number of responses), originality (novelty of responses), variability (differences between responses), flexibility (use of a stimulus for multiple purposes), and divergent thinking (problem solving) (Neuringer, 2004). By reinforcing responses with these characteristics, practitioners may be able to increase creativity. For example, Lee, McComas, and Jawor (2002) reinforced children with ASD for giving different responses to social questions and found an increase in the novelty and variability of children's answers.

Social Interaction

Problems with social interactions also are a defining feature of ASD. In young children with ASD such as Jason, a key problem is imitating actions performed by others (Rogers, 1998). From a behavior analytic viewpoint, imitation is a response that resembles the discriminative stimulus (Baer & Sherman, 1964). For example, if the instructor claps her hands (discriminative stimulus) and a child responds by performing a similar action, imitation is said to occur. Generalized imitation is demonstrated when a child gives the correct response on the first learning trial with a novel discriminative stimulus and when imitation itself appears to be a reinforcing activity (Baer & Sherman, 1964). Procedures for teaching imitation to children with autism have been studied for many years (e.g., Baer, Peterson, & Sherman, 1967; Lovaas, Freitas, Nelson, & Whalen, 1967; Kymissis & Poulson, 1990) and are now a standard part of ABA intervention programs for these children. A child with problems such as Jason's might benefit from extensive instruction to increase imitation skills. These skills in imitation can be used to teach social interactions and cooperative play (Jahr & Eldevik, 2002).

Another key problem in young children is joint attention, which involves shifting focus back and forth between another person and an object such as a toy (Mundy & Crawson, 1997). An example of joint attention is looking at an adult, then looking at a toy, and then looking back at the adult. From a behavior analytic perspective, joint attention requires that the adult and toy each function both as discriminative stimuli and as reinforcers (Dube, MacDonald, Mansfield, Holcomb, & Ahearn, 2004). ABA teaching methods for systematically establishing these functions have been shown to increase joint attention (Whalen & Schreibman, 2003).

For older or more advanced children with autism, such as Ryan, problems with social interaction are often attributed to a lack of "theory of mind" (Baron-Cohen, 1995). According to the "theory of mind" hypothesis, persons with autism lack other people's prewired ability to explain, predict, and interpret the behavior of people in terms of mental states such as desires, beliefs, feelings, and thoughts. For example, Ryan's seemingly endless discussions of trains might be explained as a failure to realize that others may want to change the topic. However, this problem may reflect an inability to respond to social cues that indicate when a listener is or is not receptive to a discussion of trains, such as facial expressions or body language. Alternatively, it may reflect an inability to converse on other topics. Thus, teaching Ryan to identify and respond to social cues or to talk about other topics may be effective interventions. Researchers have studied a variety of strategies for increasing such appropriate social behavior. Examples include employing peers as tutors or models of social behavior, arranging situations in which children with ASD are likely to mand to peers, having children learn scripts for handling common social situations, directly teaching children with ASD skills such as age-appropriate games, and using inconspicuous cues such as pagers to signal when it is time to engage in a social behavior (Weiss & Harris, 2001).

In sum, although language and some forms of social communication and reciprocal interaction are largely unique to humans, ABA has a well-developed technology that continues to expand to address problems that children with ASD have in these areas.

Current Issues and Future Directions

Soon after reports of favorable long-term outcomes appeared (Lovaas, 1987), interest in ABA for children with autism began to grow. In a book titled *Let Me Hear Your Voice*, Catherine Maurice (1993) chronicled the positive effects of an intensive ABA intervention for her two children diagnosed with autism and for the rest of the family. Maurice's book popularized ABA by presenting the intervention in an engaging and accessible format. Subsequently, many parents advocated to make ABA widely available to children with autism (Jacobson, 2000), and publication of books and manuals for practitioners working with persons with ASD increased (Leaf & McEachin, 1999; Maurice, Green, & Luce, 1996).

While parent advocacy succeeded in making ABA a standard intervention in many communities (Jacobson, 2000), the huge rise in demand for services created a shortage of qualified providers. To address this problem, many educational institutions added programs offering graduate training in ABA (see http://www.abainternational.org). Also, a system for certifying behavior analysts and associate behavior analysts was implemented, and the number of people taking and passing the examination has increased greatly in recent years: In

May 2000, there were 59 certified behavior analysts and 13 certified associate behavior analysts, but by December 2004, the numbers were 522 and 276, respectively (see http://www.bacb.com). In addition, the Autism Special Interest Group of the Association for Behavior Analysis, one of the primary affiliations for professional behavior analysts, published guidelines on competencies that consumers should look for in ABA providers for persons with autism (Autism Special Interest Group, 2004). These include certification by the Behavior Analyst Certification Board and 1,000 hours of hands-on training in supervising ABA interventions for persons with ASD. Still, the shortage of qualified behavior analysts persists, and the potential for underqualified individuals to present themselves as ABA providers is a concern.

Another challenge is that as ABA has received more attention, opposition to it appears to have amplified; at the same time, endorsement of interventions that have not been validated may have increased (Jacobson, 2000). To help parents and practitioners sort through conflicting statements about interventions and evaluate their options, several governing bodies have reviewed the available research evidence. In a comprehensive report, ABA was the only intervention recommended by the New York State Department of Health (2001). Additionally, citing many years of research supporting the efficacy of ABA teaching methods, the U.S. Surgeon General (U.S. Department of Health and Human Services, 1999) also recommended intensive, sustained educational programming based on ABA for children with ASD. However, opposition to ABA has not abated.

Despite the gains made in implementing ABA to treat problems associated with ASD, there is still much work to be done. For example, little collaboration has taken place between behavior analysts and investigators who study the neurobiology of autism; such collaborations could potentially lead to more effective interventions. Few studies have tested the combined effects of ABA and psychoactive medications (Napolitano et al., 1999). As a result, it is currently unclear whether such combinations are beneficial. Since the early 1970s, no studies have directly evaluated ABA for children with ASD against alternate educational methods such as TEACCH or the Denver Model. For this reason, comparisons between ABA and other popular intervention models are needed. Furthermore, although studies indicate that ABA can successfully address the defining features of autism such as social communication, reciprocal interactions, and repetitive behavior, many findings require replication and extension. For example, only a handful of published studies have appeared on recognizing social cues, establishing joint attention, and increasing creativity. Finally, behavior analysts must continue to address some key questions about service provision such as large-scale dissemination, long-term outcomes of intervention, and individual differences in outcomes achieved by different children with

ASD. We look forward to seeing further advancements in scientifically based treatments for persons with ASD that build on the intervention strategies reviewed in detail in subsequent chapters of this book.

Summary

This chapter has reviewed the application of ABA to the variety of challenges that children and adults with ASDs and their families may have. ABA can successfully address all three core deficits in autism and enhance a wide variety of skills. The application of ABA has gradually expanded from treatment of relatively simple behavior and continues to address progressively more and more complex and subtle behavior. Our review has several implications for parents, teachers, and caregivers, especially with regard to diagnosis, treatment, medication, and use of ABA with children and adolescents with ASD.

 ## PRACTITIONER RECOMMENDATIONS

1. Obtain an evaluation by a clinician with expertise in diagnosing autism spectrum disorder. An evaluation should
    a. include interviews with caregivers,
    b. include careful observations of the child's behavior, and
    c. be conducted as soon as social or communication delays are suspected or high rates of restricted or repetitive behavior are observed.

2. If diagnosis of an ASD is made, consider interventions carefully.
    a. Find out if scientific evidence shows intervention to be effective.
    b. Make sure child's progress will be monitored using data-based measures.

3. If medication is being considered,
    a. request information on what behavior the medication is intended to treat and find out if scientific research has shown the medication to be effective in treating the targeted behavior and

    b. find out what the side effects are and how they will be measured and monitored.

4. Intervention based on the science of ABA should be made available to the person with ASD. An ABA-based intervention should have the following characteristics:

    a. uses a variety of teaching strategies such as DTT, incidental teaching, and instruction or modeling from peers

    b. emphasizes the systematic analysis of functional relationships between the environment and behavior and prescribes interventions based on this analysis

    c. promotes generalization and maintenance of skills, including teaching across environments and having caregivers participate actively in the intervention

    d. uses objective data collection procedures to monitor an individual's acquisition of skills and reduction of problem behavior

    e. uses teaching programs that directly address areas of difficulty for persons with ASD, such as social communication, creativity, joint attention, and imitation

    f. is supervised by professionals who have Board Certification in Behavior Analysis (or equivalent education in behavior analysis) and 1,000 hours or more of specialized training in working with individuals with ASD

References

American Academy of Neurology. (2000). Practice parameter: Screening and diagnosis of autism. *Neurology, 55,* 468–479.

American Psychiatric Association. (2000). *Diagnostic and statistical manual of mental disorders* (4th ed. text revision). Washington, DC: Author.

Autism Special Interest Group: Association for Behavior Analysis. (2004). *Revised guidelines for consumers of applied behavior analysis services to individuals with autism and related disorders.* Retrieved February 4, 2005, from http://www.abainternational.org/sub/membersvcs/sig/contactinfo/Autism.asp

Baer, D. M., Peterson, R. F., & Sherman, J. A. (1967). The development of imitation by reinforcing behavioral similarity to a model. *Journal of the Experimental Analysis of Behavior, 10,* 405–416.

Baer, D. M., & Sherman, J. A. (1964). Reinforcement control of generalized imitation in young children. *Journal of Experimental Child Psychology, 1,* 37–49.

Baer, D. M., Wolf, M. M., & Risley, T. R. (1968). Some current dimensions of applied behavior analysis. *Journal of Applied Behavior Analysis, 1,* 91–97.

Bailey, A., LeCouteur, A., Gottesman, I., Bolton, P., Simonoff, E., Yuzda, E., & Rutter, M. (1995). Autism is a strongly genetic disorder: Evidence from a British twin study. *Psychological Medicine, 25,* 63–77.

Baron-Cohen, S. (1995). *Mindblindness: An essay on autism and theory of mind.* Cambridge, MA: MIT Press.

Baron-Cohen, S., Ring, H. A., Bullmore, E. T., Wheelwright, S., Ashwin, C., & Williams, S. C. (2000). The amygdala theory of autism. *Neuroscience and Biobehavioral Reviews, 24,* 355–364.

Bijou, S. W. (1993). *Behavior analysis of child development.* Reno, NV: Context Press.

Bondy, A., Tincani, M., & Frost, L. (2004). Multiply controlled verbal operants: An analysis and extension to the picture exchange communication system. *The Behavior Analyst, 27,* 247–261.

Carr, E. G., Yarbrough, S. C., & Langdon, N. A. (1997). Effects of idiosyncratic stimulus variables on functional analysis outcomes. *Journal of Applied Behavior Analysis, 30,* 673–686.

Chakrabarti, S., & Fombonne, E. (2001). Pervasive developmental disorders in preschool children. *Journal of the American Medical Association, 24,* 3093–3099.

Chiesa, M. (1994). *Radical behaviorism: The philosophy and the science.* Boston: Authors Cooperative.

Constantino, J. N., & Todd, R. D. (2003). Autistic traits in the general population: A twin study. *Archives of General Psychiatry, 60,* 524–530.

Courchesne, E., Carper, R., & Akshoomoff, N. (2003). Evidence of brain overgrowth in the first year of life in autism. *Journal of the American Medical Association, 290,* 337–393.

Courchesne, E., Yeung-Courchesne, R., Press, G. A., Hesselink, J. R., & Jernigan, T. L. (1988). Hypoplasia of cerebellar vermal lobules VI and VII in autism. *New England Journal of Medicine, 318,* 1349–1354.

Department of Developmental Services. (1999). *Changes in the population of persons with autism and pervasive developmental disorders in California's developmental services system: 1987 through 1999.* Retrieved February 4, 2005, from http://www.dds.ca.gov/autism/pdf/autism_report_1999.pdf

Dube, W. V., MacDonald, R. P. F., Mansfield, R. C., Holcomb, W. L., & Ahearn, H. (2004). Toward a behavioral analysis of joint attention. *The Behavior Analyst, 27,* 197–208.

Ferster, C. B., & DeMeyer, M. K. (1962). The development of performances in autistic children in an automatically controlled environment. *Journal of Chronic Diseases, 13,* 312–345.

Fisher, W. W., Piazza, C., Bowman, L. G., Hagopian, L. P., Owens, J. C., & Slevin, I. (1992). A comparison of two approaches for identifying reinforcers for persons with severe and profound disabilities. *Journal of Applied Behavior Analysis, 25,* 491–498.

Fombonne, E. (2003). Epidemiological surveys of autism and other pervasive developmental disorders: An update. *Journal of Autism and Developmental Disorders, 33,* 365–382.

Friman, P. C., Hayes, S. C., & Wilson, K. G. (1998). Why behavior analysts should study emotion: The example of anxiety. *Journal of Applied Behavior Analysis, 31,* 137–156.

Geier, M. R., & Geier, D. A. (2003). Thimerosal in childhood vaccines, neurodevelopment disorders and heart disease in the United States. *Journal of American Physicians and Surgeons, 8,* 6–11.

Ghaziuddin, M., & Mountain-Kimchi, K. (2004). Defining the intellectual profile of Asperger syndrome: Comparison with high-functioning autism. *Journal of Autism and Developmental Disorders, 34,* 279–284.

Green, G., Brennan, L. C., & Fein, D. (2002). Intensive behavioral treatment for a toddler at high risk for autism. *Behavior Modification, 26,* 69–102.

Greenspan, S. I. (Ed.). (2000). *ICDL guidelines for assessment, diagnosis and treatment.* Bethesda, MD: Interdisciplinary Council for Developmental and Learning Disorders.

Hagopian, L. P., Rush, K. S., Lewin, A. B., & Long, E. S. (2001). Evaluating the predictive validity of a single stimulus engagement preference assessment. *Journal of Applied Behavior Analysis, 34,* 475–486.

Hart, B., & Risley, T. R. (1975). Incidental teaching of language in the preschool. *Journal of Applied Behavior Analysis, 8*, 411–420.

Hart, B., & Risley, T. R. (1980). In vivo language intervention: Unanticipated general effects. *Journal of Applied Behavior Analysis, 13*, 407–432.

Individuals with Disabilities Education Act of 1990, 20 U.S.C. § 1400 *et seq.*

Institute of Medicine. (2004). *Immunization safety review: Vaccines and autism.* Retrieved February 4, 2005, from http://www.iom.edu/report.asp?id=20155

Iwata, B. A., Dorsey, M. F., Slifer, K. J., Bauman, K. E., Richman, G. S. (1982/1994). Towards a functional analysis of self-injury. *Journal of Applied Behavior Analysis, 27*, 197–209. (Reprinted from *Analysis and Intervention in Developmental Disabilities, 2*, 3–20, 1982)

Iwata, B. A., Vollmer, T. R., & Zarcone, J. R. (1990). The experimental (functional) analysis of behavior disorders: Methodology, applications, and limitations. In A. C. Repp & N. N. Singh (Eds.), *Perspectives on the use of nonaversive and versive interventions for persons with developmental disabilities* (pp. 301–330). Sycamore, IL: Sycamore.

Jacobson, J. W. (2000). Early intensive behavioral intervention: Emergence of a consumer-driven service model. *Behavior Analyst, 23*, 149–171.

Jacobson, J. W., Foxx, R. M., & Mulick, J. A. (Eds.). (2004). *Controversial therapies for developmental disabilities.* Mahwah, NJ: Erlbaum.

Jacobson, J. W., Mulick, J. A., & Schwartz, A. A. (1995). A history of facilitated communication: Science, pseudoscience, and antiscience. *American Psychologist, 50*, 750–765.

Jahr, E., & Eldevik, S. (2002). Teaching cooperative play to typical children utilizing a behavior modeling approach: A systematic replication. *Behavioral Interventions, 17*, 145–157.

Keller, F. S., & Schoenfeld, W. N. (1950). *Principles of psychology.* New York: Appleton-Century-Croft.

Kerr, A. M., & Ravine, D. (2003). Review article: Breaking new ground with Rett syndrome. *Journal of Intellectual Disability Research, 47*, 580–587.

Koegel, R. L., O'Dell, M. C., & Koegel, L. K. (1987). A natural language paradigm for teaching autistic children by reinforcing attempts. *Journal of Autism and Developmental Disorders, 17*, 187–189.

Kreiling, J. A., Stephens, R. E., & Reinisch, C. L. (2005). A mixture of environmental contaminants increases cAMP-dependent protein kinase in *Spisula* embryos. *Environmental Toxicology and Pharmacology, 19*, 9–18.

Kymissis, E., & Poulson, C. L. (1990). The history of imitation in learning theory: The language acquisition process. *Journal of the Experimental Analysis of Behavior, 54*, 113–127.

Leaf, R. B., & McEachin, J. J. (1999). *A work in progress: Behavior management strategies and a curriculum for intensive behavioral treatment of autism.* New York: DRL Books.

Lee, R., McComas, J. J., & Jawor, J. (2002). The effects of differential and lag reinforcement schedules on varied verbal responding by individuals with autism. *Journal of Applied Behavior Analysis, 35,* 391–402.

Lovaas, O. I. (1987). Behavioral treatment and normal educational and intellectual functioning in young autistic children. *Journal of Consulting and Clinical Psychology, 55,* 3–9.

Lovaas, O. I., Ackerman, A., Alexander, D., Firestone, P., Perkins, M., Young, D. B., et al. (1981). *Teaching developmentally disabled children: The me book.* Baltimore: University Park Press.

Lovaas, O. I., Freitag, G., Gold, V. J., & Kassorla, I. C. (1965). Recording apparatus and procedure for observation of behaviors of children in free play settings. *Journal of Experimental Child Psychology, 2,* 108–120.

Lovaas, O. I., Freitas, L., Nelson, K., & Whalen, C. (1967). The establishment of imitation and its use for the development of complex behavior in schizophrenic children. *Behaviour Research and Therapy, 5,* 171–181.

Lovaas, O. I., Koegel, R., Simmons, J. Q., & Long, J. S. (1973). Some generalization and follow-up measures on autistic children in behavior therapy. *Journal of Applied Behavior Analysis, 6,* 131–166.

Lovaas, O. I., Schreibman, L., Koegel, R. L., & Rehm, R. (1971). Selective responding by autistic children to multiple sensory input. *Journal of Abnormal Psychology, 77,* 211–222.

Lovaas, O. I., & Smith, T. (1989). A comprehensive behavioral theory of autistic children: Paradigm for research and treatment. *Journal of Behavior Therapy and Experimental Psychiatry, 20,* 17–29.

Luiselli, J. K., Putnam, R. F., & Sunderland, M. (2002). Longitudinal evaluation of behavior support intervention in a public middle school. *Journal of Positive Behavior Interventions, 4,* 182–188.

Manjiviona, J., & Prior, M. (1999). Neuropsychological profiles of children with Asperger syndrome and autism. *Autism, 3,* 327–356.

Marcus, L., Schopler, E., & Lord, C. (2001). TEACCH services for preschool children. In J. S. Handleman & S. L. Harris (Eds.), *Preschool education programs for children with autism* (2nd ed., pp. 215–232). Austin, TX: PRO-ED.

Matson, J. L., Benavidez, D. A., Compton, L. S., Paclawskyj, T., & Baglio, C. (1996). Behavioral treatment of autistic persons: A review of research from 1980 to the present. *Research in Developmental Disabilities, 17,* 433–465.

Matson, J. L., Bielecki, J. A., Mayville, E. A., Smalls, Y., Bamburg, J. W., & Baglio, C. S. (1999). The development of a reinforcer choice assessment scale for persons with severe and profound mental retardation. *Research in Developmental Disabilities, 20,* 379–384.

Maurice, C. (1993). *Let me hear your voice: A family's triumph over autism.* New York: Ballantine Books.

Maurice, C., Green, G., & Luce, S. C. (1996). *Behavioral intervention for young children with autism.* Austin, TX: PRO-ED.

McCracken, J. T., McGough, J., Shah, B., Cronin, P., Hong, D., Aman, M. G., et al. (2002). Risperidone in children with autism and serious behavior problems. *The New England Journal of Medicine, 347,* 314–321.

Michael, J. (1982). Distinguishing between discriminative and motivational functions of stimuli. *Journal of the Experimental Analysis of Behavior, 37,* 149–155.

Michael J. (1993). Establishing operations. *The Behavior Analyst, 16,* 191–206.

Miller, J., & Ozonoff, S. (2000). The external validity of Asperger disorder: Lack of evidence from the domain of neuropsychology. *Journal of Abnormal Psychology, 109,* 227–238.

Mouridsen, S. E. (2003). Review article: Childhood disintegrative disorder. *Brain & Development, 25,* 225–228.

Mundy, P., & Crawson, M. (1997). Joint attention and early social communication: Implications for research on intervention with autism. *Journal of Autism and Developmental Disorders, 27,* 653–676.

Napolitano, D. A., Jack, S. L., Sheldon, J. B., Williams, D. C., McAdam, D. B., & Schroeder, S. R. (1999). Drug–behavior interactions in persons with mental retardation and developmental disabilities. *Mental Retardation and Developmental Disabilities Research and Reviews, 5,* 322–344.

Neuringer, A. (2004). Reinforced variability in animals and people: Implications for adaptive action. *American Psychologist, 59,* 891–906.

Newsom, C. (1998). Autistic disorder. In E. J. Mash & R. A. Barkley (Eds.), *Treatment of childhood disorders* (2nd ed., pp. 416–467). New York: Guilford.

New York State Department of Health. (2001). *Clinical practice guidelines: Report of the recommendations—Autism/pervasive developmental disorders assessment and intervention for young children/age 0–3 years.* Retrieved April 20, 2006, from http://www .health.state.ny.us/community/infants_children/early_intervention/autism/index .htm

Nicolson, R., & Szatmari, P. (2003). Genetic and neurodevelopmental influences in autistic disorder. *Canadian Journal of Psychiatry, 8,* 526–537.

Prior, M., Eisenmajer, R., Leekam, S., Wing, L., Gould, J., Ong, B., et al. (1998). Are there subgroups within the autistic spectrum? A cluster analysis of a group of children with autistic spectrum disorders. *Journal of Child Psychology & Psychiatry & Allied Disciplines, 39,* 893–902.

Rafaeli-Mor, N., Foster, L., & Berkson, G. (1999). Self-reported body-rocking and other habits in college students. *American Journal on Mental Retardation, 104*, 1–10.

Reichelt, K. L., Knivsberg, A. M., Lind, G., & Nodland, M. (1991). Probable etiology and possible treatment of childhood autism. *Brain Dysfunction, 4*, 308–319.

Reid, D. H., Rotholz, D. A., Parsons, M. B., Morris, L., Braswell, B. A., Green, C. W., et al. (2003). Training human service supervisors in aspects of PBS. *Journal of Positive Behavior Interventions, 5*, 35–46.

Rodier, P. M. (2000). The early origins of autism. *Scientific American, 282*, 56–63.

Rogers, S. J. (1998). Neuropsychology of autism in young children and its implications for early intervention. *Mental Retardation & Developmental Disabilities Research Reviews, 4*, 104–112.

Rogers, S. J., Hall, T., Osaki, D., Reaven, J., & Herbison, J. (2001). The Denver Model: A comprehensive, integrated educational approach to young children with autism and their families. In J. S. Handleman & S. L. Harris (Eds.), *Preschool programs for children with autism* (2nd ed., pp. 95–134). Austin, TX: PRO-ED.

Saitoh, O., Courchesne, E., Egaas, B., Lincoln, A. J., & Schreibman, L. (1995). Cross-sectional area of the posterior hippocampus in autistic patients with cerebellar and corpus collosum abnormalities. *Neurology, 45*, 317–345.

Schultz, R. T., Gauthier, I., Klin, A., Fullbright, R. K., Anderson, A. W., Volkmar, F., et al. (2000). Abnormal ventral temporal cortical activity during face discrimination among individuals with autism and Asperger syndrome. *Archives of General Psychiatry, 57*, 331–340.

Simonoff, E. (1998). Genetic counseling in autism and pervasive developmental disorders. *Journal of Autism and Developmental Disorders, 28*, 447–456.

Skinner, B. F. (1938). *The behavior of organisms.* New York: Appleton-Century-Crofts.

Skinner, B. F. (1950). Are theories of learning necessary? *Psychological Review, 57*, 193–216.

Skinner, B. F. (1953). *Science and human behavior.* New York: Macmillan.

Skinner, B. F. (1957). *Verbal behavior.* Englewood Cliffs, NJ: Prentice Hall.

Skinner, B. F. (1981). Selection by consequences. *Science, 213*, 501–504.

Smith, T. (1999). Outcome of early intervention for children with autism. *Clinical Psychology: Science & Practice, 6*, 33–49.

Smith, T. (2001). Discrete trial training for children with autism. *Focus on Autism and Related Disorders, 16*, 86–92.

Smith, T., & Antolovich, M. (2000). Parental perceptions of supplemental interventions received by young children in intensive behavior analytic treatment. *Behavioral Interventions, 15*, 83–97.

Stokes, T., & Baer, D. M. (1977). An implicit technology of generalization. *Journal of Applied Behavior Analysis, 10*, 349–367.

Strain, S., Shores, R. E., & Timm, M. A. (1977). Effects of peer social initations on the behavior of withdrawn preschool children. *Journal of Applied Behavior Analysis, 10,* 289–298.

Sturmey, P. (2004). Secretin is an ineffective treatment for pervasive developmental disabilities: A review of 15 double-blind randomized controlled trials. *Research in Developmental Disabilities, 26,* 87–97.

Sundberg, N., & Partington, J. W. (2001). *Teaching language to children with autism and other developmental disabilities.* Pleasant Hill, CA: Behavior Analysts.

Szatmari, P., Archer L., Fisman, S., Streiner, D. L., & Wilson, F. (1995). Asperger's syndrome and autism: Differences in behavior, cognition and adaptive functioning. *Journal of the American Academy of Child and Adolescent Psychiatry, 34,* 1662–1671.

Treffert, D. A. (1988). The idiot savant: A review of the syndrome. *American Journal of Psychiatry, 145,* 563–572.

U.S. Department of Education. (2002). *Twenty-fourth annual report to Congress on the implementation of the Individuals with Disabilities Education Act.* Retrieved February 4, 2005, from http://www.ed.gov/about/reports/annual/osep/2002/appendix-a-pt1.pdf

U.S. Department of Health and Human Services. (1999). *Mental health: A report of the surgeon general—Executive summary.* Retrieved February 4, 2005, from http://www.surgeongeneral.org/library/mentalhealth/home.html

Vitiello, B., & Wagner, A. (2004). Government initiatives in autism clinical trials. *CNS Spectrums, 9,* 66–70.

Volkmar, F. R., Cicchetti, D. V., Bregman, J., & Cohen, J. (1992). Three diagnostic systems for autism: DSM–III, DSM–III–R, and ICD–10. *Journal of Autism & Developmental Disorders, 22,* 483–492.

Volkmar, F. R., & Pauls, D. (2003). Autism. *Lancet, 362,* 1133–1141.

Volkmar, F. R., & Weisner, L. A. (2004). *Topics in autism: Healthcare for children on the autism spectrum.* Bethesda, MD: Woodbine House.

Wacker, D. P., & Berg, W. K. (2002). PBS as a service delivery system. *Journal of Positive Behavior Interventions, 4,* 25–28.

Wakefield, A. J., Murch, S. H., Anthony, A., Linnell, J., Casson, D. M., Malik, M., et al. (1998). Ileal-lymphoid-nodular hyperplasia, non-specific colitis, and pervasive developmental disorder in children. *Lancet, 351,* 637–641.

Weiss, M. J., & Harris, S. L. (2001). *Reaching out, joining in: Teaching social skills to young children with autism.* Bethesda, MD: Woodbine House.

Whalen, C., & Schreibman, L. (2003). Joint attention training for children with autism using behavior modification procedures. *Journal of Child Psychology & Psychiatry & Allied Disciplines, 44,* 456–468.

Wing, L. (1988). The continuum of autistic characteristics. In E. Schopler & G. Mesibov (Eds.), *Diagnosis and assessment in autism* (pp. 91–110). New York: Plenum.

Wing, L. (1992). Manifestations of social problems in high-functioning autistic people. In E. Schopler & G. B. Mesibov (Eds.), *High-functioning individuals with autism* (pp. 129–142). New York: Plenum.

Wolf, M. M., Risley, T. R., & Mees, H. (1964). Application of operant conditioning procedures to the behaviour problems of an autistic child. *Behaviour Research and Therapy, 1,* 305–312.

World Health Organization. (1994). *International classification of diseases* (ICD–10). Geneva: Author.

Yeargin-Allsopp, M., Rice, C., Karapurkar, T., Doernberg, N., Boyle, C., & Murphy, C. (2003). Prevalence of autism in a US metropolitan area. *Journal of the American Medical Association, 289,* 49–55.

CHAPTER

BEHAVIOR ANALYTIC TEACHING PROCEDURES: BASIC PRINCIPLES, EMPIRICALLY DERIVED PRACTICES

William H. Ahearn, Rebecca MacDonald, and Richard B. Graff
The New England Center for Children

William V. Dube
University of Massachusetts Medical School Shriver Center

The purpose of this chapter is to describe the conceptual framework, methods, and teaching practices that are applied behavior analysis (ABA). In a paper considered to serve as a definition of the field, Baer, Wolf, and Risley (1968) stated that Applied Behavior Analysis is the application of the principles of learning to address socially meaningful behavioral challenges. Autism clearly qualifies as a challenge for society in that persons with this disorder often require special services. We define this spectrum of disorders by the behaviors, both present and absent, that set these persons apart from their typically developing peers. The principles being applied in developing effective educational and clinical solutions to these behavioral deficits and excesses are grounded in the science of behavior analysis, but behavior analysis is widely misunderstood, misinterpreted, and misrepresented.

Why Do People Not Understand Behavior Analysis?

ABA has garnered a great deal of attention in the past two decades or so, largely due to the successful outcomes produced by its practitioners with children diagnosed with autism. In the first chapter of this book by Smith, McAdam, and Napolitano, the scientific status of this evidence is detailed and evaluated. Many will rightly point out that identifying critical aspects of ABA procedures as intervention for Autism Spectrum Disorders (e.g., optimal intensity of service, best setting in which to provide service, best practices for establishing communicative and social skills) requires further investigation (e.g., Kasari, 2002). However, ABA is the most comprehensive and effective means of teaching children with autism because it involves an assessment of each individual's behavior and its relationship to the environment, with intervention based on this individualized assessment.

Still, the efficacy of ABA is often either grudgingly acknowledged or referred to as a simplistic approach of limited value. There are many reasons why ABA is not readily accepted, but the main one is that it is not well understood. Behavior analysis is an approach within psychology that assumes that human behavior can be explained by a detailed analysis of the current environments in which behavior occurs, the past environments in which it has occurred, and the motivational conditions affecting the person at the time he or she is acting. B. F. Skinner was the founder of this scientific approach to investigating behavior, and psychologists and persons in the lay community hold and, in some cases, have propagated many false assumptions about Skinner and behavior analysis.

Many incorrectly associate Skinner's behavior analysis with the behaviorism of Watson (e.g., Chomsky, 1959; Koch, 1964; Rogers, 1964). Watson (1913, 1924) claimed that a person's mind, thoughts, and feelings either did not exist or were irrelevant. From Watson's perspective, a person's behavior can be defined by its form, and it is mechanistically determined. He suggested that stimulus–response associations between environmental stimuli and human responses are what are expressed when a person acts. Though all behavioral approaches have sought to bring a scientific approach to psychology, Skinner's "radical behaviorism" was a departure from Watson's behaviorism. The term *radical* seems unfortunate because it may imply to some that Skinner proposed an even more extreme version of behaviorism than Watson. However, Skinner intended it as a means of describing a radical or fundamental *departure* from the behaviorist manifesto of Watson and his followers. Skinner's assumptions about the cause of behavior are better characterized as contextual (Morris, 1988). That is, it is the events or consequences that are occurring now and that have occurred for the behavior in the past that determine how likely behavior will be in future similar situations. Behavior and its consequences are said to be functionally related and this functional relation is dynamic, ever changing due to life experience.

The following is a simplified example: The social greeting "Hello, Lisa" occurs and is followed by a specific consequence, "Hi, Bill. Nice to see you today." However, the same behavior may meet a different consequence when it occurs in the future (e.g., saying hello to Lisa again a few minutes later or on another day may be ignored). Each instance of behavior occurs under specific conditions or contexts. Although present behavior is ultimately caused by a history of consequences, the conditions under which a given behavior occurs and comes into contact with a particular consequence (i.e., the return of the social greeting) relative to another (i.e., the ignored social greeting) are also critically important. Conditions that are the same as or similar to those that have in the past resulted in a desirable consequence will make that response more probable. If the conditions are not the same or if Lisa begins to ignore all of Bill's social greetings, then this behavior becomes less probable. In this case, other behavior that has met positive consequences (e.g., greeting other persons, drinking coffee, whistling) or that avoids undesirable consequences will be more likely to occur.

Many of the misconceptions about behavior analysis stem from a misunderstanding of how behavior analysis interprets private or covert behavior. Skinner's (1945) position on thinking and feelings is also quite different from Watson's. He stated that these private, unobservable events exist and are just as important as publicly observable behavior. However, Skinner (1953, 1977) noted that psychologists give special explanatory status to thinking and other private events. Skinner's position was that we can assume that other people think but that thoughts and feelings are not always or necessarily a cause of an action. Skinner argues that when we treat thinking routinely as a cause of behavior, we say the thought caused the behavior and look no further into the matter. His argument was that the thinking is behavior, not its cause, and like any other behavior, it must also be explained. Thinking, at least in words, does not preexist in a person. As children acquire the ability to communicate, the social community teaches them how to talk about thinking and feeling. Talking about thinking changes or underlies how we think at least as much, if not more, than our genetic endowment.

Nevertheless, many still characterize behavior analysis as stimulus–response psychology, simplistic and involving rote learning rather than complex cognitive processing. Associating behavior analysis with the mechanistic stimulus–response psychology that was the dominant school of thought in American psychology through the late 1950s is incorrect (Lana, 1991). The sweeping dismissal of behavior analysis as a viable means of investigating human behavior flies in the face of its successful application for addressing complex phenomena like autism, drug dependency (Hursh, 1991; Johnson & Bickel, 2003), safety (Alavosius & Sulzer-Azaroff, 1985; Fox, Hopkins, & Anger, 1987), organizational management (Gikalov, Baer, & Hannah, 1997; Wittkopp, Rowan, & Poling, 1990), at-risk youth (Friman et al., 1996; Thompson et al., 1996), and many other social issues (Austin & Carr, 2000).

The Environment as a Causal Agent

Psychological investigations seek to provide extraordinary and reliable explanations of our behavior; unfortunately, explanations of behavior already exist within our vernacular. Our everyday language leads us to readily assume private events as causes of behavior. We say a person goes to a vending machine and acquires a granola bar because he or she is hungry. If someone were to ask us, however, why we went to the vending machine and procured a granola bar, we might find ourselves describing our actions in a bit more detail. We would perhaps note how long it had been since we had eaten and the fact that we missed lunch because of an important meeting and needed to eat something because we felt we were coming down with a hunger headache. We might then go on to extol the virtues of granola as a food source.

Both of these explanations flow from our membership in a verbal community (Hineline, 1992). When describing our own actions, we are more likely to refer to the ambient conditions in the environment, but when explaining the actions of others, our language predisposes us to summarize the agent of their actions as something existing inside the skin, in this case "hunger." However, explaining that person's behavior in this situation as being caused by hunger is inexact and simplistic. Hunger, including discrimination of the impending hunger headache, is perhaps the motivating condition resulting in a switch in activities from working to going to the vending machine. Making one's way to the vending machine is determined by previous experience in foraging and moving through space in that office building. Discriminating among the alternatives in the vending machine requires that arbitrary stimuli, namely the food items and the alphanumeric symbols corresponding to them, be acted upon as if they are equivalent to each other. Finally, the selection of granola involves the expression of an individual's preference.

The goal of behavior analysis is to formulate scientific explanations of the individual's behavior. To develop extraordinary and reliable knowledge of an individual's behavior, it was necessary to develop a science of the individual.

Skinner and those who have followed in his footsteps have done just that. This approach assumes that psychological investigations should be scientific and should be in continuity with the natural sciences. Explanation in the natural sciences assumes that the laws of nature determine physical events. We have no preexisting knowledge of these laws; they must be discovered through empirical investigation.

The science closest to psychology is biology. Biological science is continuous with chemistry, chemistry with physics, and psychology should be in continuity with biology. It is well accepted as scientific explanation that a species evolves over time because of natural selection. In simple terms, genes that express traits or characteristics related to survival and reproduction become better represented in the gene pool of the species. These contingencies of survival and reproduction are the ultimate cause of the species as we see them at a point in time. The anatomy and physiology of a species change over time due to these contingencies. Behavior is also similarly selected during the life of an individual (Skinner, 1981).

Environments are not static, and natural selection has also prepared species to be susceptible to the consequences following behavior. As Skinner (1981) stated,

> When members of a species eat a certain food simply because eating it has had survival value, the food does not need to be … a reinforcer. Similarly, when sexual behavior is simply a product of natural selection, sexual contact does not need to be … a reinforcer. But when, through the evolution of special susceptibilities, food and sexual contact become reinforcing, new forms of behavior can be set up. New ways … of behaving … can be shaped and maintained…. In summary, then, human behavior is the joint product of (1) the contingencies of survival responsible for the natural selection of the species and (2) the contingencies of reinforcement responsible for the repertoires acquired by its members, including (3) the special contingencies maintained by an evolved social environment. (p. 502)

Behavior analysis is then an approach that can be characterized as an extension of natural selection. That behavior is sensitive to consequences is part of our genetic endowment. The environment or context in which behavior occurs determines the events that follow behavior. Appetitive or rewarding consequences make behavior that produces them more probable, and aversive consequences make behavior that produces them less probable. (How these consequence operations work are briefly described in the following section.) The context in which behavior is possible, the context in which behavior has occurred in the past, and the current motivating conditions affecting the person converge to determine one's actions.

A Science of the Individual

Behavior analysis assumes that reliable scientific observation combined with direct and systematic replication to confirm the generality of these observations must be conducted with individuals in order to understand the causes of behavior. "Science, it is argued, proceeds by manipulating variables in a systematic fashion, and by unifying the results of such manipulation within a conceptual framework" (Sidman, 1960, p. 23). This conceptual framework and the underlying assumptions of behavior analysis are briefly described. From this point on, the focus of this chapter will be to detail its general methods.

Behavior, before it can be studied, must be defined, and the behavior analyst defines behavior precisely in terms of observable actions. These definitions must be reliable in that independent observers must be able to accurately identify the occurrence and nonoccurrence of the behavior of interest. To illustrate, consider one of the core deficits of autism, communication skills. In developing a definition that we could reliably record, we would need to select one class of communicative behavior. Let us say we are interested in a child's ability to express wants or needs. Requesting, or manding, is behavior that identifies the event or thing that the child currently wants to have. This behavior can involve vocalizations or gestures, and it must be distinguished from the child labeling an object. Thus, an accurate definition, for example, a vocal or gestural response not directed by another person that specifies a desired item or event, will take into account what will count and not count as an instance of this behavior.

The methods of behavior analysts are concerned with studying repeated instances of behavior across time and across imposed changes in the environmental conditions under which behavior is studied. As an example, Bob was a child diagnosed with autism who engaged in self-injurious behavior (SIB) in many situations and at varying intensities. These conditions included academic task (demand) presentation where SIB produced a break from tasks; an adult providing attention every time SIB occurred; play in which the child was given activities to play with and SIB was ignored; and a condition in which Bob was alone. Each environmental condition mimicked situations in which problem behavior had been found to commonly occur (see Figure 2.1). Bob was exposed to each condition five times in what is referred to as a *multielement design.* In this multielement design each of the four conditions was presented in randomized order once every four sessions for five blocks of four sessions. Bob was most likely to self-injure when academic demands were removed contingent upon SIB, and much less likely to do so in any other situation. This multielement design allowed the isolation of the likely cause and suggested possible treatment plans for his SIB.

ABA also uses other well-established single-subject designs including the *withdrawal or reversal design.* With this design, one variable such as a skill build-

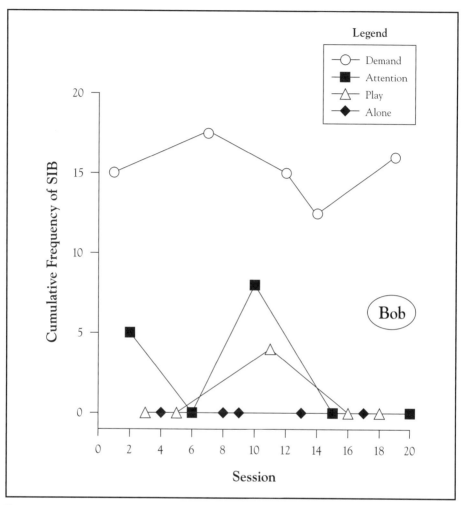

Figure 2.1. Total number of occurrences of self-injurious behavior (SIB) recorded in each environmental setting during a multielement design.

ing technique or behavior deceleration strategy is manipulated to determine whether the introduction and subsequent withdrawal of this variable causes a change in behavior. If the introduction of the variable results in a change in behavior, then the variable is removed to determine whether the behavior reverts to its baseline level. If it does, then the variable is reintroduced to determine whether the originally obtained effect on behavior is replicated.

As an example, staff taught Bob to request a break by pointing to a stop sign. To determine whether teaching Bob to request a break would replace SIB as an escape response during academic task performance, Bob was first presented with an academic task every 30 s during a baseline condition for three sessions (see Figure 2.2). Then, the stop sign was introduced into this academic demand setting and Bob was given a break for 30 s every time he pointed to the stop sign. Bob's SIB became infrequent when the stop sign was present but remained quite probable when it was not. Additional procedures were necessary to motivate Bob to spend more time working than taking breaks, but providing him with an efficient response to escape from demands without hitting himself caused a change in his SIB. In academic or therapeutic situations where severe problem behavior such as head banging or aggression toward others is being addressed, the use of a reversal design raises ethical concerns. In most cases, if a treatment has been shown to decrease or eliminate problem behavior, many would argue that reversing or removing the treatment to demonstrate experimental control is not in the best interest of the consumer. However, it is appropriate to use other experimental designs in those situations.

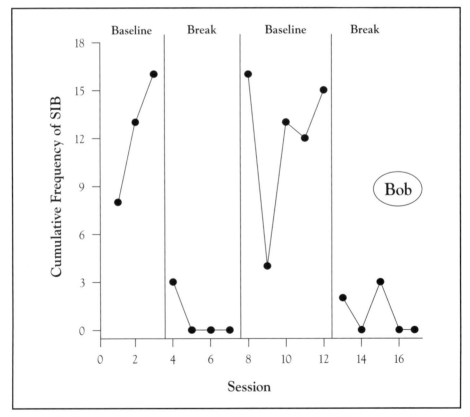

Figure 2.2. Total number of occurrences of self-injurious behavior (SIB) recorded when academic demands were presented in baseline and break conditions during a withdrawal design.

Some behavior will not revert back to a baseline level of occurrence after it has been changed by a procedure or some new relevant behavior has been learned. When a child learns to read a word, it is likely that he or she will continue to learn to read new words in the absence of the skill acquisition program that produced this outcome. In such cases, the effectiveness of the teaching program can be evaluated by staggering the training across various sets of words in what is called a *multiple baseline design*. Tim was an 8-year-old child with autism who could not identify various three-letter words. Prior to implementing a sight-word identification program, a number of target words were presented to him in a baseline condition (see Figure 2.3). Three sets, each consisting of three words, were presented for 18 trials per set, and correct or incorrect selection of the word presented on each trial was recorded. A delayed cue procedure, described in more detail later in this chapter, was then used to teach correct word identification, one set at a time. In this example, Tim learned to correctly identify words across each set because of the delayed cue procedure. The multiple-baseline design is also appropriate to use when a reversal design is not recommended, for example when treating severe problem behavior.

These basic designs and the many other validated procedures of behavior analysis are the core methods of this science of behavior. When discussing the empirical support for behavior analysis it is necessary to understand how these designs identify the causes or functional relations between behavior and the environments in which it occurs. Only after understanding these causes and relations is it possible to evaluate the principles of behavior analysis. These demonstrations must be recognized as the science underlying the effective teaching and behavior deceleration strategies for treating autism.

Basic Principles of Behavior Analysis

Behavior is complexly determined. When we watch an adult eating a granola bar, we are witnessing the seamless coming together of multiple behavioral processes and biological inheritance. When this person was born, the brush of a breast or bottle against the cheek, the sucking reflex, and complementary events resulted in food ingestion. We know that eating is not purely reflexive (i.e., an automatic or innate response to a stimulus) because the child that is not exposed to higher textures of food during early childhood does not readily acquire these responses later (Illingworth & Lister, 1964). Over time, an individual's mouth cavity changes, he or she is exposed to other foods like jarred baby foods, and he or she acquires developmentally advanced eating. Social influences such as the foods regularly presented at home then modifies and establishes the person's

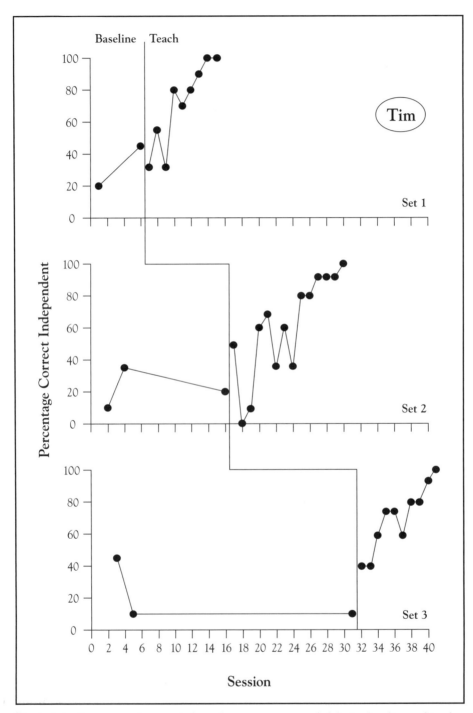

Figure 2.3. Percentage of correct independent responses recorded during baseline and teaching conditions across three sets of stimuli during a multiple-baseline design.

food preferences. However, these histories are typically not readily apparent. Furthermore, understanding how these responses came to exist as we now see them requires that we understand how behavior develops from its initial occurrence onward.

Some behavior we exhibit is reflexive. The origin of reflexive behavior is well understood to be caused by environmental stimuli that our bodies react to in an automatic fashion. Dust in the eye leads to a blink; a loud sudden noise results in a startle. Yet, some reflexes lead to consequences that then alter the nature of the response. The child who sucks jarred baby food as he would his bottle will gag. The child learns to process a novel food differently through the consequences that follow behavior, and these consequences come to establish the new eating behavior. Behavior controlled by its consequences is referred to as *operant* behavior (i.e., behavior that operates on the environment and produces consequences).

Operant behavior is not reflexive. Broadly speaking, it is said to be caused by consequences, but this is a simplification. The cause or explanation for any single occurrence of behavior involves consequences that have or have not followed behavior in the past and the environmental conditions presently influencing the individual. The first time a response leads to reinforcement, something new is created. Imagine that you gave a child a pop-up toy that has several buttons that when pressed causes an animal to pop up. Then you visit a month later and watch the child play with it. The child presses the buttons and animals pop up, she puts the animals down, and then she starts pressing the buttons again. When she was first given the toy, she may have held the toy as she would other objects, but then perhaps her arm happened to touch one of the buttons and an animal popped up. The child may have been startled, looked to her mother who was smiling, looked back at the toy, smiled, and laughed. These responses are *induced* by reinforcement; they are brought forth by this consequence of her action. Reinforcing, appetitive, or rewarding stimuli have this effect of leading to more behavior. The reinforcing event will also lead to similar responding again, but this time the response is not accidental. Subsequent instances of behavior are often very different from the initial response, and the behavior becomes more efficient. Over time the behavior selected becomes more refined and is emitted with little effort. Thus, the child comes to press the button slightly to the right with the right index finger, even though an infinite number of other behaviors could effectively produce the same consequence.

But if the animal is still up, pressing that same button will not produce the same consequence until the animal is put down. Responding differentiates from the unreinforced response. We say that this button pressing when the animal is up extinguishes. *Extinction* occurs when a previously reinforced response becomes less likely because it does not lead to reinforcement. More responses then are directed at the other buttons on the toy, leading to other reinforced responses. Once all of the animals are up, button pressing will not be reinforced again until the animals are put down. Next, imagine that the mother puts the animals down for the child and the child starts pressing the buttons again. Eventually the child will learn how to put the animals down. Then the child will press buttons when the animals are down and put the animals down when they are up. Thus, two repertoires of behavior are acquired—one that is reinforced in the presence of one context (button pressing is reinforced when animals are down) and another, putting the animals down, that is reinforced by the opportunity to press buttons. This process of *differential reinforcement* has caused the behavior that we observe when we visit the child.

Discrimination and Generalization

In the preceding example, pressing the button when the animal was already up was not effective in producing the reinforcing consequence. This led to variation in responding. The variation in responding then led to the occurrence of another effective response when a second button was pressed and the animal popped up. Pushing the first button was only reinforced when the first animal was down; when the first animal was up, pressing this button was extinguished and was reinforced again only after this animal was pushed down. Pressing the button when the animal is down and putting the animal down when it is up demonstrates *discrimination.*

The process of discrimination involves responding differently in different situations (Hineline, 1992). The animal down is one situation that occasions or establishes that button pressing will be reinforced, and the animal up is another situation that occasions or establishes that button pressing will not be reinforced unless the animal is pushed down. That the child learns to push each of the buttons demonstrates *generalization* of responding. After pushing one button, pushing the other buttons will be similarly reinforced. Generalization involves responding similarly in different situations. Each button can be considered a different situation: The buttons are in different locations, but the consequences for pressing the first button makes pressing the other buttons more likely.

Discrimination and generalization are processes that underlie all operant learning. Consider how a child learns the concept *dog.* At first, the child may identify all four-legged furry creatures as dogs. With experience the child comes to discriminate between dogs, cats, cows, pigs, and other animals but generalizes across very different kinds of dogs such as poodles and Labradors. These concepts are similar to Piaget's (1929) observations of assimilation and accommodation during child development, but *discrimination* and *generalization* are more precise terms.

Establishing Discriminative and Generalized Responding

Over the past 30 years, much has been learned about the way that individuals with autism and other developmental disabilities acquire new skills. A majority of the research on discrimination learning has been conducted in laboratory settings, and this technology has been translated into effective educational curricula. One of the most fundamental aspects of this teaching technology is often referred to as *stimulus control.* Stimulus control refers to the ways in which features of the learning environment—the presence of certain stimulus conditions but not others—influence the likelihood of behavior. For instance, if a child reliably says "cat" when the letters "C-A-T" are presented during instruction, we say that the combination of these three letters *controls* the vocal response "cat." Serna, Dube, and McIlvane (1997) suggested that discrimination learning often involves coming to respond to some sets of different (i.e., physically dissimilar) stimuli as if they were the same and coming to respond to other sets of different stimuli as if they were different. For example, the written word "C-A-T," a picture of a cat, and an actual cat all produce the same vocal response "cat," whereas different stimuli, such as pictures of dogs or cows, produce other responses (see Figure 2.4). Most typically developing children acquire such behavior seamlessly, but children with developmental difficulties often require more

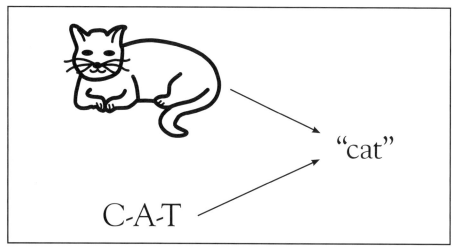

Figure 2.4. Physically dissimilar yet conceptually related stimuli.

time and focused instruction that helps to direct them to the relevant features of the environment.

Serna et al. (1997) described a taxonomy for organizing discrimination and stimulus control as a model for learning. Their model begins with a distinction between *simple* (nonrelational) and *conditional* (relational) discriminations. When a response always occurs reliably in the presence of one stimulus and not in the presence of others as a result of differential reinforcement, the discrimination is nonrelational. For example, saying "cat" when given a picture of a cat will produce the teacher's approval, and no other response will do so. In this case, a single feature of the environment or stimulus (the picture) becomes the discriminative stimulus or signal that reinforcement will follow a certain response (saying "cat"), and it is therefore called a discriminative stimulus (S^d). Simple discriminations describe many situations, such as orienting to one's name when called but not at other times, or picking up a phone only when it rings.

In a conditional discrimination situation, the stimuli still function as discriminative stimuli, but this function is conditional upon the presence of other stimuli. For example, suppose a set of animal pictures is placed before the child. If the teacher says, "Point to the cat," the cat picture becomes the S^d for a pointing response (see Figure 2.5). But if the teacher then says, "Now point to the dog," the cat picture is no longer the S^d—the S^d is now the dog picture. That is, the discriminative functions of the pictures are *conditional* upon the teacher's verbal cue. In conditional discriminations, the contingencies for reinforcement depend on relations between two or sometimes more stimuli. Matching-to-sample instructional procedures are a common format for teaching conditional discriminations. Relational or conditional discriminations underlie much of the complex behavior involved in communication, reading, and math.

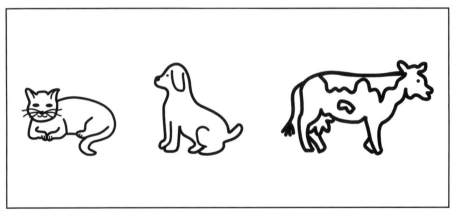

Figure 2.5. Physically dissimilar, conceptually unrelated stimuli arranged as comparisons for matching-to-sample training.

Attending and Session Behavior

Efficient learning requires many responses coming together at one time. The most critical responses are observing or attending to the relevant features of the learning task and engaging in appropriate behavior for the learning task while simultaneously not engaging in disruptive behavior. These responses are sometimes referred to as *session behavior*, prereadiness, or readiness skills. Attending and session behavior increase the likelihood of learning, and they are ordinarily considered to be behavioral prerequisites for any teaching situation. (See Chapter 3 by Rehfeldt and Rosales for an extensive discussion on session behavior and readiness skills.) *Attention* is behavior-indicative learning (Terrace, 1966). It specifically refers to a person's behavior with respect to some aspect of the environment. A child's sitting when he is asked to sit by an adult implies that he has attended to the adult's instruction.

For many children who have Autism Spectrum Disorders, session behavior cannot be assumed. Rather, it must be taught explicitly; otherwise the teacher will not know whether failure to acquire discriminations reflects problems in attending and session behavior, or whether it indicates a true deficit in the actual discrimination performance. Therefore, it is necessary to ensure that attending and session behavior are established first. Session behavior can be viewed as a chain of responses that include sitting, eye contact, waiting until stimuli are presented, scanning and observing the relevant stimuli, and emitting the appropriate response such as touching or pointing to a stimulus. These responses should first be established in the context of already mastered tasks. For example, if a child is able to select between two preferred toys, one might teach session behavior in the context of opportunities to point to and play with a toy. After these responses are established, then the child is ready to begin discrimination training.

Simple Discrimination Training Procedures

As indicated earlier, the most basic form of discrimination is a simple or nonrelational discrimination in which one response comes under the discriminative control of one stimulus. In one of the most basic simple discriminations for the instructional situation, and one that is a useful starting point for many children with severe disabilities, the S^d is a visual form on the tabletop and the response is pointing to it. This is sometimes referred to as a "form versus no-form" task (see Figure 2.6). A single form, for example a black cross, is presented alone on a page in either the left, right, or middle position. Touching the form is reinforced, and touching anywhere else on the page is not. The position of the form should vary irregularly from left to right to the middle across trials. The child

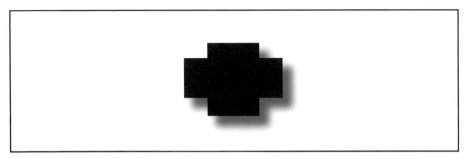

Figure 2.6. A stimulus, or form, which would vary in location, used during a simple discrimination training procedure.

learns to touch the form and to not touch any other position on the page. To teach this skill, we often use a stimulus board with three positions: left, right, and middle, marked by pieces of Velcro. We place the stimulus card with the S+ on the board (attached by Velcro) in the position designated for the correct response, making sure that the position of the S+ varies across trials. After this discriminative performance has been established with a variety of stimuli, the student has learned some basic skills for instructional sessions, and the teacher can move on to more complex discriminations.

Conditional Discriminations

Conditional discriminations are used to establish relational stimulus control between two distinct stimuli (Saunders & Spradlin, 1989, 1990, 1993; Saunders, Williams, & Spradlin, 1995). In other words, when the word "cat" is spoken, pointing to the cat is followed by reinforcement and pointing to the dog picture is not followed by reinforcement (see Figure 2.7). At other times, when the word "dog" is spoken, pointing to the cat is not followed by reinforcement and pointing to the dog is. The matching-to-sample procedure is often used to teach conditional discriminations. In matching-to-sample, the conditional stimuli (in this case, the spoken words) are called "samples," and the discriminative stimuli (in this case the pictures) are called the "comparison" stimuli.

 Match-to-sample learning trials involve the presence of a sample or conditional stimulus followed by the presentation of two or preferably more comparison stimuli (Sidman, 1980). A sample stimulus does not control responding in isolation, but rather determines the control that other stimuli may exert over responding. For each sample stimulus, one comparison stimulus is designated as the correct stimulus, or S+, to which responding will be followed by reinforcement, and the other stimuli are designated as incorrect, or S−, and responding

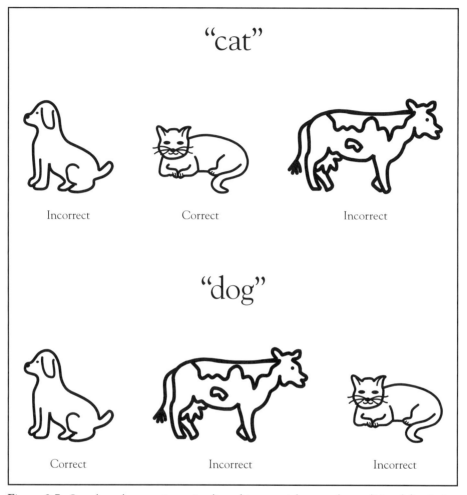

Figure 2.7. Sample and comparison stimuli used in two trial types of a conditional discrimination training procedure.

to S— will not be followed by reinforcement. The sample stimulus changes from trial to trial, and each comparison stimulus will be designated as S+ in the presence of a different sample stimulus. Therefore, the S+ (correct) and S— (incorrect) functions of the comparison stimuli change from trial to trial, making accuracy conditional on the sample. Additionally, on any given trial the comparison stimuli are presented in different positions.

Conditional *identity matching* and conditional *arbitrary matching* refer to different types of conditional performances (Dube, Iennaco, & McIlvane, 1993; McIlvane, Dube, Green, & Serna, 1993). These skills underlie symbolic functioning and communication. They are thus fundamental to teaching individuals with autism and other developmental disabilities. Identity matching-to-sample requires the child to be able to match based on the physical appearance of the stimuli, for example a matching-to-sample task in which the samples and comparisons are all pictures of animals and so the correct comparison on every trial is identical to the sample. Most would agree that the critical performance is accurately matching stimuli that have never been trained. This is known as *generalized identity matching*. Generalized identity matching is a useful skill because it allows the teacher to pretest the student's ability to discriminate between new sets of stimuli prior to teaching. Conditional arbitrary matching is matching two related but physically distinct stimuli, for example pointing to a picture of a ball in the presence of the spoken word "ball." This type of performance is fundamental to the development of conceptual behavior.

Identity Matching-to-Sample

Teaching procedures for establishing identity matching-to-sample begin with the presentation of a sample stimulus followed by the presentation of several comparison stimuli (see Figure 2.8). One of those comparison stimuli is physically identical to the sample stimulus. It is designated as the S+ on that trial. Responding to the physically identical comparison stimulus is followed by reinforcement. Responding to comparison stimuli that are not physically identical to the sample (S−) on that trial is not followed by reinforcement. Trials should be arranged to ensure that each stimulus is presented an equal number of times as S+ and S− within a learning set.

When teaching identity matching performance, we often begin by using stimuli that are very different from each other, such as a large ball and a small ball. Once these matching performances have been acquired, we move to stimuli that look more similar in form, such as knives, forks, and spoons. In addition, we teach matching objects first and then progress through a hierarchy of stimulus types, from line drawings, to photographs, and then to printed forms such as words, letters, and numerals. Identity matching-to-sample is considered mastered when matching performance generalizes to stimuli that are physically similar but have never been directly trained.

An alternative procedure for assessing and teaching identity matching is through use of a sorting task. Sorting involves the presentation of multiple bins, each of which has a stimulus in it. The child is then given an object that is physically identical to one of the objects in the bins and is required to place the object in the matching bin. The object given to the child is analogous to the sample stimulus, and the array of objects in the bins is analogous to the comparison or discriminative stimuli. Because sorting is often present in the repertoires of individuals with disabilities, Serna and McIlvane (1996) developed a

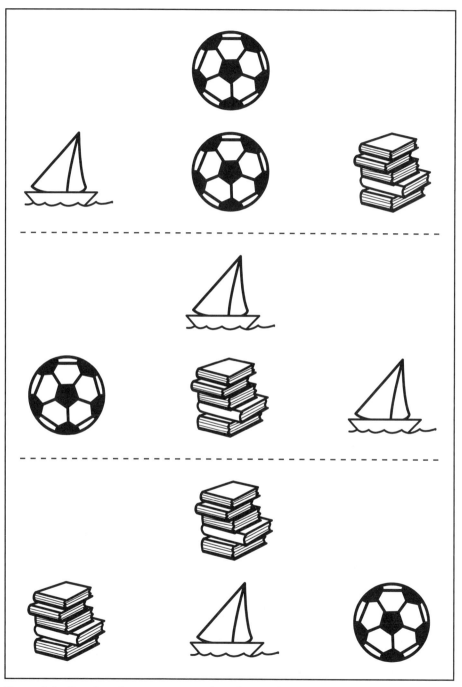

Figure 2.8. Sample and comparison stimuli used in an identity matching-to-sample training procedure.

protocol for using sorting to teach traditional matching-to-sample performance with two-dimensional stimuli.

Arbitrary Matching-to-Sample

The teaching procedures for arbitrary matching-to-sample are similar to those used in identity matching-to-sample. They begin with the presentation of a sample stimulus, for example the spoken word "ball," followed by the presentation of several comparison stimuli (see Figure 2.9a). One of those comparison stimuli is related to the sample stimulus, but is dissimilar in form (e.g., a picture of a ball). This related stimulus is designated as the S+ on that trial. Responding to the related comparison stimulus is followed by reinforcement. Responding to any other comparison stimulus that is not related (S−) to the sample on that trial is not reinforced. As with identity matching-to-sample, trials should be arranged so that each stimulus is presented an equal number of times as S+ and S− within a learning set.

There are a variety of different types of arbitrary matching performances used in educational tasks. *Auditory–visual* arbitrary matching tasks present spoken words as sample stimuli and visual stimuli such as objects, photos, or printed words as the comparison stimuli. *Visual–visual* arbitrary matching tasks involve matching visual stimuli such as objects, photos, or printed words to other visual stimuli (see Figure 2.9b). For example, when teaching the concept *ball,* one might teach a child to match a picture of a basketball with a picture of a soccer ball. The range of combinations of visual stimuli is virtually limitless.

Conditional discrimination performance in the form of arbitrary matching-to-sample is an important means to encourage the development of concepts such as color, shape, vehicles, clothing, and so on. Language, reading, spelling, and money use are just a few of the skills that have been evaluated experimentally using matching-to-sample discrimination procedures. Published curricula like the Edmark reading program incorporate the procedures of match-to-sample into a systematic and comprehensive sight word reading program (Conners, 1992). This has resulted in widespread availability and use of these teaching procedures across many educational settings.

Equivalence Class Formation

The development of concepts using conditional discrimination matching-to-sample procedures can be expanded using the *stimulus equivalence* model (see Figure 2.10). Sidman (1971) introduced this approach. Later Sidman and Tailby (1982) described it in terms of mathematical equivalence and its three properties of reflexivity, symmetry, and transitivity. Reflexivity is demonstrated by matching identical stimuli (e.g., matching object to object). Symmetry is shown when

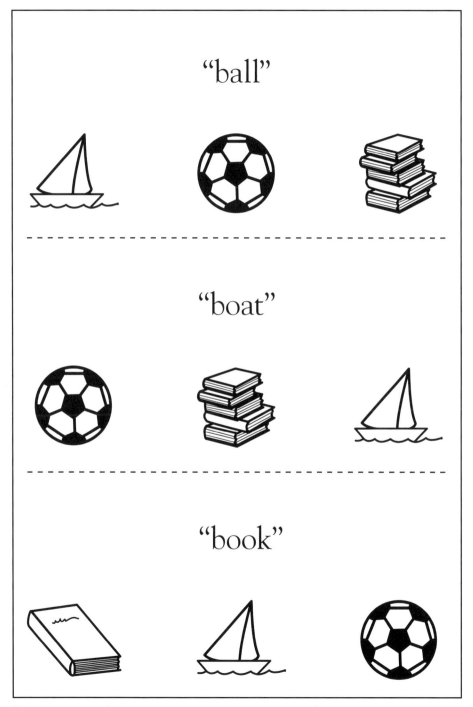

Figure 2.9a. Sample and comparison stimuli used in three trial types of an auditory–visual arbitrary matching-to-sample training procedure.

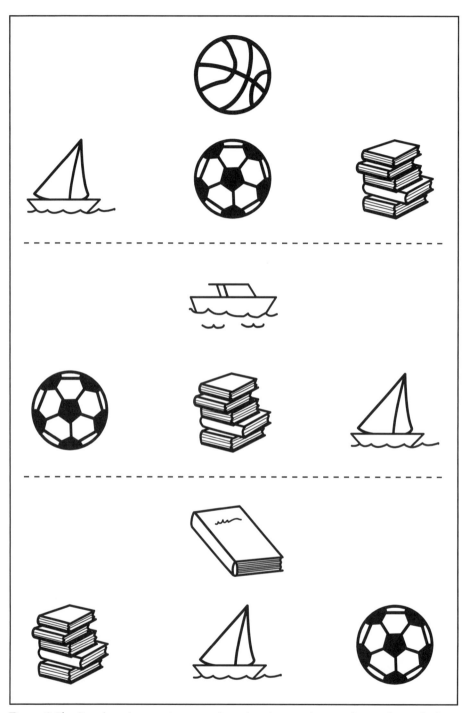

Figure 2.9b. Sample and comparison stimuli used in three trial types of a visual–visual arbitrary matching-to-sample training procedure.

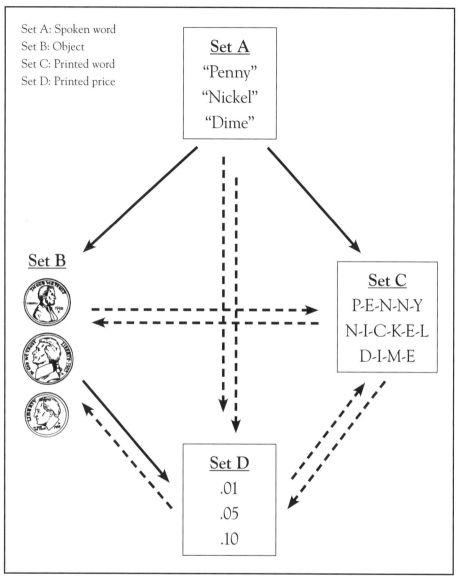

Figure 2.10. Diagram depicting the relations that are trained (solid lines) and that emerge (dashed lines) as a result of instruction when conditional discrimination training procedures are arranged to produce stimulus equivalence.

the sample and comparison stimuli within a matching-to-sample discrimination can be reversed while maintaining the same functional relation (e.g., after learning to match object to picture, matching picture to object without explicit training). Transitivity is shown by the emergence of untrained relations following training of two conditional discriminations with one set of stimuli in common (e.g., after learning to match object to printed word and printed word to picture, matching object to picture). Other training arrangements may permit more elaborate tests for untrained relations. For example, after learning to match a spoken word to a picture, and the same spoken word to a printed word, the student may be able to match the picture to the printed word and vice versa (e.g., Sidman, 1971). In this example the emergent behavior of matching the picture to the printed word may be called a combined test for symmetry and transitivity (e.g., Fields & Verhave, 1987) or a test for equivalence.

Equivalence classes that are taught in educational settings include objects, pictures, letters, words, or numerals and their corresponding spoken words (Mackay, 1985; Stoddard, Brown, Hurlbert, Manoli, & McIlvane, 1989; Stromer, Mackay, & Stoddard, 1992). The instructional sequence one can use to establish and test for equivalence class formation may begin with three-member classes that include visual stimuli only (objects, pictures, and printed words). For example, given a book as a sample, the child would be taught to point to a picture of a book. On other trials, given the same sample book the child would be taught to point to the printed word "B-O-O-K." The resulting test for untrained equivalence class formation would determine whether the child matches the picture of a book with the printed word "B-O-O-K" and vice versa. The results of such teaching may be described as all-visual three-member equivalence classes in which each class consists of an object, picture, and printed word. Other instructional sequences may be used to establish three-member equivalence classes that include both auditory and visual stimuli, for example by substituting the spoken word "book" for the book object in the training described above.

After three-member equivalence classes have been established, training only one additional relation may expand them to include four members (Johnson, White, Green, Langer, & MacDonald, 2000). For example, money-skills instruction might establish a three-member equivalence class by (a) teaching the relation of the spoken word "dime" to an actual dime (A-B relation), (b) teaching the relation of the spoken word "dime" to the written word "D-I-M-E" (A-C relation), and then (c) testing for the written word "D-I-M-E" to actual dime relation (C-A relation). If emergent matching verifies the three-member class, then one might teach the student to match the printed price of 10 cents to the dime and then test for all other relations between the printed price and the other stimuli within the class (McDonagh, McIlvane, & Stoddard, 1984).

Stimulus Overselectivity

A well-documented learning problem in children with autism is a tendency for the stimulus control to be unusually narrow or restricted. For example, a student learning to identify her printed name may respond to the initial letter only. Although such a student could discriminate "SUE" from "FAY" or "BOB," she would fail to discriminate "SUE" from "SAM" reliably. Lovaas, Koegel, and Schreibman (1979) called this *stimulus overselectivity*. They first described this problem of atypically limited learning with complex stimuli in detail. Procedures for assessing stimulus overselectivity have traditionally involved discrimination training with a complex stimulus that has at least two elements (e.g., auditory and visual) that have been presented simultaneously. Each element is then tested individually to assess stimulus control. Overselectivity is found if only one element exerts discriminative control. Overselectivity can be particularly problematic when the controlling element is not relevant to the criterion performance. For example, Schreibman and Lovaas (1973) used dolls to teach the discrimination between male and female. They discovered that some of the children made the discrimination based on a doll's belt rather than the face or other more socially relevant features.

Although there has been a plethora of research identifying overselectivity as a problem, there have been relatively few experimental demonstrations of effective remedial procedures. One approach has been to provide preliminary discrimination training with the individual stimuli or stimulus components before introducing the stimulus components together. Component pretraining has sometimes been reported effective in increasing the number of relevant stimulus dimensions that gain control of responding (Huguenin, 1985; Schneider & Salzberg, 1982).

A second promising approach to remediation comes from studies of *multiple-cue training*. In multiple-cue training, participants were given extended practice with tasks where high accuracy on simultaneous discrimination of two or more stimuli was taught. In three of these studies the correct response would be to select on every trial the compound stimulus A+B, and to reject the incorrect alternatives A+C and A alone (Allen & Fuqua, 1985; Koegel & Schreibman, 1977; Schreibman, Charlop, & Koegel, 1982). Burke and Cerniglia (1990) employed a matching task with multiple verbal cues, for example "[touch the] big red pencil," where the incorrect alternatives included a small red pencil, big blue pencil, and other variations. In all four studies, the stimulus sets were arranged so that responding based on only one cue would not be consistently reinforced. Many children who were overselective on initial assessments improved at least to some extent with multiple-cue training.

Probably the most effective remedial technique is to change the task requirements to include *differential observing responses*. This type of procedure is related to multiple-cue training, but it has the addition of explicit response requirements for each of the cues. For example, in a matching-to-sample task the student would be required to make observing responses that verify discrimination of all relevant sample–stimulus elements. The students would make the observing responses *before* selecting a comparison stimulus. For example, if the sample stimuli were printed words, a child who can spell could be required to name all of the sample letters aloud before selecting a comparison stimulus. Similar requirements might be to name pictures (Gutowski, Geren, Stromer, & Mackay, 1995), repeat spoken words, or perform an identity-matching task with complex samples (Dube & McIlvane, 1999).

Prompting Procedures

Discrimination training procedures do not stand alone. Instructional techniques must be tailored to a child's specific learning style. The following section details instructional techniques used in structured learning environments. However, the techniques are not only relevant for teaching discrimination skills but also apply in other situations such as teaching communication skills, activities of daily living, and other chains of behavior. *Prompts* are defined as ancillary stimuli that are effective in establishing the appropriate behavior in the presence of the target or new discriminative stimulus (Foxx, 1982; MacDuff, Krantz, & McClannahan, 2001; Snell, 1993). Prompts are introduced either before or after the target stimuli that will eventually set the occasion for the correct response. They must be stimuli that already control responding. The terminal goal is always for responding to occur in the presence of natural environmental cues in the absence of prompts (Etzel & LeBlanc, 1979).

Discrimination learning is established through the systematic manipulation of stimulus and response prompts. Prompts facilitate learning and rapid acquisition of new discriminations. They can also reduce errors. Errors can be problematic for children with autism (Stella & Etzel, 1986). They can interfere with acquisition of new skills (Albin & Horner, 1988), establish error patterns that are difficult to correct (Demchak, 1990), and lead to decreased motivation to perform and increases in challenging behavior during learning (Carr & Durand, 1985). The careful and systematic use of prompting is an important ingredient in the development of effective instructional teaching procedures.

The use of prompting procedures involves two decisions. The first is to decide what types of prompts to use. The two major types of instructional prompts are response prompts and stimulus prompts. Both types of prompts direct the child's responding to the critical features of the discriminative stimuli during acquisition. The second decision concerns the method of transfer from the prompt to the target discrimination. For example, if the child is learning to say the word "book" in the presence of a book, the teacher may begin by presenting a point prompt to the book simultaneously with the spoken word "book." Over trials the teacher will delay the onset of the point prompt until the child points to the book in the presence of the spoken word alone. This is referred to as the *transfer of control* from an extrastimulus prompt, a point cue, to the target discriminative stimulus, in this case a book (Schreibman et al., 1982). The type of prompt and the method of fading the prompt both deserve careful consideration when designing a discrimination learning program.

Types of Instructional Prompts

Response Prompts

Response prompts are supplementary stimuli that guide the child's response during learning. The major types of response prompts include verbal prompts (instructions), textual prompts, modeling, gestures, and physical prompts.

Verbal Prompts

Verbal prompts include one-word directions or complete phrases with very specific information. For example, when teaching a child to wash his or her hands, a teacher might say, "Turn on the water" to prompt the next step in the task. Verbal prompts are perhaps the most commonly used prompts in educational instruction. The instruction "turn on the water" is considered a verbal prompt because the goal is for the previous step in the task (e.g., approaching the sink) to become the discriminative stimulus that occasions the response of turning on the faucet, and the instruction "turn on the water" to be faded.

A number of studies have investigated the use of verbal prompts to increase social interactions between children with autism and peers or siblings (James & Egel, 1986; Odom & Strain, 1986; Shafer, Egel, & Neef, 1984). Odom and Strain used the verbal prompt "Today I want you to play with John" to increase social interactions with typical peers. They found that verbal prompts to the child with autism were more effective at increasing social initiations than prompts to the peer. In some cases, children need more specific strategies for how to play with peers. For instance, one may use the verbal cue "Play what a friend is playing" to prompt a child to join in play with peers. Verbal prompts can be very specific or can cue the child to engage in behavior she has previously learned.

Textual Prompts

Textual prompts include written words, lists, or instructions. These prompts can be used to set the occasion for completing a list of tasks (Cuvo, Davis, O'Reilly,

Mooney, & Crowley, 1992), for example an after-school routine that includes putting away a lunch box, getting a snack, and playing the piano. Textual prompts have also been used to prompt a conversation with a peer (Krantz & McClannahan, 1993).

Krantz and McClannahan (1998) used written scripts to teach children with autism to initiate conversations with teachers. They presented the printed words "Look" and "Watch" in the context of an activity, and children were taught to read the word, approach a teacher, and say the word(s) to the teacher. This written prompt then set the occasion for a teacher to comment on what the child had done or watch the child perform an activity. Scripted and unscripted verbal interactions increased using the procedure and generalized to new activities. Solicitations of this kind can make important contributions to the development of social repertoires in children with autism.

Another type of textual prompt involves scripted statements that set the occasion for conversational interactions with peers. For example, children with autism were taught to engage in scripted conversations within the context of an art activity (Krantz & McClannahan, 1993). Several children sat at an art table and each child was given a list of scripted statements to read such as "(Name), would you like to use one of my crayons?" Children were prompted to check off each script once it was used and to say each statement or question once during the activity. Over time, these scripts were faded and children continued to have social conversations during these art activities and began to vary their conversations to include novel unscripted information. Textual cues can reduce reliance on teacher presence during activities that involve independent performance or social interactions.

Picture Prompts

Pictures can prompt a variety of tasks including self-help (Spellman, DeBriere, Jarboe, Campbell, & Harris, 1978), meal preparation (Johnson & Cuvo, 1981), and leisure activity schedules (MacDuff, Krantz, & McClannahan, 1993; Pierce & Schreibman, 1994). Early in training, picture prompts are often paired with other types of prompting procedures to establish the target responses. Over time, picture prompts can be very effective in establishing long chains of behavior.

MacDuff et al. (1993) used photo activity schedules and graduated guidance to teach children with autism to engage in lengthy periods of independent play. After training to engage in a series of after-school activities using a picture schedule, children generalized the strategy to new activities and across different settings in their group home. Picture schedules are frequently used as prompts to establish responding in the absence of a teacher; in such cases the pictures are typically not faded out and continue to control performance.

Modeling

Modeling involves the demonstration of a response so the child imitates the model's behavior to produce reinforcement. For example, if a child is learning to sort objects by categories, the teacher might model placing a car in the vehicle bin and an apple in the food bin so that the child can imitate the model by placing identical or similar items in the correct category bins. Modeling is effective only when the child has the prerequisite skill of generalized imitation (Young, Krantz, McClannahan, & Poulson, 1994) and the motor ability to imitate the modeled behavior.

Observational learning is a form of modeling that can include demonstrations by the teacher, a peer, or a video. It has been an effective instructional prompting strategy to teach equivalence relations (MacDonald, Dixon, & LeBlanc, 1986; Rehfeldt, Latimore, & Stromer, 2003), receptive labeling (Charlop, Schreibman, & Tryon, 1983), sight words (Schoen & Ogden, 1995), and food preparation (Griffen, Wolery, & Schuster, 1992). Chronological age and level of disability correlate with learning through observation for children with autism (Varni, Lovaas, Koegel, & Everett, 1979).

Teacher modeling is often used in the context of discrete trial teaching. For example, if a child is learning body parts, the teacher says, "Touch nose" and immediately demonstrates by touching his or her own nose. It is important during this type of instruction to teach several different body parts simultaneously (i.e., a conditional discrimination). In this way, the teacher can verify that the child listens to the whole instruction. Modeling can include demonstrations of a motor response, a vocal response, or a written demonstration (e.g., for the child to copy text).

Peer models have been used extensively in inclusive educational settings. Learning in a traditional classroom environment requires that children are able to watch their peers and imitate the modeled actions (Johnson, Meyer, & Taylor, 1996). Egel, Richman, and Koegel (1981) used typically developing peer models to teach discrimination tasks to children with autism and found rapid acquisition and maintenance of the tasks.

In *video modeling,* a model demonstrating the target behavior is videotaped, and the child watches the video model of scripted actions, verbalizations, or both. The videotape may be edited to highlight desirable behavior and to remove maladaptive behavior. Video modeling is typically used to teach longer chains of behavior such as community purchasing skills (Haring, Kennedy, Adams, & Pitts-Conway, 1987) and daily living skills (Rehfeldt, Dahman, Young, Cherry, & Davis, 2003; Shipley-Benamou, Lutzker, & Taubman, 2002). In addition, video modeling has been effective in teaching social conversational skills (Charlop & Milstein, 1989; Charlop-Christy, Le, & Freeman, 2000; Sherer, Pierce, Paredes, Kisacky, Ingersoll, & Schreibman, 2001), perspective taking

(LeBlanc et al., 2003), play initiation skills (Charlop-Christy et al., 2000; Nikopoulos & Keenana, 2004), and pretend play (Cota et al., 2003; D'Ateno, Mangiapanello, & Taylor, 2003; MacDonald, Clark, Garrigan, & Vangala, 2005). Some studies have shown that video modeling is superior to in-vivo modeling (Charlop-Christy et al., 2000). Sherer et al. (2001) found that with video modeling it does not appear to make a difference whether the model is the child or another person, although the relative merits of different forms of video modeling procedures are still being evaluated. (Rehfeldt and Rosales discuss video modeling in more detail in Chapter 4.)

Gestures

Gestures are a straightforward means to prompt a child to look at a stimulus. A point prompt is the most commonly used gesture. Gestures differ from modeling in that they do not show the student how to perform the correct response. Rather, they show the child which stimulus is correct. In a conditional discrimination task such as touching a book in the presence of the spoken word "book," a point prompt is usually presented when both the sample and the comparison stimuli are available. Point prompts can also be used to prompt a child to interact with a more complex environment. For example, when washing hands, the teacher points to the faucet to direct the child to turn on the water. Again, the child is not shown how to turn on the water; the gesture merely serves to call attention to the faucet.

Physical Prompts

Physical prompts are the most intrusive of the response prompts. Physical prompts involve "putting the child through" the response by touching him and directing his body to perform a specific action. When teaching a child to brush her teeth, the teacher may start by holding the child's hand to her mouth and hand-over-hand guiding the brushing motions. Physical prompts can be used in the context of discrimination tasks or longer chains of behavior. In making the decision to use physical prompting, it is important to be sure that the child is not resistant to being touched. Physical prompts are often used in combination with other less restrictive prompts.

Stimulus Prompts

Stimulus prompts are supplementary stimuli that are used to guide the child to respond correctly to a stimulus. There are two major types of stimulus prompts: position cues and within-stimulus prompts. *Position cues* involve arranging the comparison stimuli such that the S+ is closer to the child than the other stimuli. For example, in teaching a child to identify letters, the teacher might present the letter M followed by the presentation of three comparison letters, M, S, and T. However, the letter M would be closer to the child than the incorrect stimuli. This procedure increases the likelihood of the child selecting the correct stimulus on each trial.

A *within-stimulus* prompt, sometimes referred to as a redundancy cue, is a distinctive manipulation of color, shape, or size within the target discriminative stimulus. Schreibman (1975) found that exaggerating the relevant component of a training stimulus resulted in more rapid acquisition of the discrimination than other types of prompts that were placed outside of the stimulus. Nelson, Holt, and Etzel (1976) taught children to label numbers by pairing cue words and pictures that started with the same sound as the numeral name. For example, the numeral zero was presented with the cue "zip zero" and a picture of a zero with a zipper in the middle. Other numerals were introduced in a similar fashion. After training, children labeled the numerals without the picture or verbal cues. Within-stimulus prompts are often preferred for children with autism because they may minimize the problem of stimulus overselectivity discussed above.

Transfer of Stimulus Control and Fading Prompts

Transfer of Response Prompts

Prompts must be faded or removed so that stimulus control can be transferred from the prompts, which are effective but inappropriate discriminative stimuli, to the appropriate discriminative stimuli. There are a variety of ways to accomplish this transfer of control.

Touchette (1971) introduced the *delayed cue* procedure, which is perhaps the most widely used prompt-elimination strategy. The prompt is initially presented simultaneously with the discriminative stimulus. Then, across trials, the onset of the prompt is gradually delayed beyond the onset of the discriminative stimulus. This delay gives the child an opportunity to respond before the prompt is presented. For example, when teaching a child to match a picture of a car with a toy car, the teacher presents a toy car as a sample stimulus followed by three pictures of comparison stimuli, which include a car. Simultaneously with the presentation of the comparisons, the teacher points to the picture of the car. The child responds by pointing to the picture of the car, and a reinforcer is delivered. On subsequent trials, the point prompt is delayed in time using either a progressive or fixed delay procedure. A progressive delay involves increasing the delay, for example in 1-s increments, up to some maximum value such as 5 s (Clark &

Green, 2004; Gast, Doyle, Wolery, Ault, & Farmer, 1991; Godby, Gast, & Wolery, 1987). Guidelines for increasing the delay vary. In general accurate performance on three to five consecutive trials is recommended prior to increasing the delay interval. With a fixed delay, the prompt-onset delay remains constant across training sessions (Ault, Wolery, Gast, Doyle, & Eizenstat, 1988; Doyle, Wolery, Gast, Ault, & Wiley, 1990; Wolery et al., 1992). In both cases, mastery is achieved when the child reliably responds correctly prior to the prompt.

Oppenheimer, Saunders, and Spradlin (1993) used the delayed cue method of transferring stimulus control to teach a wide variety of skills. Godby et al. (1987) compared a progressive delayed cue procedure to a least-to-most response prompt hierarchy to teach children to identify objects. They found that acquisition required fewer teaching trials and was accomplished with fewer errors with the delayed cue procedure relative to least-to-most prompting. The delayed cue method is often a useful procedure for transferring stimulus control but can also produce prompt dependency (Glat, Gould, Stoddard, & Sidman, 1994). Some children will always wait for the prompt to be delivered prior to responding. When this happens an alternative transfer procedure is necessary.

Graduated guidance involves the systematic fading of physical prompts. Typically, graduated guidance procedures begin with full hand-over-hand physical guidance, using only as much assistance as necessary to produce accurate responding. Then, the degree of assistance is reduced over successive trials to partial prompting, shadowing (keeping the hand near but not touching the child), and finally no prompts. During the prompt-elimination sequence, the teacher must continuously monitor the accuracy of the child's responses in order to determine the appropriate level of prompt during each trial, providing more assistance when the child begins to make an error and reducing the level of support when the child is correct.

Graduated guidance has been used to teach children to follow photo activity schedules (MacDuff et al., 1993). A photo activity schedule involves teaching a chain of behavior occasioned by a picture or written schedule in order to develop long sequences of independent responding. For example, with a book that has one picture of a previously mastered activity on each page, the child is taught the following behavior chain: point to the picture, obtain the materials, play with the materials, put the materials away, turn to next page, and then repeat this sequence with the next picture. As the child moves through the chain, physical assistance is provided initially and gradually reduced across steps of the chain as the child begins to respond more independently. Graduated guidance can be a relatively quick procedure for establishing such repeated chains of behavior. However, it requires a great deal of proficiency on the part of the teacher. If this procedure is going to be used across multiple teachers, it is necessary that they all implement the procedure in a consistent manner.

Most-to-Least Prompt Fading

Most-to-least prompt fading is another errorless procedure for transferring stimulus control from the response prompt to the target discriminative stimulus. This procedure is similar to graduated guidance; however, the criterion for fading to less intrusive prompts is determined by performance across trials and sessions. For instance, when teaching a child to imitate motor actions, the teacher models the action of clapping hands and immediately provides hand-over-hand guidance for the child to complete this action. Once the child has performed this response at that level of prompting across several repetitions, a less intrusive prompt is used. Next a physical prompt is provided at the child's wrist until the performance is stable and so on until the child performs the response without prompting. Mastery criteria can vary. For example, the skill may be considered mastered when the child responds independently in eight of nine performance opportunities.

Most-to-least prompt fading procedures have been shown effective with a variety of prompts including physical guidance, gestural cues, verbal models, and verbal instructions (MacDuff et al., 2002). In many cases, we transfer control from the prompt to the terminal stimulus by using prompt hierarchies that include a combination of prompt types. For example, if we are teaching a child to fold a shirt, we may begin by giving the instruction "fold your shirt" in the context of an unfolded shirt. The teacher can begin by initially providing physical guidance to perform the task, and across trials this prompt is faded to a gesture, then a point, and finally no prompt.

Most-to-least prompting can be used for teaching skills such as motor imitation, following directions, self-feeding, and other self-care skills (Snell, 1993). One variation of most-to-least prompting that has been found to be effective is to begin with immediate presentation of the most intrusive prompt, and once the child responds correctly with prompting for several successive trials, introduce a 2-s delay between the discriminative stimulus and the prompt. The less intrusive prompts can then be introduced, maintaining the 2-s delay for the remainder of the training trials. This procedure allows for the child to respond prior to the prompt and may foster more rapid prompt fading. Most-to-least fading is a generally effective procedure and acquisition can occur with a minimum of errors. However, proficient learners may acquire skills more rapidly with graduated guidance or least-to-most prompting.

Least-to-Most Prompt Fading

Least-to-most prompt fading is another procedure for transferring stimulus control from the response prompt to the target discriminative stimulus. Least-to-most prompting is not an errorless procedure, but it is perhaps the most commonly used type of prompt fading procedure across educational settings and skills. Using this procedure, the learner is given the terminal discriminative stimulus and then provided with the least intrusive prompt that will result in the correct response. This is accomplished by providing an interval of about 5 s between the discriminative stimulus for responding, for example saying, "stand up," and giving a gestural cue. If the child does not respond within 5 s, the prompt is provided. Unlike the most-to-least fading procedure, with least-to-most fading the initial prompt is one of the less intrusive prompts, such as the gesture. If the child responds correctly to this prompt, reinforcement follows and the next trial is introduced. If the child does not respond to the less intrusive prompt, then more intrusive prompts within the prompt hierarchy (e.g., light physical assistance at the shoulder, manually guiding standing up) are delivered until the child responds correctly. This procedure is repeated on subsequent trials until the performance criterion is met.

This prompt fading procedure is most effective when the child has the prerequisites to perform the target response, or when he has a history of acquiring skills rapidly. Because this procedure is not errorless, children who are likely to make errors are not good candidates for this prompt fading procedure. The basic premise of least-to-most prompt fading is that the child is given an opportunity to respond to the natural target stimulus on every trial and provided prompts only if necessary. In addition, when assistance is provided, the student is given only as much assistance as is needed to perform the task correctly. Though this procedure appears less restrictive than most-to-least fading, studies have shown that least-to-most prompting may produce more errors, require more prompted trials than other procedures like a delayed cue, and ultimately result in a slower rate of acquisition (Doyle et al., 1990; Godby et al., 1987).

Effective Reinforcers

The preceding section of this chapter highlighted the basic procedures for teaching new skills. One point that was not covered was the necessity to provide the proper motivation for individuals with severe learning difficulties. Typically developing children are often readily motivated by the social feedback, and other natural consequences of behavior they receive from their parents, teachers, and peers are all that is necessary for learning to take place. However, these natural or *intrinsic reinforcers* are sometimes not effective in establishing appropriate behavior for persons with autism and others with developmental or learning disabilities. For persons with autism, insensitivity to social consequences and other social signals is at the core of the disorder. In these cases relatively dense schedules of potent reinforcers might be necessary for skill acquisition. Thus, identifying potent reinforcers is crucial for effective intervention. Yet, the concept of reinforcement seems to be misunderstood by many.

Over the years, we have heard many negative comments from parents and educators about using positive reinforcement such as, "I don't want you using bribes with my child." However, reinforcement is one of the most basic and crucial mechanisms in learning. So, what exactly is reinforcement? Simply put, reinforcement is a consequence that follows a behavior that increases the future probability of that behavior. In other words, reinforcement strengthens behavior. For example, suppose a young child is learning to brush her teeth, and the first time she passes the brush over her teeth, the parent says, "I'm so proud of you, what a nice job." This enthusiastic praise is natural or intrinsic to the situation, and if the child is more likely to brush her teeth in the future, the social praise of the parent was likely a reinforcer. Most parents and teachers praise children for appropriate behavior, but we rarely think of this in terms of delivering reinforcement. The reality is that reinforcement and other feedback determine our behavior, but because they occur in the natural course of events, we rarely see or evaluate these consequences. These consequences do become apparent though when learning that should take place does not.

Not all reinforcement for our behavior is intrinsic. Why do we go to work? Although our employers may think we do this out of the goodness of our hearts, the reality is that we go to work to earn money. Money allows us to access other reinforcers, and working to earn money is *extrinsic reinforcement*. Our job is to teach children, and the natural consequence of our actions is that children learn. Certainly we find this quite pleasurable and delight in the progress of our students, but we would not be able to do this without pay unless we were independently wealthy. Extrinsic reinforcement is often necessary to teach a child who is not learning by the natural consequences for his or her behavior. However, the goal of behavior analysis is to prepare the child to be sensitive to the consequences that should naturally follow behavior. Baer et al. (1968) state that "application typically means producing … behavior; valuable behavior usually meets [intrinsic] reinforcement in a social setting; thus valuable behavior, once set up, may no longer be dependent upon the … technique which created it." (We substitute the word *intrinsic* for a synonymous term to contrast with *extrinsic*.)

Consequence Operations

Extrinsic reinforcement is crucial for establishing (and sometimes necessary for maintaining) appropriate behavior and teaching new skills. Reinforcement is also sometimes necessary for maintaining behavior change. However, the ultimate goal of the applied behavior analyst is to prepare behavior for the natural consequences it will meet. Reinforcement can be thought of as a law of nature, like the law of gravity. Gravity works for all people, animals, and inanimate objects in the same way, no matter where you are—it is a lawful phenomenon. Reinforcement is similar; it works the same way for all individuals. Reinforcement refers to events that are produced by a behavior that make behavior more likely to happen. If a *positive reinforcer* follows a behavior, the likelihood of that behavior occurring again will maintain at its current level or increase; if a reinforcer does not follow a behavior at least occasionally, it will not maintain or increase.

Negative reinforcement also involves behavior that increases, but it involves responding that makes an aversive event less aversive. When a parent hears a child crying, the child's crying is an unpleasant or aversive event. Let us imagine that the parent enters the child's room, picks him up, and gently rocks him, and the crying stops. The discontinuation of crying negatively reinforces the behavior of the parent, and the parent is more likely to pick up and rock the child in a similar manner the next time he cries. Much of our behavior is determined by the lessening of aversive events. Both positive and negative reinforcement result in an increase in the future probability of behavior.

Applying aversive events contingent upon undesirable behavior occurs frequently in most societies. When a behavior is followed by an aversive consequence or an appetitive consequence is withheld because of a behavior and the behavior occurs less frequently, this is called *punishment.* There is much controversy about punishment. Skinner (1953) was a long-standing opponent to the use of punishment. Punishment is a process that occurs in nature and is applied by social institutions. Nevertheless, punishment is not the most direct or functionally appropriate and is the least desirable means of changing behavior. If a behavior occurs that is problematic because it is harmful to the person who engages in it or to the social community, it occurs because of some relation it has to the environment. The most efficient way of changing undesirable behavior is to discover its cause and develop a functionally appropriate intervention (see Chapter 7 by Smith, Vollmer, and St. Peter Pipkin for a discussion of this issue). On the other hand, because punishment is a process that occurs in nature and is applied by society, it is important to understand the process of punishment and its implications. This issue is, however, beyond the scope of this book (see Van Houten et al., 1988 for an extensive discussion of this topic). The remainder of our discussion of consequence operations will focus on positive reinforcement procedures.

Identifying Reinforcers

A few children with autism may make progress just as fast as or faster than their typical peers, without any extrinsic or arranged reinforcement. Obviously, this is the ideal scenario. However, for some children or for specific skills, arranged reinforcement will be necessary in order for learning to take place. Failure to do so will result in learning occurring slowly or not at all. So how do many parents, teachers, and clinicians determine the preferences of the children they work with? In many cases, the parents or caregivers are asked what they think the child prefers. If children communicate, we may ask them what they would like to earn. There is some evidence to suggest that these techniques may not identify effective reinforcers for some individuals.

Green et al. (1988) addressed the question of whether simply asking caregivers what a child preferred would identify reinforcers as reliably as a systematic preference assessment. Adults were asked to rank items they thought would be most preferred by the children. This ranking was then compared to a systematic assessment. For many children, there was little to no correspondence between what the adults thought were preferred and what actually ranked as preferred on a systematic assessment. This discrepancy demonstrated that simply asking caregivers what children like is not an effective way to determine a child's preferences. Another technique that is frequently used to assess preferences is simply to ask the children themselves what they prefer. Northup (2000) asked children to rate how much they liked various items and compared their responses to systematic assessment. Asking children to identify their own reinforcers was successful in identifying reinforcers in less than 60% of cases.

One sound means of identifying potential reinforcers is through the use of a *stimulus preference assessment* (SPA). In most SPA procedures, potential reinforcers like activities and edible items are repeatedly presented to a child singly, in pairs, or in groups, and what the child approaches is recorded. "Approach" needs to be defined for each item or activity, but in general, approach refers to interacting with a stimulus, for example picking up and manipulating a toy or consuming a food or drink. When many stimuli are assessed, they are typically ranked from most to least preferred. This is called a *preference hierarchy.*

We are interested in the level of preference an individual has for various stimuli because high-preference stimuli are the most likely to function as effective reinforcers. However, it is crucial to note that high-preference stimuli are not guaranteed to function as reinforcers for all responses. Some tasks may be beyond the child's current abilities and they will need to learn prerequisite skills before succeeding at higher level skills. Nevertheless, you increase the chances that the child is properly motivated to learn if you use high-preference stimuli.

Preference Assessment Procedures

There have been several different types of SPA procedures developed over the years. Which SPA procedure may be the most effective and efficient for any given individual probably depends on the skills that the individual possesses. One of the first systematic preference assessments developed was the *single-stimulus preference assessment* (Pace, Ivancic, Edwards, Iwata, & Page, 1985). With this procedure, a series of stimuli are placed one at a time in front of the child, and the teacher records which items were approached and which were not. Across several sessions, all stimuli are presented more than once. Then, approach toward each item is calculated by determining the number of times each stimulus was approached and dividing by the number of times that stimulus was presented. Pace et al. (1985) considered high-preference stimuli to be those approached on at least 80% of opportunities, and low-preference stimuli were those approached on 50% or fewer of opportunities. This preference assessment can generate distinct preference hierarchies for each individual, but it is necessary to show that preferred items will reinforce behavior, and a *reinforcer assessment* can be used to verify a reinforcer's effectiveness. The reinforcer assessment involves a high preference or a low preference being provided for responding on a task (e.g., sorting different colored objects). Pace and colleagues found that when stimuli were made contingent on responding, high-preference stimuli generally led to higher response rates than low-preference stimuli. Thus, the single-stimulus preference assessment is generally effective in identifying reinforcers. One potential drawback of this procedure is that only one stimulus is presented on each trial, and some individuals may approach all stimuli at high rates. This results in little differentiation in preferences across stimuli.

Fisher et al. (1992) developed the *paired-stimulus assessment.* This procedure solved the potential problem of having an individual select each stimulus on 100% of opportunities by placing two stimuli in front of the person on each trial and allowing him to select only one. Fisher et al. (1992) selected 16 stimuli, but the procedure can be done with any number of items. On each trial, two items are presented and placed about 0.3 m apart and 0.3 m in front of the individual, who selects one. Across a series of trials, each stimulus is paired with every other stimulus an equal number of times, and each stimulus falls on the participant's left and right 50% of the trials. For most individuals, distinct preference hierarchies were generated, and high-preference stimuli were generally effective reinforcers. For success with this assessment, individuals must scan an array of two stimuli and must have appropriate session behavior (i.e., they must select only one stimulus on each trial). If the participant has these skills, the paired-stimulus assessment can be a very effective way to identify effective reinforcers. However, if the individual does not possess these skills, the single-stimulus assessment may be preferable.

Although the paired stimulus assessment identifies effective reinforcers for many individuals, it can be time-consuming to complete. *Multiple stimulus preference assessments* offer a time-efficient alternative. One commonly used multiple stimulus assessment is the multiple stimulus without replacement assessment (MSWO; DeLeon & Iwata, 1996). DeLeon and Iwata placed seven stimuli in a straight line in front of a child, who selected one. They recorded the selection, and the selected item was not replaced in the array. They changed the positions of the remaining items in the array. The child then selected from the remaining items. They continued the procedure until all stimuli were selected or the child stopped approaching items. The procedure was typically repeated five times.

The MSWO can be scored by calculating the percentage of times an item was selected over the number of trials that item was available; since items are not replaced following a selection, not all stimuli are available on each trial. Ciccone, Graff, and Ahearn (2005) developed a point weighting method of scoring the MSWO that places more importance on items selected early in a session. The item selected first from a seven-item array would be assigned a value of 7 points, whereas an item selected last, when it is the only remaining item in the array, would receive a value of 1 point. Following MSWO preference assessments, reinforcer assessments have been conducted to verify that items identified as high preference function as reinforcers.

The MSWO is an efficient SPA method because it can be completed in less time than a paired stimulus assessment. Participants should have the appropriate prerequisite skills (e.g., scanning large arrays, not grabbing items between trials). Additionally, brief MSWO assessments have also been shown to be effective. Although DeLeon and Iwata (1996) conducted five-preference assessment sessions, one recent study demonstrated that effective reinforcers could be identified if only three-preference assessments were conducted (Carr, Nicolson, & Higbee, 2000). Similarly, although DeLeon and Iwata continued each preference assessment session until all stimuli had been selected or the participant stopped responding, Graff and Ciccone (2002) have shown that similar preference hierarchies are generated if each preference assessment is terminated after only three trials.

Although many SPA procedures involve placing tangible items in front of an individual and measuring approach responses, researchers have measured the duration of time spent interacting with stimuli as a measure of preference. In *duration-based preference assessments*, it is possible to assess preference for larger items that are difficult to place on the tabletop (e.g., board or computer games) or community-based activities (e.g., going to the movies, eating out, shopping, or vocational tasks). Roane, Vollmer, Ringdahl, and Marcus (1998) used brief, 5-min sessions in which individuals had free access to a variety of stimuli, and the duration of engagement with items was measured. During this assessment, participants differentially engaged with stimuli. Subsequent reinforcer assessments demonstrated that high-preference stimuli functioned as reinforcers. Additionally, the brief duration-based assessment was quicker to administer than a paired-stimulus assessment. Brief duration-based assessments have also been shown to be effective in clarifying ambiguous results from approach-based assessments (DeLeon, Iwata, Conners, & Wallace, 1999) and for predicting preference for vocational tasks (Worsdell, Iwata, & Wallace, 2002).

Recently, there has been an interest in developing alternative methods to assess preferences. *Verbal preference assessments*, either asking individuals to rate how much they like stimuli when presented with the name of a single item (Northup, 2000) or conducting a verbal paired-stimulus assessment (Cohen-Almeida, Graff, & Ahearn, 2000), effectively identify reinforcers for some, but not all, individuals. Similarly, *pictorial paired-stimulus assessments* (Graff & Gibson, 2003) have been shown to effectively identify reinforcers for individuals who possess the appropriate discrimination skills (e.g., Clevenger & Graff, 2005; Conyers et al., 2002). Both verbal and pictorial preference assessments yield similar preference hierarchies compared to tangible assessments for items that can easily be delivered on the tabletop. However, to date there are no published studies assessing the efficacy of verbal and tangible assessments for identifying preferences for stimuli that are difficult to present on the tabletop, such as social or community-based stimuli.

The literature has clearly demonstrated that SPAs can identify effective reinforcers, although there are some factors that can impact the results of these assessments. How much access an individual has to the stimuli prior to a preference assessment may have an impact on what he selects during the preference assessment (Gottschalk, Libby, & Graff, 2000). Similarly, it may be beneficial not to mix edible items with activities during a preference assessment, as edible items tend to displace preference for activities (DeLeon, Iwata, & Roscoe, 1997).

SPAs provide us with a technology to identify high-preference stimuli that we can present contingently to teach new skills. To use reinforcement, in addition to identifying potential reinforcers, we must deliver them effectively. One potential way to increase the effectiveness of reinforcers is to manipulate motivating operations (Laraway, Snycerski, Michael, & Poling, 2003). For some individuals, performance on simple tasks may be influenced by the amount of access that is available prior to sessions (Vollmer & Iwata, 1991; Zhou, Iwata, & Shore, 2002). Restricting access to reinforcers may enhance reinforcement effects for some individuals, and repeated consumption of highly preferred edibles may result in a decrease in reinforcer effectiveness for some individuals (North & Iwata, 2005). Thus, varying reinforcers may have beneficial effects (Egel, 1980, 1981). One potential method for varying reinforcers would be to allow the individual to choose his or her own reinforcer. Although some studies have suggested that there may be beneficial effects of allowing choice of reinforcers (Graff & Libby, 1999; Graff, Libby, & Green, 1998), other studies have suggested that access to a choice of reinforcer may not enhance reinforcer effectiveness relative to an adult presenting a high-preference stimulus (Lerman et al., 1997).

Conclusion

In this chapter, we have outlined some of the principles and practices that define applied behavior analysis. What should be apparent is that underlying these practices and procedures are countless scientific studies of learning. Any parent or teacher helping a child with autism to learn should become fluent in these core principles. Teaching a child to communicate requires that they function symbolically. If a strong communicative repertoire does not exist, then the child is going to need precise instruction to develop the prerequisite skills for communication. The child is going to need to respond to different stimuli, for example the written word "B-A-L-L," the spoken word "ball," and an actual ball, as if these stimuli are the same at some times and different at other times. They will need to say, "ball," in the presence of the written word and the object but they will also need to kick or catch the ball and not the written word. Such differences may seem quite obvious, and they certainly are for the typically developing child who readily learns from others in a social environment. Autism, though, is associated with profound difficulties in socialization. Therefore, detailed instruction producing discrimination and generalization is often necessary for producing behavior that is sensitive to the social context in which it needs to occur.

For similar reasons, extrinsic reinforcement is a critical component of learning for children with autism. Social consequences such as praise and reprimands are incredibly potent motivators for typically developing children. Children with autism often seem insensitive to these consequences. We could speculate that this insensitivity to social consequences causes impairments in learning to communicate, but the important point here is that effective consequences are needed to teach these skills. If praise is ineffective, whatever is reinforcing for that child needs to be discovered and used in teaching. While reinforcing responses with extrinsic reinforcers, pairing them with social consequences might result in the child becoming more sensitive to social consequences. A thorough discussion of this topic is, however, beyond the scope of this chapter.

Any concise description of discrimination learning, and the prompting and reinforcement procedures necessary for supporting such instruction, will necessarily omit important research. The general framework provided here and the supporting literature referenced, however, should provide the reader the resources needed to contact these other relevant works. In our discussion of discrimination learning, we specifically describe procedures that could be termed discrete trial instruction. It is important to note that while discrete trial instruction is often needed to teach skills, the child will also need to learn to perform these skills consistently in the settings in which they are needed. Incidental instruction, or learning opportunities in less structured settings, is a necessary complement to discrete trial instruction.

 ## PRACTITIONER RECOMMENDATIONS

TEACHING DISCRIMINATION SKILLS

1. Does the child attend to task materials and exhibit session behavior (e.g., sitting, waiting, eye contact with the teacher, and responding when appropriate)?

   a. If yes, go to 2.

   b. If not, then teach *attending and session behavior.* Use a familiar task like selecting a toy. Begin by sitting at a table or desk and prompt the child to place his hands in lap and display eye contact. Then, present two toys, say, "choose one," prompt scanning, and let the child pick one. Ensure that each session behavior occurs before the child responds.

2. Is the child able to match identical objects, pictures, or letters?

   a. If yes, then go to 3.

   b. If not, then consider teaching *identity match-to-sample* using objects or pictures. Initially teach using three distinctly different stimuli. Then proceed to similar stimuli. If initial training does not result in rapid acquisition, you may need to teach a *simple discrimination* first. Using one stimulus and a board with three locations, require the child to point to the stimulus on the board. Be sure to unsystematically rotate the position of the stimulus across trials so that it is presented in each location equally often.

3. Once the child is able to match identical stimuli, teach *arbitrary match-to-sample* (e.g., visual-to-visual stimuli, auditory-to-visual stimuli). These skills can be taught sequentially or simultaneously.

   a. Teach *visual–visual match-to-sample* with objects or pictures using stimuli that are similar but have different features, for example matching cups, which could include cups with and without handles, cups of different colors, and cups that are shaped differently (tall, short, wide). Then proceed to categories of visually dissimilar stimuli, for example vehicles (i.e., cars, planes, buses, trucks).

b. *Auditory–visual match-to-sample* instruction can then be used to teach a label for the item presented in mastered visual–visual discriminations. When presenting auditory samples, consider repeating the auditory sample until the child responds to facilitate accurate responding.

4. When the child has established a wide repertoire of arbitrary matching performances, benefits from instruction designed to foster equivalence relations can be identified.

a. Begin with 3-member equivalence classes. Identify three stimulus classes that are relevant to the child's instructional program and select three forms of the stimuli in each class (e.g., penny, nickel, and dime are the classes, and the forms are spoken words, pictures, and printed words). Teach spoken-word-to-picture equivalences and spoken-word-to-printed-word equivalences. Test for printed-word-to-picture performance.

b. Once 3-member classes form, then consider adding a stimulus to the class. For example, teach the child to match the picture to the printed value (.01, .05, .10). Once acquired, the relations between the new member of the class, value, and all other stimulus forms (picture, printed word, and spoken word) should emerge.

ASSESSING PREFERENCES

1. Can the items being assessed be placed on a table in front of the learner?

a. If not, go to 2.

b. If yes, can the learner scan an array of stimuli and make a selection (i.e., select only one item) from two or more alternatives?

- If they cannot scan an array of stimuli, use a *single-stimulus preference assessment*. Use items approached on the highest percentage of trials as potential reinforcers.

- If they can scan an array of two or more stimuli, but attempt to select more than one item at a time, consider using a *paired-stimulus preference assessment*. Use items approached on the highest percentage of trials as potential reinforcers.

- If they can scan more than two items and do not select more than one at a time, consider using a *multiple stimulus without replacement preference assessment* (MSWO). Use items approached on the highest percentage of trials or items scoring the most points on a point weighting scoring system as potential reinforcers. Conduct a brief MSWO preference assessment and compare results to a full MSWO assessment. If similar preference hierarchies are generated, use brief MSWOs to assess preferences more often.

2. If the items cannot be placed on a table (e.g., using a computer, swinging on a swing set), follow these steps.

   a. If the learner has vocal speech and can label all of the stimuli to be assessed, consider conducting a *verbal preference assessment*. Use items named on the highest percentage of trials as potential reinforcers.

   b. If the learner can match objects and pictures for all the stimuli to be assessed, or if the learner has difficulty labeling all stimuli that need to be assessed, consider conducting a *pictorial preference assessment*. Use items corresponding to pictures selected on the highest percentage of trials as potential reinforcers.

   c. If the learner does not have vocal speech and cannot match objects and pictures, consider a *duration-based preference assessment*, where you give the learner access to various items, and record the duration of time spent appropriately engaged with each item.

References

Alavosius, M. P., & Sulzer-Azaroff, B. (1985). An on-the-job method to evaluate patient lifting techniques. *Applied Ergonomics, 16*, 307–311.

Albin, R. W., & Horner, R. H. (1988). Generalization with precision. In R. H. Horner, G. Dunlap, & R. L. Koegel (Eds.), *Generalization and maintenance: Life-style changes in applied settings* (pp. 99–120). Baltimore: Brookes.

Allen, K. D., & Fuqua, R. W. (1985). Eliminating selective stimulus control: A comparison of two procedures for teaching mentally retarded children to respond to compound stimuli. *Journal of Experimental Child Psychology, 39*, 55–71.

Ault, M. J., Wolery, M., Gast, D. L., Doyle, P. M., & Eizenstat, V. (1988). Comparison of response prompting procedures in teaching numeral identification to autistic subjects. *Journal of Autism and Developmental Disorders, 18*, 627–636.

Austin, J., & Carr, J. E. (Eds.). (2003). *Handbook of applied behavior analysis.* Reno, NV: Context Press.

Baer, D. M., Wolf, M. M., & Risley, T. R. (1968). Some current dimensions of applied behavior analysis. *Journal of Applied Behavior Analysis, 1*, 91–97.

Burke, J. C., & Cerniglia, L. (1990). Stimulus complexity and autistic children's responsivity: Assessing and training a pivotal behavior. *Journal of Autism and Developmental Disorders, 20*, 233–253.

Carr, E. G., & Durand, V. M. (1985). Reducing behavior problems through functional communication training. *Journal of Applied Behavior Analysis, 18*, 111–126.

Carr, J. E., Nicolson, A. C., & Higbee, T. S. (2000). Evaluation of a brief multiple-stimulus preference assessment in a naturalistic context. *Journal of Applied Behavior Analysis, 33*, 353–357.

Charlop, M. H., & Milstein, J. P. (1989). Teaching autistic children conversational speech using video modeling. *Journal of Applied Behavior Analysis, 22*, 275–285.

Charlop, M. H., Schreibman, L., & Tryon, A .S. (1983). Learning through observation: the effects of peer modeling on acquisition and generalization in autistic children. *Journal of Abnormal Child Psychology, 11*, 355–366.

Charlop-Christy, M. H., Le, L., & Freeman, K. A. (2000). A comparison of video modeling with in vivo modeling for teaching children with autism. *Journal of Autism and Developmental Disorders, 30*, 537–552.

Chomsky, N. (1959). A review of B. F. Skinner's *Verbal Behavior. Language, 35*, 26–58.

Ciccone, F. J., Graff, R. B., & Ahearn, W. H. (2005). An alternate scoring method for the multiple stimulus without replacement preference assessment. *Behavioral Interventions, 20*, 1–7.

Clark, K., & Green, G. (2004). Comparison of two procedures for teaching dictated-work/symbol relations to learners with autism. *Journal of Applied Behavior Analysis, 37,* 503–507.

Clevenger, T., & Graff, R. B. (2005). Assessing object-to-picture and picture-to-object matching as prerequisite skills for pictorial preference assessments. *Journal of Applied Behavior Analysis, 38,* 543–547.

Cohen-Almeida, D., Graff, R. B., & Ahearn, W. H. (2000). A comparison of verbal and tangible stimulus-choice preference assessments. *Journal of Applied Behavior Analysis, 33,* 329–334.

Conners, F. A. (1992). Reading instruction for students with moderate mental retardation: Review and analysis of research. *American Journal of Mental Retardation, 96,* 577–597.

Conyers, C., Doole, A., Vause, T., Harapiak, S., Yu, D. C. T., & Martin, G. L. (2002). Predicting the relative efficacy of three presentation methods for assessing preferences of persons with developmental disabilities. *Journal of Applied Behavior Analysis, 35,* 49–58.

Cota, S., DeBar, R., Geckeler, A., MacDonald, R., Mansfield, R., O'Flaherty, C., et al. (May, 2003). *Using video modeling to teach pretend play to children with autism and typically developing peers.* Presented at the annual meeting of the Association for Behavior Analysis, San Francisco.

Cuvo, A. J., Davis, P. K., O'Reilly, M. F., Mooney, B. M., & Crowley, R. (1992). Promoting stimulus control with textual prompts and performance feedback for persons with mild disabilities. *Journal of Applied Behavior Analysis, 25,* 477–489.

D'Ateno, P., Mangiapanello, K., & Taylor, B. (2003). Using video modeling to teach complex play sequences to a preschooler with autism. *Journal of Positive Behavior Interventions, 5,* 5–11.

DeLeon, I. G., & Iwata, B. A. (1996). Evaluation of a multiple-stimulus presentation format for assessing reinforcer preferences. *Journal of Applied Behavior Analysis, 29,* 519–532.

DeLeon, I. G., Iwata, B. A., Conners, J., & Wallace, M. D. (1999). Examination of ambiguous stimulus preferences with duration-based measures. *Journal of Applied Behavior Analysis, 32,* 111–114.

DeLeon, I. G., Iwata, B. A., & Roscoe, E. M. (1997). Displacement of leisure reinforcers by food during preference assessments. *Journal of Applied Behavior Analysis, 33,* 475–484.

Demchak, M. (1990). Response prompting and fading methods: A review. *American Journal on Mental Deficiency, 94,* 603–615.

Doyle, P. M., Wolery, M., Gast, D. L., Ault, M. J., & Wiley, K. (1990). Comparison of constant time delay and system of least prompts in teaching preschoolers with developmental delays. *Research in Developmental Disabilities, 11,* 1–22.

Dube, W. V., Iennaco, F. M., & McIlvane, W. J. (1993). Generalized identity matching to sample of two-dimensional forms in individuals with intellectual disabilities. *Research in Developmental Disabilities, 14,* 457–477.

Dube, W. V., & McIlvane, W. J. (1999). Reduction of stimulus overselectivity with non-verbal differential observing responses. *Journal of Applied Behavior Analysis, 24,* 305–317.

Egel, A. L. (1980). The effects of constant vs. varied reinforcer presentation on respond-ing by autistic children. *Journal of Experimental Child Psychology, 30,* 455–463.

Egel, A. L. (1981). Reinforcer variation: Implications for motivating developmentally disabled children. *Journal of Applied Behavior Analysis, 14,* 345–350.

Egel, A. L., Richman, G. S., & Koegel, R. L. (1981). Normal peer models and autistic children's learning. *Journal of Applied Behavior Analysis, 14,* 3–12.

Etzel, B. C., & LeBlanc, J. M. (1979). The simplest treatment alternative: The law of parsimony applied to choosing appropriate instructional control and errorless learning procedures for the difficult-to-teach child. *Journal of Autism and Develop-mental Disorders, 9,* 361–382.

Fields, L., & Verhave, T. (1987). The structure of equivalence classes. *Journal of the Ex-perimental Analysis of Behavior, 48,* 317–332.

Fisher, W., Piazza, C. C., Bowman, L. G., Hagopian, L. P., Owens, J. C., & Slevin, I. (1992). A comparison of two approaches for identifying reinforcers for persons with severe and profound disabilities. *Journal of Applied Behavior Analysis, 25,* 491–498.

Fox, D. K., Hopkins, B. L., & Anger, W. K. (1987). The long-term effects of a token economy on safety performance in open-pit mining. *Journal of Applied Behavior Analysis, 22,* 131–141.

Foxx, R. M. (1982). *Increasing behaviors of severely retarded and autistic individuals* (pp. 81–96). Champaign, IL: Research Press.

Friman, P., Osgood, D., Shanahan, D., Thompson, R., Larzelere, R., & Daly, D. (1996). A longitudinal evaluation of prevalent negative beliefs about residential placement for troubled adolescents. *Journal of Abnormal Child Psychology, 24,* 299–324.

Gast, D. L., Doyle, P. M., Wolery, M., Ault, M. J., & Farmer, S. A. (1991). Assessing the acquisition of incidental information by secondary age students with mental retar-dation: Comparison of response prompting strategies. *American Journal of Mental Retardation, 96,* 63–80.

Gikalov, A. A., Baer, D. M., & Hannah, G. T. (1997). The effects of work task manipu-lation and scheduling on patient load revenue, eyewear turnover, and utilization of staff and doctor time. *Journal of Organizational Behavior Management, 17,* 3–35.

Glat, R., Gould, K., Stoddard, L. T., & Sidman, M. (1994). A note on transfer of stimulus control in the delayed-cue procedure: Facilitation by an overt differential response. *Journal of Applied Behavior Analysis, 27,* 699–704.

Godby, S., Gast, D. L., & Wolery, M. (1987). A comparison of time delay and system of least prompts in teaching object identification. *Research in Developmental Disabilities, 8,* 283–305.

Gottschalk, J. M., Libby, M. L., & Graff, R. B. (2000). The effects of establishing operations on preference assessment outcomes. *Journal of Applied Behavior Analysis, 33,* 81–84.

Graff, R. B., & Ciccone, F. (2002). A post-hoc analysis of multiple-stimulus preference assessment results. *Behavioral Interventions, 17,* 85–92.

Graff, R. B., & Gibson, L. (2003). Using pictures to assess reinforcers in individuals with developmental disabilities. *Behavior Modification, 27,* 470–483.

Graff, R. B., & Libby, M. E. (1999). A comparison of presession and within-session reinforcement choice. *Journal of Applied Behavior Analysis, 32,* 161–173.

Graff, R. B., Libby, M. E., & Green, G. (1998). The effects of reinforcer choice on rates of challenging behavior and free operant responding in individuals with severe disabilities. *Behavioral Interventions, 13,* 249–268.

Green, C. W., Reid, D. H., White, L. K., Halford, R. C., Brittain, D. P., & Gardner, S. M. (1988). Identifying reinforcers for persons with profound handicaps: Staff opinion versus systematic assessment of preferences. *Journal of Applied Behavior Analysis, 21,* 31–43.

Griffen, A. K., Wolery, M., & Schuster, J. W. (1992). Triadic instruction of chained food preparations responses: Acquisition and observational learning. *Journal of Applied Behavior Analysis, 25,* 193–204.

Gutowski, S. J., Geren, M., Stromer, R., & Mackay, H. A. (1995). Restricted stimulus control in delayed matching to complex samples: A preliminary analysis of the role of naming. *Experimental Analysis of Human Behavior Bulletin, 13,* 18–24.

Haring, T. G., Kennedy, C. H., Adams, M. J., & Pitts-Conway, V. (1987). Teaching generalization of purchasing skills across community settings to autistic youth using videotape modeling. *Journal of Applied Behavior Analysis, 19,* 159–171.

Hineline, P. N. (1992). A self-interpretive behavior analysis. *American Psychologist, 47,* 1274–1286.

Huguenin, N. H. (1985). Attention to multiple cues by severely mentally retarded adults: Effects of single-component pretraining. *Applied Research in Mental Retardation, 6,* 319–335.

Hursh, S. R. (1991). Behavioral economics of drug self-administration and drug abuse policy. *Journal of the Experimental Analysis of Behavior, 56,* 377–393.

Illingworth, R. S., & Lister, J. (1964). The critical or sensitive period with special reference to certain feeding problems in infants and children. *Journal of Pediatrics, 65,* 839–848.

James, S. D., & Egel, A. L. (1986). A direct prompting strategy for increasing reciprocal interactions between handicapped and nonhandicapped siblings. *Journal of Applied Behavior Analysis, 19,* 173–186.

Johnson, B., & Cuvo, A. J. (1981). Teaching mentally retarded adults to cook. *Behavior Modification, 5,* 187–202.

Johnson, C., White, D., Green, G., Langer, S., & MacDonald, R. (2000, May). A discrimination and stimulus equivalence curriculum for students with severe learning difficulties. In R. Stromer, *Discrete trial assessment and instruction: Innovative tabletop and technological strategies.* Symposium paper presented at the annual convention of the Association for Behavior Analysis, Washington, DC.

Johnson, M. W., & Bickel, W. K. (2003). The behavioral economics of cigarette smoking: The concurrent presence of a substitute and an independent reinforcer. *Behavioural Pharmacology, 14,* 137–144.

Johnson, S. C., Meyer, L., & Taylor, B. A. (1996). Supported inclusion. In C. Maurice, G. Green, & S. C. Luce (Eds.), *Behavioral intervention for young children with autism* (pp. 331–342). Austin, TX: PRO-ED.

Kasari, C. (2002). Assessing change in early intervention programs for children with autism. *Journal of Autism and Developmental Disorders, 32,* 447–461.

Koch, S. (1964). Psychology and emerging conceptions of knowledge as unitary. In T. W. Wann (Ed.), *Behaviorism and phenomenology: Contrasting bases for modern psychology.* Chicago: The University of Chicago Press.

Koegel, R. L., & Schreibman, L. (1977). Teaching autistic children to respond to simultaneous multiple cues. *Journal of Experimental Child Psychology, 24,* 299–311.

Krantz, P. J., & McClannahan, L. E. (1993). Teaching children with autism to imitate to peers: Effects of a script-fading procedure. *Journal of Applied Behavior Analysis, 26,* 121–132.

Krantz, P. J., & McClannahan, L. E. (1998). Social interaction skills for children with autism: A script-fading procedure for beginning readers. *Journal of Applied Behavior Analysis, 31,* 191–202.

Lana, R. E. (1991). *Assumptions of social psychology: A reexamination.* Hillsdale, NJ: Erlbaum.

Laraway, S., Snycerski, S., Michael, J., & Poling, A. (2003). Motivating operations and terms to describe them: Some further refinements. *Journal of Applied Behavior Analysis, 36,* 407–414.

LeBlanc, L., Coates, M., Daneshvar, S., Charlop-Christy, M., Morris, C., & Lancaster, B. (2003). Using video modeling and reinforcement to teach perspective-taking skills to children with autism. *Journal of Applied Behavior Analysis, 36,* 253–257.

Lerman, D. C., Iwata, B. A., Rainville, B., Adelinis, J. D., Crosland, K., & Kogan, J. (1997). Effects of reinforcement choice on task responding in individuals with developmental disabilities. *Journal of Applied Behavior Analysis, 30,* 411–422.

Lovaas, O. I., Koegel, R. L., & Schreibman, L. (1979). Stimulus overselectivity in autism: A review of research. *Psychological Bulletin, 86,* 1236–1254.

MacDonald, R., Clark, M., Garrigan, E., & Vengala, M. (2005). Using videomodeling to teach pretend play to children with autism. *Behavioral Interventions, 20,* 225–238.

MacDonald, R. F., Dixon, L. S., & LeBlanc, J. M. (1986). Stimulus class formation following observational learning. *Analysis and Intervention of Developmental Disabilities, 6,* 73–87.

MacDuff, G. S., Krantz, P. J., & McClannahan, L. E. (1993). Teaching children with autism to use photographic activity schedules: Maintenance and generalization of complex response chains. *Journal of Applied Behavior Analysis, 26,* 89–97.

MacDuff, G. S., Krantz, P. J., & McClannahan, L. E. (2001). Prompts and prompt-fading strategies for people with autism. In C. Maurice, G. Green, & R. Foxx (Eds.), *Making a difference: Behavioral intervention for autism.* Austin, TX: PRO-ED.

Mackay, H. A. (1985). Stimulus equivalence in rudimentary reading and spelling. *Analysis and Intervention in Developmental Disabilities, 5,* 373–387.

McDonagh, E. C., McIlvane, W. J., & Stoddard, L. T. (1984). Teaching coin equivalences via matching to sample. *Applied Research in Mental Retardation, 5,* 177–197.

McIlvane, W. J., Dube, W. V., Green, G., & Serna, R. W. (1993). Programming conceptual and communication skill development: A methodological stimulus class analysis. In A. P. Kaiser & D. B. Gray (Eds.), *Enhancing children's communication* (pp. 243–285). Baltimore: Brookes.

Morris, E. K. (1988). Contextualism: The world view of behavior analysis. *Journal of Experimental Child Psychology, 46,* 289–323.

Nelson, A., Holt, W. J., & Etzel, B. C. (1976, April). *A description of programs to teach beginning math skills.* Paper presented at the Council for Exceptional Children, Chicago.

Nikopoulos, C. K., & Keenana, M. (2004). Effects of video modeling on social initiations by children with autism. *Journal of Applied Behavior Analysis, 37,* 93–96.

North, S. T., & Iwata, B. A. (2005). Motivational influences on performance maintained by food reinforcement. *Journal of Applied Behavior Analysis, 38,* 317–333.

Northup, J. (2000). Further evaluation of the accuracy of reinforcer surveys: A systematic replication. *Journal of Applied Behavior Analysis, 33,* 335–338.

Odom, S. L., & Strain, P. S. (1986). A comparison of peer-initiation and teacher-antecedent interventions for promoting reciprocal social interaction of autistic preschoolers. *Journal of Applied Behavior Analysis, 19,* 59–71.

Oppenheimer, M., Saunders, R. R., & Spradlin, J. E. (1993). Investigating the generality of the delayed-prompt effect. *Research in Developmental Disabilities, 14,* 425–444.

Pace, G. M., Ivancic, M. T., Edwards, G. L., Iwata, B. A., & Page, T. J. (1985). Assessment of stimulus preference and reinforcer value with profoundly retarded individuals. *Journal of Applied Behavior Analysis, 18,* 249–255.

Piaget, J. (1929). *The child's conception of the world*. New York: Harcourt.

Pierce, K. L., & Schreibman, L. (1994). Teaching daily living skills to children with autism in unsupervised settings through pictorial self-management. *Journal of Applied Behavior Analysis, 27,* 471–481.

Rehfeldt, R. A., Dahman, D., Young, A., Cherry, H., & Davis, P. (2003). Teaching a simple meal preparation skill to adults with moderate and severe mental retardation using video modeling. *Behavioral Interventions, 18,* 209–218.

Rehfeldt, R. A., Latimore, D., & Stromer, R. (2003). Observational learning and the formation of classes of reading skills by individuals with autism and other developmental disabilities. *Research on Developmental Disabilities, 24,* 333–358.

Roane, H. S., Vollmer, T. R., Ringdahl, J. E., & Marcus, B. A. (1998). Evaluation of a brief stimulus preference assessment. *Journal of Applied Behavior Analysis, 31,* 605–620.

Rogers, C. R. (1964). Toward a science of the person. In T. W. Wann (Ed.), *Behaviorism and phenomenology: Contrasting bases for modern psychology*. Chicago: The University of Chicago Press.

Saunders, K. J., & Spradlin, J. E. (1989). Conditional discrimination in mentally retarded adults: The effect of training the component simple discriminations. *Journal of the Experimental Analysis of Behavior, 52,* 1–12.

Saunders, K. J., & Spradlin, J. E. (1990). Conditional discrimination in mentally retarded adults: The development of generalized skills. *Journal of the Experimental Analysis of Behavior, 54,* 239–250.

Saunders, K. J., & Spradlin, J. E. (1993). Conditional discrimination in mentally retarded subjects: Programming acquisition and learning set. *Journal of the Experimental Analysis of Behavior, 60,* 571–586.

Saunders, K. J., Williams, D. C., & Spradlin, J. E. (1995). Conditional discrimination by adults with mental retardation: Establishing relations between physically identical stimuli. *American Journal on Mental Retardation, 99,* 558–563.

Schneider, H. C., & Salzberg, C. L. (1982). Stimulus overselectivity in a match-to-sample paradigm by severely retarded youth. *Analysis and Intervention in Developmental Disabilities, 2,* 273–304.

Schoen, S. F., & Ogden, S. (1995). Impact of time delay, observational learning, and attentional cuing upon word recognition during integrated small-group instruction. *Journal of Autism and Developmental Disorders, 25,* 503–519.

Schreibman, L. (1975). Effects of within-stimulus and extra-stimulus prompting on discrimination learning in autistic children. *Journal of Applied Behavior Analysis, 87,* 91–112.

Schreibman, L., Charlop, M. H., & Koegel, R. L. (1982). Teaching autistic children to use extra-stimulus prompts. *Journal of Experimental Child Psychology, 33,* 475–491.

Schreibman, L., & Lovaas, O. I. (1973). Overselective response to social stimuli by autistic children. *Journal of Abnormal Child Psychology, 1,* 152–168.

Serna, R. W., Dube, W. V., & McIlvane, W. J. (1997). Assessing same/different judgments in individuals with severe intellectual disabilities: A status report. *Research in Developmental Disabilities, 18,* 343–368.

Serna, R. W., & McIlvane, W. J. (1996, March). A model for integrating research and practice in teaching basic discrimination skills. *Proceedings of the 29th Annual Gatlinburg Conference on Research and Theory in Mental Retardation and Developmental Disabilities,* Gatlinburg, TN.

Shafer, M. S., Egel, A. L., & Neef, N. A. (1984). Training mildly handicapped peers to facilitate changes in the social interaction skills of autistic children. *Journal of Applied Behavior Analysis, 17,* 461–476.

Sherer, M., Pierce, K. L., Paredes, S., Kisacky, K. L., Ingersoll, B., & Schreibman, L. (2001). Enhancing conversational skills in children with autism via video technology: Which is better, "self" or "other" as a model? *Behavior Modification, 25,* 140–158.

Shipley-Benamou, R., Lutzker, J., & Taubman, M. (2002). Teaching daily living skills to children with autism through instructional video modeling. *Journal of Positive Behavior Interventions, 4,* 165–175.

Sidman, M. (1960). *Tactics of scientific research.* New York: Basic Books.

Sidman, M. (1971). Reading and auditory-visual equivalences. *Journal of Speech and Hearing Research, 14,* 5–13.

Sidman, M. (1980). A note on the measurement of conditional discrimination. *Journal of the Experimental Analysis of Behavior, 33,* 285–289.

Sidman, M., & Tailby, W. (1982). Conditional discrimination vs. matching to sample: An expansion of the testing paradigm. *Journal of the Experimental Analysis of Behavior, 37,* 5–22.

Skinner, B. F. (1945). The operational analysis of psychological terms. *Psychological Review, 52,* 270–277.

Skinner, B. F. (1953). *Science and human behavior.* New York: Macmillan.

Skinner, B. F. (1977). Why I am not a cognitive psychologist. *Behaviorism, 5,* 1–10.

Skinner, B. F. (1981). Selection by consequences. *Science, 213,* 501–504.

Snell, M. E. (1993). *Instruction of students with severe disabilities.* New York: Merrill.

Spellman, C., DeBriere, T., Jarboe, D., Campbell, S., & Harris, C. (1978). *Pictorial instructions: Training daily living skills.* Columbus, OH: Merrill.

Stella, M. E., & Etzel, B. C. (1986). Stimulus control of eye orientations: Shaping S+ only versus shaping S− only. *Analysis and Intervention in Developmental Disabilities, 6,* 137–153.

Stoddard, L. T., Brown, J., Hurlbert, B., Manoli, C., & McIlvane, W. J. (1989). Teaching money skills through stimulus class formation, exclusion, and component matching methods: Three case studies. *Research in Developmental Disabilities, 10,* 413–439.

Stromer, R., Mackay, H. A., & Stoddard, L. T. (1992). Classroom applications of stimulus equivalence technology. *Journal of Behavioral Education, 2,* 225–256.

Terrace, H. S. (1966). Stimulus control. In W. K. Honig (Ed.), *Operant behavior: Areas of research and application* (pp. 271–344). New York: Appleton-Century-Crofts.

Thompson, R., Smith, G., Osgood, D., Dowd, T., Friman, P., & Daly, D. (1996). Residential care: A study of short and long-term effects. *Children and Youth Services Review, 18,* 139–162.

Touchette, P. (1971). Transfer of stimulus control: Measuring the moment of transfer. *Journal of the Experimental Analysis of Behavior, 15,* 347–354.

Van Houten, R., Axelrod, S., Bailey, J. S., Favell, J. E., Foxx, R. M., Iwata, B. A., et al. (1988). The right to effective behavioral treatment. *Journal of Applied Behavior Analysis, 21,* 381–384.

Varni, J. W., Lovaas, O. I., Koegel, R. L., & Everett, N. L. (1979). An analysis of observational learning in autistic and normal children. *Journal of Abnormal Child Psychology, 7,* 31–43.

Vollmer, T. R., & Iwata, B. A. (1991). Establishing operations and reinforcement effects. *Journal of Applied Behavior Analysis, 24,* 279–291.

Watson, J. B. (1913). Psychology as the behaviorist views it. *Psychological Review, 20,* 158–177.

Watson, J. B. (1924). *Behaviorism.* New York: Norton.

Wittkopp, C. J., Rowan, J. F., & Poling, A. (1990). Use of a feedback package to reduce machine set-up time in a manufacturing setting. *Journal of Organizational Behavior Management, 11,* 7–22.

Wolery, M., Holcombe, A., Cybriwsky, C., Doyle, P. M., Schuster, J. W., Ault, M., et al. (1992). Constant time delay with discrete responses: A review of effectiveness and demographic, procedural, and methodological parameters. *Research in Developmental Disabilities, 13,* 239–266.

Worsdell, A. S., Iwata, B. A., & Wallace, M. D. (2002). Duration-based measures of preference for vocational tasks. *Journal of Applied Behavior Analysis, 35,* 287–290.

Young, J. M., Krantz, P. J., McClannahan, L. E., & Poulson, C. L. (1994). Generalized imitation and response-class formation in children with autism. *Journal of Applied Behavior Analysis, 27,* 685–697.

Zhou, L., Iwata, B. A., & Shore, B. A. (2002). Reinforcing efficacy of food on performance during pre- and postmeal sessions. *Journal of Applied Behavior Analysis, 35,* 411–414.

CHAPTER

3

READINESS SKILLS

Ruth Anne Rehfeldt and Rocio Rosales
Southern Illinois University

Readiness skills are rudimentary skills that prepare an individual for intensive instruction in a number of other curriculum areas. These skills are often considered prerequisites that must be mastered before more advanced skills are established (Lovaas, 1981; Zager, Shamow, & Schneider, 1999), the rationale being that more complex learning objectives are often not attainable without the prior mastery of these minimum requirements. The absence of readiness skills may thus impede the acquisition of other skills. For this reason, readiness skills are often targeted early in intervention as a first step in teaching individuals with autism. Among these are sitting at a table, making eye contact and orienting to one's name, displaying joint attention, demonstrating generalized imitation, and complying with instructions. The purpose of this chapter is to provide an overview of instructional strategies for establishing readiness skills. We discuss the relevant research literature with regard to each skill and provide recommendations for practitioners who wish to adopt the strategies defined. Because the effective use of positive reinforcement is paramount, we also include a brief section on reinforcement control.

Discrete trial teaching procedures are often used to teach readiness skills. Discrete trial instruction is typically led by the instructor, who presents short and clear instructions (e.g., "Look at me"), follows a carefully planned procedure for prompting correct responses and fading those prompts, and provides immediate, high-magnitude consequences, often edible or tangible items coupled with praise, for correct responses. If the individual does not respond or responds incorrectly, a correction procedure is often employed. Instruction is frequently carried out at a table, and massed trials of the same skill may be presented until mastery occurs (Lovaas, 1981; Sundberg & Partington, 1999; see also Sarokoff & Sturmey, 2004, for a task analysis of discrete trial teaching). Lovaas and colleagues emphasized the importance of planning for the generalization of skills to new situations by varying the instructor, teaching materials, and settings in which instruction is carried out (Lovaas, Koegel, Simmons, & Long, 1973; Lovaas, Schreibman, & Koegel, 1974). Naturalistic or incidental instruction may also be employed to teach readiness skills. With this form of instruction, situations that are interesting to the learner are identified, and instruction is carried out in those situations. Less structured prompt and prompt reduction strategies are employed, and consequences for correct responses are typically related to the individual's immediate interests. A disadvantage of naturalistic teaching is that there may be fewer opportunities for instructional trials than with discrete trial teaching, and initial acquisition may be slower. Given that instruction is carried out in a less structured manner, naturalistic teaching may facilitate the generalization of newly acquired skills across slightly varied stimuli and settings. For learners who are new to intensive instruction, we recommend using discrete trial teaching initially and employing more naturalistic approaches as skills are acquired.

Sitting

Learning to sit at a table or on the floor upon the instructor's request may be the first learning experience for many children with autism (Lovaas, 1981). Depending on the child's age, it may be more desirable to teach sitting at a table as opposed to sitting on the floor, in preparation for future instruction in a classroom setting. Teaching the child to sit is an important prerequisite for many academic and preacademic skills that are demonstrated while working at a table or desk. Sitting is easy to prompt physically and is readily acquired by most learners.

Several instructional techniques are commonly used to teach sitting. One of the most familiar approaches is to establish discriminative control over sitting using a verbal instruction such as "sit down" (Lovaas, 2003; Taylor & McDonough, 1996). Physical prompts are often used to facilitate correct responses and are ultimately faded. Once responding is under control of these instructions, discriminative control may also be established for the instructions to "face forward" and "sit up straight" (Lovaas, 1981). During the initial stages of instruction, it is important to keep instructions concise and consistent across instructors. Once the individual responds correctly when instructions are presented, instructions may be gradually changed to promote generalization across instructions (e.g., "take a seat," or "sit in your chair"). Whereas physical prompts are often used in conjunction with verbal instructions, it may also be desirable to use such prompts in the absence of verbal instructions to increase the likelihood that the child will sit spontaneously rather than perform the behavior only when a direct instruction is given. Verbal praise and access to edible or tangible items should be delivered contingent upon independent sitting.

When teaching readiness behavior such as sitting, it is important to avoid inadvertently reinforcing any behavior that may lead to an interruption in teaching. When the time to work on sitting has been designated by the instructor or parent, the child should be physically prompted to remain in the chair in an upright position. All efforts should be made to pair sitting at the table with access to positive reinforcers. It may also be important to gradually increase the time for which the child must remain seated before access to a preferred activity is granted. Sitting at a table or on the floor for the purpose of instruction may be monotonous and aversive for some children. Therefore, the child should not be expected to sit for a long period of time during the early stages of instruction, but the required time period can be increased in small increments. As a last resort, if the child gets out of the chair repeatedly, we suggest that the instructor place his or her legs around the chair, but we strongly suggest using other teaching procedures to teach sitting before this technique is used.

Efforts must be made early on in instruction to promote generalization of sitting across different settings and stimuli. As previously mentioned, naturalistic approaches may be more likely to promote the generalization of skills than discrete trial instruction. Strategies that will promote generalization using either instructional approach include varying the adults who provide the instructions to sit, varying the furniture used during instruction, varying the number of other people present in the instructional setting, and performing instruction in a variety of settings.

Eye Contact

As a rudimentary skill, eye contact involves looking directly into the eyes of another individual, either in response to one's name, when directly instructed to do so, or in response to another person's eye contact or facial or bodily orientation. Failure to establish eye contact with others is a common characteristic of individuals with autism (Margolies, 1977). Making eye contact with one's task materials and shifting eye contact between different task materials is also an important readiness skill. At a basic level, these responses suggest that the learner is attentive and oriented to the task at hand. At a more complex level, eye contact with other people is indicative of an interest in and awareness of others. Making eye contact with others is often considered a prerequisite skill for simple social interactions such as social greetings or answering social questions. In addition, teaching eye contact upon request has been shown to improve compliance with instructor requests (Hamlet, Axelrod, & Kuerschner, 1984). For these reasons, it is important to target eye contact as a goal early on in an intervention program. Lovaas (1981) suggested that eye contact be well established before the instruction of other preacademic skills is initiated, while Foxx (1977) and Margolies (1977) advised teaching eye contact simultaneously with other skills. Whichever position is adopted, several strategies have been shown to be effective for teaching eye contact.

Lovaas (1981) developed instructional strategies that are now conventional practices for teaching and improving eye contact in young children. To teach eye contact, the learner should be seated in a chair directly in front of the instructor, and the instructor should present a verbal discriminative stimulus (e.g., "Look at me," or the learner's name) while simultaneously physically or visually prompting eye contact. Physical prompts include moving the individual's head until he or she directly faces the instructor or gently guiding his or her chin upward. A danger in using physical prompts is that the individual's eye contact may come under the stimulus control of physical prompts, rather than other people calling his or her name. Although eye contact may increase during discrete trial teaching using this strategy, eye contact outside of teaching sessions may remain limited. Nonphysical prompting procedures consist of placing a preferred item or a visually stimulating object directly in the line of vision between the individual's eyes and the instructor's eyes at the same time the verbal instruction is given. Once eye contact is made, the teacher should deliver a positive reinforcer immediately. Physical and visual prompts are often faded using a graduated time-delay procedure, which involves waiting for successively longer periods of time before delivering a prompt until the learner eventually makes eye contact independently. It may be desirable to gradually increase the duration of eye contact required for reinforcement so that the individual learns to make eye contact for progressively longer periods of time. Because an ultimate goal is for the individual to make eye contact independently during ongoing daily activities, the distance between the learner and instructor should be gradually increased over the course of instruction. Likewise, the verbal instruction "Look at me" should be gradually eliminated so that the individual does not make eye contact only upon the command to do so.

Matson, Manikam, Coe, Raymond, and Taras (1988) exemplified these strategies when they used discrete trial instruction to improve eye-contact, in-seat, and on-task behavior in children with autism, mental retardation, and hearing impairment. These authors used a combination of social and edible reinforcers and performance feedback. When the children displayed the desired target behaviors, they received verbal praise, were informed of the appropriate responses emitted, and were allowed to select from an array of reinforcers. When the target behaviors were not emitted, the children were reminded of the desired behaviors and physical, verbal, or modeled prompts were presented.

Some children with autism may be unresponsive to social praise and even to preferred items when presented contingent upon correct responding. Foxx (1977) reported an alternative approach for teaching eye contact. In this study, the effectiveness of overcorrection plus edible items and social praise was compared to that of edible items and social praise alone in establishing eye contact following the instruction "Look at me" in children with autism and mental retardation. The overcorrection procedure consisted of functional movement training, in which the child was required to move his or her head in one of three positions under a teacher's manual guidance, maintaining each position for 15 s. The procedure was used whenever a child failed to respond to the verbal prompt "Look at me," and established eye contact as a discriminated avoidance response. Verbal praise or edibles were always delivered contingent upon eye contact that occurred within 5 s of the instructions. The combination of overcorrection plus verbal praise and edibles was more effective in developing eye contact, but verbal praise and edibles alone nonetheless resulted in an increase in eye contact. This procedure is recommended only as a last resort when positive reinforcement procedures have failed.

To facilitate attention to task materials, practitioners may find it helpful to initially present visually stimulating items alongside the task materials and to immediately praise the learner for "good looking." Gestural prompts, such as tapping on the table proximally to task materials, may also be helpful to facilitate attention to task materials. Once the individual learns that reinforcement will be provided contingent upon attending to and engaging with task materials, such prompts will be unnecessary.

Joint Attention

A more sophisticated form of eye contact is involved in what developmental and cognitive psychologists identify as "joint attention." Joint attention is defined as the coordination of attending behaviors between a social partner and an environmental object or event using conventional gestures and gaze alternations (Kasari, Freeman, & Paparella, 2001). For example, a child assembling a puzzle demonstrates joint attention when, upon completion of the puzzle, he or she proudly looks from the puzzle to a nearby parent or caregiver and back to the puzzle. In everyday language, it might be said that this action invites the parent to "share the experience" of the completed puzzle (Dube, MacDonald, Mansfield, Holcomb, & Ahearn, 2004). Likewise, a child responds to a parent's bid for joint attention when he or she follows the caregiver's shift in gaze to a nearby object or event. This action demonstrates that the child is "sharing an awareness" for the particular object or event (Dube et al., 2004). Recent research has confirmed that persons with autism have deficits in the area of joint attention (Jones & Carr, 2004; Whalen & Schreibman, 2003). When compared to typically developing children and children with other developmental disabilities, only children with autism but not other developmental disabilities showed deficits in joint attention (Charman et al., 1998). Thus, the absence of joint attention is considered by many researchers to be an early predictor of autism and is considered pivotal to deficits in language, play, and social development. Because this skill plays a critical role in social development, it should be made a priority in early intervention efforts once basic eye contact is established (Jones & Carr, 2004). Behavioral strategies for ameliorating joint attention deficits have been the focus of very recent research endeavors. (See Dube et al. [2004] for a behavioral analysis of joint attention, and Jones and Carr [2004] for a review.)

Whalen and Schreibman (2003) used a combination of discrete trial and naturalistic teaching to teach 4-year-old children with autism to follow the gaze of an adult to a nearby toy. The specific purpose of the intervention was to establish the experimenter's shift in gaze to a nearby object as a discriminative stimulus for gaze following. Instruction proceeded through six levels, all of which targeted the prerequisite skills necessary for the children to ultimately respond to the experimenter's bids for joint attention. The levels included (a) teaching the child to engage with a toy after the child's hand was physically placed on that toy, (b) teaching the child to engage with a new toy when already engaged with another toy following the experimenter's tapping the new toy, (c) teaching the child to engage with a new toy shown to the child by the experimenter while already engaged with another toy, (d) teaching the child to make eye contact with the experimenter in order to gain access to a new toy, (e) teaching the child to shift his or her gaze to a new toy when pointed to by the experimenter and when engaged with another toy, and (f) teaching the child to shift his or her gaze to a new toy following the experimenter's gaze alone. Physical prompts were primarily used throughout all levels, and access to desired toys was provided contingent upon correct responses. Improvements in joint attention were observed for all of the children, and the skills were shown to generalize to novel settings. Consequently, some of the children were rated as not being significantly different from their typically developing peers by novel observers following this intervention (Whalen & Schreibman, 2003).

Generalized Imitation

Imitation refers to the emission of a behavior that is topographically similar and temporally proximal to the behavior of a model (Baer, Peterson, & Sherman, 1967). Reinforcement contingencies are often arranged for imitating, as in the case of a child who receives verbal praise contingent upon clapping her hands shortly after her parent claps her hands, or the adult with a developmental disability who receives social reinforcement contingent upon performing a self-help skill in a manner identical to that modeled by a caregiver. Imitation skills have been shown to generalize to novel response topographies for which reinforcement has never been provided (Garcia, Baer, & Firestone, 1971). For example, the child may also pat the table shortly after her mother pats the table, solely on the basis of her history of reinforcement for imitating hand clapping. Likewise, the adult may imitate a new skill modeled by a staff person in the absence of social reinforcement for doing so. Once a generalized imitation repertoire is established, the learner has acquired an overarching response class of "doing as the model does" (Poulson, Kymissis, Reeve, Andreatos, & Reeve, 1991). These skills play a powerful role in behavioral development, as the emergence of language, social, daily living, and play skills are often products of generalized imitation (see Bijou & Baer, 1961, 1965).

Whereas generalized imitation skills have been demonstrated in typically developing infants as young as 10 months (Poulson & Kymissis, 1988), much research suggests that individuals with autism show marked deficits in the acquisition of imitation skills when compared to their age-matched typically developing peers and individuals with other types of developmental disabilities, such as mental retardation or Down syndrome (Smith & Bryson, 1994). The nature of these deficits is not clear, however. Some studies have shown that persons with autism have deficits in symbolic imitation, such as imaginary play, but not functional imitation, including the imitation of actions with objects. Other studies have suggested that the deficits are limited to multistep tasks, while additional research suggests that the imitation of single-step tasks is problematic for learners with autism. The reader is referred to Ingersoll, Schreibman, and Tran (2003) for a review. These deficits may be closely tied to the impairments in social functioning exhibited by persons with autism, as the individual who does not comprehend the social intent of others may lack motivation to imitate their actions (Whiten & Brown, 1998; Ingersoll et al., 2003).

It is important for individuals with autism to acquire generalized imitation skills because these skills can promote further developments in language, play, and self-help skills. Several decades of research in applied behavior analysis have specified instructional techniques that can be implemented with learners with autism and related disorders to ameliorate imitation deficits. In an early seminal study by Peterson and Whitehurst (1971), typically developing preschool-age children were taught to imitate simple motor movements displayed by an adult that were accompanied by the instruction, "Do this." Generalized imitative responses were shown to be durable in the absence of programmed reinforcement, and responses persisted as the delay before reinforcement was increased. More recent research with typically developing infants has confirmed the effectiveness of behavior analytic strategies for establishing generalized imitation. In a study by Poulson and Kymissis (1988), mothers taught their 10-month-old infants to imitate simple actions using objects, such as tossing a ball and pushing a truck. The presentation of a toy marked the onset of each trial, after which the mother instructed the infant to "Do this," modeled the action, and provided praise contingent upon responses that were identical to or were close approximations of the modeled response. Physical guidance was not necessary to establish imitation for any of the infants. Unreinforced probe trials were presented intermittently, which tested whether the infants would imitate response topographies that had not been explicitly trained. All of the infants showed generalized imitation. A similar procedure was used to establish generalization of simple vocal sounds such as "oh" and "wow" in infants in the same age group (Poulson et al., 1991).

There may be learning situations in which it is not desirable for the learner to immediately imitate a model. For example, if a learner climbing the ladder on a slide observes another child jumping on a trampoline, it would not be appropriate for the child to imitate jumping while about to go down the slide. Therefore, delayed imitation should be targeted as a goal once generalized immediate imitation has developed. Garcia (1976) established both generalized and delayed imitation in children with mental retardation. Immediate imitation was defined as the occurrence of a motor response that was identical to or closely matched that of a model's within 5 s after the response was modeled. Delayed imitation was defined as the occurrence of a motor response that was identical to or closely matched that of a model's between 5 and 25 s after the response was modeled. Physical prompts were initially necessary to establish correct responding, but the prompts were ultimately faded, and the children all developed delayed generalized imitation.

It may appear that generalized imitation was readily established in the aforementioned studies. Yet, there may be a limit to the size of a generalized response class that may develop. In a study conducted at the Princeton Child Development Institute by Young, Krantz, McClannahan, and Poulson (1994), four children with autism between the ages of 2 and 4 years were taught to imitate vocal, toy-play, and pantomime responses that consisted of motor movements resembling activities performed with objects or movements of the body, such as blowing a kiss. After receiving training trials in one of these three topographies, unreinforced probe trials were presented. The probe trials evaluated generalization to untrained response topographies. Generalized imitation of vocal responses was found only following vocal imitation training, but not following toy-play or pantomime imitation training. Likewise, generalized imitation of toy play was found only following toy-play imitation training, but not following vocal or pantomime imitation training. The same was true for the generalized imitation of pantomime responses. Thus, generalization occurred only within, but not across, functional response classes. Poulson, Kyparissos, Andreatos, Kymissis, and Parnes (2002) made similar findings. They taught mothers to train their infants to imitate motor-with-toy, motor-without-toy, and vocal responses. Generalization to untrained response topographies was tested, and generalization was shown to have occurred only to untrained responses of a particular topography following imitation training in that particular topography, but not following training in other topographies. Thus, if generalized imitation of a particular response topography is desired, one should train other imitative responses in that same topography.

When a learner demonstrates generalized imitation it facilitates acquisition of numerous other skills, either naturalistically or over the course of explicit programming. Once an individual learns to do as the model does, modeled prompts can be incorporated into instructional programs. Ingenmey and Van Houten (1991) used vocal imitation to increase spontaneous speech during toy play in a child with autism, for example, and speech skills were shown to generalize across multiple settings. Motor imitation can also be used to establish daily living skills. A promising area of instruction in schools and clinics for children is to systematically arrange for a child to imitate other children. A child who has learned to imitate other children may be more attentive to and curious about the actions of other children, such that he or she spontaneously imitates their actions in the absence of direct training.

Popular behavior analytic curriculum guides for children with autism provide specific recommendations for conducting imitation training. Lovaas (1981) suggested that imitation be taught after the child has learned to sit quietly in a chair for up to 5 min without displaying disruptive behaviors, but well-established eye contact is not a prerequisite. Lovaas (1981) also suggested presenting the instruction, "Do this," while simultaneously displaying the model, and physically guiding the correct response if necessary. Gross motor imitation should be taught prior to fine motor imitation, which should be taught prior to oral motor imitation. Once gross and fine motor imitation of one-step actions are established, the imitation of two-step, three-step, and more complex combinations of actions can be taught (Taylor & McDonough, 1996). When oral motor imitation is mastered, the imitation of single syllables followed by more complex words as well as sentences can be taught. An ideal outcome following imitation training is for the individual to spontaneously imitate, in the absence of direct instruction and direct reinforcement for doing so. For this reason, it may be helpful to fade the verbal instruction, "Do this," as progress occurs. This way, the individual's behavior is less likely to be under discriminative control of the instructions to imitate. Practitioners can arrange for the generalization of imitation across settings, stimuli, and people by using multiple instructors and stimuli during training and by conducting training in multiple locations.

Reinforcement Control

It is important that those working with learners who are new to a teaching situation ensure that the items used to sustain desired responses during teaching sessions are in fact preferred by the learner. Several procedures exist for conducting formal preference assessments (Fisher et al., 1992; Pace, Ivancic, Edwards, Iwata, & Page, 1985). Such assessments should be conducted routinely so that changes in preferences can be accommodated by changing the selection of items used as reinforcers during teaching sessions (see Chapter 2 for an extensive review of these procedures). Changes in the individual's deprivation and satiation levels should also be taken into consideration over the course of teaching (Michael, 1988). A variety of reinforcers should be used to prevent satiation on any one item throughout the session. If food items are used as reinforcers, it may be important to conduct teaching sessions prior to mealtime when deprivation levels are high. Zhou, Iwata, and Shore (2002) found that preferred food items maintained higher response rates in adults with severe and profound mental retardation when sessions were conducted prior to meals. Similarly, Gottschalk, Libby, and Graff (2000) found that when children with autism were deprived of preferred edible items several hours prior to a preference assessment, preference for those items was increased during the assessment. If access to tangible items or preferred activities is used as a reinforcer, access to those items should be restricted outside of teaching sessions so the learner remains motivated to respond for those items during the session.

Using reinforcement procedures effectively may also establish the instructor as a positive conditioned reinforcer. For very young children, it is often the parent who assumes this role. To establish themselves as conditioned reinforcers, parents and other instructors should identify the child's preferred items or activities. If the child is allowed to consume an item or engage in an activity contingent upon interacting with the parent or complying with requests, the parent or instructor will be established as a conditioned reinforcer. Initially the presence of the adult may not be a discriminative stimulus that signals the presentation of preferred items, but over time the child is likely to approach and seek interaction with the adult (Lovaas, 2003; Lovaas, Schaeffer, & Simmons, 1965).

Eventually it will become important to establish social praise as a reinforcer so the continuous delivery of preferred items for correct responses can be gradually reduced. Although social praise may not be inherently reinforcing for many individuals with autism, repeatedly pairing it with the delivery of preferred items will establish praise as an effective conditioned reinforcer. Over time, it will be ideal for the individual to emit a prescribed number of correct responses for social praise alone before a preferred item or activity is made available. Presenting a neutral cue, such as a token, during the delay before which the primary reinforcer is available may help the individual tolerate the delay. Grindle and Remington (2002) taught three children with autism to identify pictures using delayed reinforcement. Picture discrimination was most accurate when a compound stimulus consisting of a light and a buzzer was presented following correct responses prior to the delivery of reinforcement. Thus, presenting neutral stimuli, such as tokens or social comments, during delays before reinforcer deliveries may establish those stimuli as conditioned reinforcers. Such stimuli may help bridge the delay before primary reinforcement becomes available (Stromer, McComas, & Rehfeldt, 2000). These strategies will prepare the learner for the naturally occurring contingencies of reinforcement outside of the teaching session.

Establishing Compliance

Attempts must be made early in teaching to prevent noncompliance from impeding learning progress. Initially, teaching sessions should be for minimal time periods—no longer than 1 min—and short periods of complying with task demands should be reinforced with the opportunity to engage in a preferred activity. Session duration should be increased gradually, no more than 1 min at a time, as task compliance increases. Likewise, sessions should never end when the individual is protesting task demands. Sessions should always end following the occurrence of desirable behavior, even if the behavior must be prompted to occur. Several strategies have been reported for decreasing escape-maintained behavior and increasing compliance with task demands, including interspersing easy and difficult tasks (Ebanks & Fisher, 2003), allowing the learner opportunities to escape task demands contingent upon appropriate escape behavior, differentially reinforcing other behavior such as remaining on task (Kodak, Miltenberger, & Romaniuk, 2003), and teaching a simple functional communicative response that serves the same function as the challenging behavior, such as teaching the individual to use a picture card to request a break from tasks (Hagopian, Wilson, & Wilder, 2001).

Conclusion

A great deal of empirical support exists for using applied behavior analysis to teach readiness skills. These skills must be intact prior to the establishment of preacademic and academic skills. Some individuals may have advanced skills, but learning may be disrupted because they do not display readiness skills. In these situations practitioners must reestablish readiness behaviors so that instruction of more sophisticated skills can resume. Appropriate measures must be taken to ensure that effective positive reinforcers are used and that behaviors that interrupt teaching sessions are addressed.

 ## PRACTITIONER RECOMMENDATIONS

TEACHING SITTING

1. Initially use physical guidance coupled with the instruction, "Sit down."
2. Vary instructions after initial acquisition to promote generalization.
3. Gradually eliminate verbal instruction, "Sit down."
4. Provide access to preferred items contingent upon short periods of sitting, and gradually increase the period of sitting required for reinforcement.
5. Promote generalization by varying instructors, furniture, people present, and settings.

TEACHING EYE CONTACT

1. Use physical prompts minimally.
2. Visually prompt by presenting a preferred item in the line of vision between the learner's and instructor's eyes simultaneously with the instruction, "Look at me," and reinforce immediately.
3. Fade prompts using graduated time delay.
4. Gradually increase the duration of eye contact required for reinforcement.
5. Present visually stimulating items or gestural prompts alongside task materials to facilitate eye contact with task materials.

TEACHING JOINT ATTENTION

Teach the child to follow another person's shift in gaze by

1. reinforcing engagement with toy with child's hand placed on toy;
2. reinforcing engagement with a new toy after the instructor taps on the new toy while child is engaged with another toy;
3. reinforcing engagement with a new toy after the instructor shows the child the new toy while the child is engaged with another toy;
4. reinforcing eye contact with the instructor to gain access to a new toy;
5. reinforcing shifts in gaze to a new toy when pointed to by the instructor while child is engaged with another toy; and
6. reinforcing shift in gaze to a new toy following a shift in the instructor's gaze (Whalen & Schreibman, 2003).

TEACHING GENERALIZED IMITATION

1. Begin teaching once the learner sits in a chair for up to 5 min.
2. Present instruction, "Do this," while modeling the response.
3. Use physical guidance initially as necessary.
4. Gradually reduce instruction to "do this."
5. Teach gross motor imitation followed by fine motor imitation followed by oral–motor imitation.
6. Train imitative responses in the particular topography in which generalization to novel responses is desired.
7. Promote generalization by varying the settings, stimuli, and people present during training.
8. Incorporate modeled prompts into other instructional programs once imitative repertoire is established.
9. Arrange for the imitation of other children in naturalistic settings.

TEACHING REINFORCEMENT CONTROL

1. Conduct routine reinforcer preference assessments.
2. Use a variety of reinforcers to prevent satiation.
3. Take learner's current deprivation and satiation levels into account.
4. Restrict access to reinforcing items outside of teaching sessions.
5. Establish the instructor as a conditioned reinforcer by pairing his or her presence with the presentation of preferred items.
6. Establish social praise as a reinforcer by pairing its delivery with preferred items, and gradually reduce the delivery of preferred items for correct responses.

7. Present stimuli such as tokens or social comments during delays preceding reinforcement availability to facilitate tolerance for delayed reinforcement.

ESTABLISHING COMPLIANCE

1. Conduct initial teaching sessions for minimal time periods, and gradually increase the amount of time required before the learner is allowed to engage in a preferred activity.
2. Do not terminate sessions if the individual is protesting task demands.
3. Intersperse easy with difficult tasks.
4. Provide opportunities for breaks that are noncontingent upon challenging behaviors.

References

Baer, D. M., Peterson, R. F., & Sherman, J. A. (1967). The development of imitation by reinforcing behavioral similarity to a model. *Journal of the Experimental Analysis of Behavior, 10*, 405–416.

Bijou, S., & Baer, D. M. (1961) *Child development: Vol. 1. A systematic and empirical theory.* Oxford, England: Appleton-Century-Crofts.

Bijou, S., & Baer, D. M. (1965). *Child development: Vol. II. Universal stage of infancy.* Oxford, England: Appleton-Century-Crofts.

Charman, T., Swettenham, J., Baron-Cohen, S., Cox, A., Baird, G., et al. (1998). An experimental investigation of social–cognitive abilities in infants with autism: Clinical implications. *Infant Mental Health Journal, 19*, 260–275.

Dube, W. V., MacDonald, R. P. F., Mansfield, R. C., Holcomb, W. L., & Ahern, W. H. (2004). Toward a behavioral analysis of joint attention. *The Behavior Analyst, 27*, 197–207.

Ebanks, M. E., & Fisher, W. W. (2003). Altering the timing of academic prompts to treat destructive behavior maintained by escape. *Journal of Applied Behavior Analysis, 36*, 355–359.

Fisher, W., Piazza, C. C., Bowman, L. G., Hagopian, L. P., Owens, J. C., & Slevin, I. (1992). A comparison of two approaches for identifying reinforcers for persons with severe and profound disabilities. *Journal of Applied Behavior Analysis, 25*, 491–498.

Foxx, R. M. (1977). Attention training: The use of overcorrection avoidance to increase the eye contact of autistic and retarded children. *Journal of Applied Behavior Analysis, 10*, 489–499.

Garcia, E. E. (1976). The development and generalization of delayed imitation. *Journal of Applied Behavior Analysis, 9*, 499.

Garcia, E., Baer, D. M., & Firestone, I. (1971). The development of generalized imitation within topographically determined boundaries. *Journal of Applied Behavior Analysis, 4*, 101–112.

Gottschalk, J. M., Libby, M. E., & Graff, R. B. (2000). The effects of establishing operations on preference assessment outcomes. *Journal of Applied Behavior Analysis, 33*, 85–88.

Grindle, C. F., & Remington, B. (2002). Discrete-trial training for autistic children when reward is delayed: A comparison of conditioned cue value and response marking. *Journal of Applied Behavior Analysis, 35*, 187–190.

Hagopian, L. P., Wilson, D. M., & Wilder, D. A. (2001). Assessment and treatment of problem behavior maintained by escape from attention and access to tangible items. *Journal of Applied Behavior Analysis, 34*, 229–232.

Hamlet, C. C., Axelrod, S., & Kuerschner, S. (1984). Eye contact as an antecedent to compliant behavior. *Journal of Applied Behavior Analysis, 17,* 553–557.

Ingenmey, R., & Van Houten, R. (1991). Using time delay to promote spontaneous speech in an autistic child. *Journal of Applied Behavior Analysis, 24,* 591–596.

Ingersoll, B., Schreibman, L., & Tran, Q. H. (2003). Effect of sensory feedback on immediate object imitation in children with autism. *Journal of Autism and Developmental Disorders, 35,* 673–683.

Jones, E. A., & Carr, E. G. (2004). Joint attention in children with autism: Theory and intervention. *Focus on Autism and Other Developmental Disabilities, 19,* 13–26.

Kasari, C., Freeman, S. F., & Paparella, T. (2001). Early intervention in autism: Joint attention and symbolic play. *International Review of Research in Mental Retardation, 23,* 207–237.

Kodak, T., Miltenberger, R. G., & Romaniuk, C. (2003). The effects of differential negative reinforcement of other behavior and noncontingent escape on compliance. *Journal of Applied Behavior Analysis, 36,* 379–382.

Lovaas, O. I. (1981). *Teaching developmentally disabled children: The me book.* Austin, TX: PRO-ED.

Lovaas, O. I. (2003). *Teaching individuals with developmental delays.* Austin, TX: PRO-ED.

Lovaas, O. I., Koegel, R., Simmons, J. Q., & Long, J. S. (1973). Some generalization and follow-up measures on autistic children in behavior therapy. *Journal of Applied Behavior Analysis, 6,* 131–165.

Lovaas, O. I., Schaeffer, B., & Simmons, J. Q. (1965). Building social behavior in autistic children by use of electric shock. *Journal of Experimental Research in Personality, 1,* 99–109.

Lovaas, O. I., Schreibman, L., & Koegel, R. L. (1974). A behavior modification approach to the treatment of autistic children. *Journal of Autism and Childhood Schizophrenia, 4,* 111–129.

Margolies, P. J. (1977). Behavioral approaches to the treatment of early infantile autism: A review. *Psychological Bulletin, 84,* 249–264.

Matson, J. L., Manikam, R., Coe, D., Raymond, K., & Taras, M. (1988). Training social skills to severely mentally retarded multiply handicapped adolescents. *Research in Developmental Disabilities, 9,* 195–208.

Michael, J. (1988). Establishing operations and the mand. *The Analysis of Verbal Behavior, 6,* 3–9.

Pace, G. M., Ivancic, M. T., Edwards, G. L., Iwata, B. A., & Page, T. J. (1985). Assessment of stimulus preference and reinforcer value with profoundly retarded individuals. *Journal of Applied Behavior Analysis, 18,* 249–255.

Peterson, R. F., & Whitehurst, G. J. (1971). A variable influencing the performance of generalized imitative behaviors. *Journal of Applied Behavior Analysis, 4,* 1–9.

Poulson, C. L., & Kymissis, E. (1988). Generalized imitation in infants. *Journal of Experimental Child Psychology, 46,* 324–336.

Poulson, C. L., Kymissis, E., Reeve, K. F., Andreatos, M., & Reeve, L. (1991). Generalized vocal imitation in infants. *Journal of Experimental Child Psychology, 51,* 267–279.

Poulson, C. L., Kyparissos, N., Andreatos, M., Kymissis, E., & Parnes, M. (2002). Generalized imitation within three response classes in typically developing infants. *Journal of Experimental Child Psychology, 81,* 341–357.

Sarokoff, R. A., & Sturmey, P. (2004). The effects of behavioral skills training on staff implementation of discrete-trial teaching. *Journal of Applied Behavior Analysis, 37,* 535–538.

Smith, I., & Bryson, S. (1994). Imitation and action in autism: A critical review. *Psychological Bulletin, 116,* 259–272.

Stromer, R., McComas, J., & Rehfeldt, R. A. (2000). Designing interventions that include delayed reinforcement: Implications of recent laboratory research. *Journal of Applied Behavior Analysis, 33,* 359–371.

Sundberg, M. L., & Partington, J. W. (1999). The need for both discrete trial and natural environment language training for children with autism. In P. M. Ghezzi, W. L. Williams, & J. E. Carr (Eds.), *Autism: Behavior analytic perspectives* (pp. 139–156). Reno, NV: Context Press.

Taylor, B. A., & McDonough, K. A. (1996). Selecting teaching programs. In C. Maurice, G. Green, & S. C. Luce (Eds.), *Behavioral intervention for young children with autism: A manual for parents and professionals* (pp. 63–177). Austin, TX: PRO-ED.

Whalen, C., & Schriebman, L. (2003). Joint attention training for children with autism using behavior modification procedures. *Journal of Child Psychology and Psychiatry, 44,* 456–468.

Whiten, A., & Brown, J. (1998). Imitation and the reading of other minds: Perspectives from the study of autism, normal children, and non-human primates. In S. Braten (Ed.), *Intersubjective communication and emotion in early ontogeny* (pp. 260–280). New York: Cambridge University Press.

Young, P. J., Krantz, P. J., McClannahan, L. E., & Poulson, C. L. (1994). Generalized imitation and response-class formation in children with autism. *Journal of Applied Behavior Analysis, 27,* 685–697.

Zager, D. B., Shamow, N. A., & Schneider, H. C. (1999). Teaching students with autism. In D. B. Zager (Ed.), *Autism: Identification, education, and treatment* (pp. 111–139). Mahwah, NJ: Erlbaum.

Zhou, L., Iwata, B. A., & Shore, B. A. (2002). Reinforcing efficacy of food on performance during pre- and postmeal sessions. *Journal of Applied Behavior Analysis, 35,* 411–414.

C H A P T E R

SELF-HELP SKILLS

Ruth Anne Rehfeldt and Rocio Rosales
Southern Illinois University

elf-help skills are skills that enable individuals to care independently for their own bodily needs (Taras & Matese, 1990). They comprise several daily living skills that are necessary for achieving maximum independence (Matson, Benavidez, Compton, Paclawskyj, & Baglio, 1996). Self-help skills are often categorized into the following curricular areas: personal maintenance (e.g., toileting, grooming, and dressing), integrated community living (e.g., self-preservation, meal preparation, and grocery shopping), and vocational preparation (e.g., public transportation and finance management) (Belfiore & Mace, 1994, p. 203). It is not unusual for persons with developmental disabilities to have deficits in self-help skills, although interestingly, self-help skills have been shown to be a relative strength for adolescents and adults with autism (Belfiore & Mace, 1994). Because considerable time and effort on the part of parents, staff, and teachers are required to care for individuals who lack these skills, intensive instruction in this area is imperative. Furthermore, the inability to care for one's bodily needs may promote stigmatization of individuals with disabilities in many settings. Finally, individuals who are proficient in self-help skills are more likely to participate in integrated community work and recreational activities, thus experiencing an enhanced quality of life (Christian & Luce, 1985).

The purpose of this chapter is to describe research-based recommendations for establishing and maintaining self-help skills in individuals with autism. Space does not permit us to discuss strategies for establishing personal maintenance, integrated community living, and vocational preparation skills in full detail. For a more exhaustive review on all three subcurricula, the reader is referred to Belfiore and Mace (1994). We discuss toileting, task analysis and response chaining, pictorial cues and schedules, observational learning and video modeling, self-instructions, and unique strategies for teaching integrated community skills.

Toileting

Toileting is a self-help skill that is of concern to many parents and caregivers of individuals with autism. A child who cares for his or her own toileting needs is more likely to participate in integrated educational classrooms. The now-famous procedure developed by Azrin and Foxx (1971) was originally successful in reducing toilet-related accidents in adults with profound mental retardation and has continued to meet with considerable success over the past few decades. Lovaas (1981) modified Azrin and Foxx's (1971) procedure and subsequently marketed it for parents of children with autism. The procedure consists of four steps: (a) the child is to sit on the toilet, and reinforcement is provided contingent upon appropriate sitting and eliminating; (b) the child is to be seated in a chair next to the toilet and reinforcement is delivered for not eliminating for a 5-min period, as well as for asking to go to the toilet and eliminating; (c) the chair is to be moved a distance from the toilet so that the child learns to go to the toilet in the bathroom, remove his or her clothing, and eliminate, with reinforcement again provided contingent upon eliminating; and (d) the parent or caregiver is to check the child's pants every 15 to 30 minutes and ask if the child is dry. The child is to be verbally praised if dry. The child should consume a lot of liquid during all phases to ensure a high frequency of urination.

Task Analysis and Response Chaining

Many self-help skills are behavior chains that are made up of a large number of different discrete responses that must be performed in a set sequence. To identify the response units comprising a chain and the order in which they must occur, the practitioner must conduct a task analysis in which the skill is broken down into a detailed listing of its component subskills in sequential order. In this way, the task is organized into teachable steps. The behaviors delineated in the task analysis must be stated in observable, measurable terms. Task analyses are typically validated by observing the performance of skilled experts, or individuals whose performance already meets some acceptable standard (Cuvo, 1978). Consideration must be granted to how finely detailed the skill breakdown is. As Cuvo (1978) noted, it is unnecessary to have a task analyzed so finely that the learner performs a number of the steps accurately prior to training, yet a task analysis that includes steps containing several responses is unlikely to be effective. Tables 4.1 and 4.2 show examples of validated task analyses, which were used to teach leisure and daily living skills to adults with severe mental retardation.

Physical, gestural, verbal, and modeled prompts can all be used to occasion a particular step in a task analysis, the goal being to eventually eliminate the prompts. Acquisition may also be facilitated if response-specific verbal praise is delivered contingent upon accurate performance of each step (e.g., "Nice job turning off the faucet"). This, too, is gradually eliminated as the steps are mastered, until eventually reinforcement is provided only contingent upon completion of the entire chain.

A considerable amount of research has acknowledged the utility of teaching self-help skills using task analytic procedures with individuals with autism. For

TABLE 4.1
Task Analysis for Making a Sandwich

Steps in the Task Analysis

1. Go to refrigerator
2. Get jar of jelly out of refrigerator
3. Get bread out of refrigerator
4. Bring jar of jelly and bread to table
5. Get butter knife from counter
6. Get plate from counter
7. Get peanut butter from counter
8. Bring knife, plate, and peanut butter to table
9. Remove two slices of bread from bag
10. Place one or both slices on plate
11. Open jar of peanut butter
12. Scoop out peanut butter with knife
13. Spread peanut butter onto slice of bread
14. Open jar of jelly
15. Scoop out jelly with knife
16. Spread jelly onto slice of bread
17. Place two slices of bread together

Materials needed: Jar of jelly, jar of peanut butter, sliced bread, butter knife, plate

TABLE 4.2
Task Analysis for Playing a Compact Disc on a Portable Walkman

Steps in the Task Analysis

1. Select Walkman from array of items
2. Open Walkman to insert disc
3. Select disc from array of items
4. Open CD case
5. Insert disc into Walkman
6. Close Walkman
7. Select headphones
8. Plug headphones into Walkman
9. Push "play" button on Walkman

Materials needed: Portable disc player, compact disc, headphones

example, Smith and Belcher (1985) trained house counselors of residential fa-cilities to use task analyses and a least-to-most prompt hierarchy to teach adults with autism to brush their teeth, comb their hair, wash their faces, and cook simple meals (see Chapter 2 for more on this prompting procedure). Likewise, Blew, Schwartz, and Luce (1985) combined task analysis training with peer tu-tors to teach children with autism such community skills as checking out a library book, buying an item at a convenience store, purchasing a snack, and crossing a street.

Once a task analysis has been established, a forward, backward, or total task chaining procedure will be used to teach the skill. With *forward chaining*, the first response of the chain is taught in isolation until mastery, after which the first and second responses of the chain are linked together and are taught until the link has been mastered, after which the first, second, and third responses of the chain are linked together and taught until mastery, and so forth, until the entire chain is mastered. An advantage of forward chaining is that it is con-ducted according to the natural order in which the responses within the chain occur in everyday situations. Richman, Reiss, Bauman, and Bailey (1984) used forward chaining to teach menstrual care skills to women with mild to severe mental retardation. They used verbal prompts over the course of the chaining procedure, and verbal praise was provided for each step in the chain that was performed correctly. When a step was prompted, the participant was allowed to perform the step and was then required to start the chain over; only after the previous step was performed correctly without prompting was she allowed to progress to the next step. This training continued until a participant performed all of the steps in the task analysis independently. All participants mastered the task, and importantly, the skills were shown to be intact at 5-month follow-up.

With *backward chaining,* the response chain is constructed by teaching re-sponse links in the opposite order from which the skill will eventually be per-formed. The last response to occur is taught first, then the second-to-the-last response and the last response are linked together and taught next, and so forth, until the entire chain is mastered. Backward chaining is thought to be effective because the stimuli that are produced by responses at the end of the chain are more proximal with reinforcement than stimuli that are produced by responses at the beginning of the chain. Additionally, unlike forward chaining, back-ward chaining does not involve extinction of previously reinforced responses, which might disrupt learning. Thus, stimuli that are produced by responses near the end of the chain may be established as effective conditioned reinforc-ers, which maintain the responses emitted earlier in the chain as instruction proceeds backward (Rehfeldt, 2002). For these reasons, a backward-chaining procedure may be effective for individuals who have trouble tolerating lengthy delay-to-reinforcement intervals. Sulzer-Azaroff and Mayer (1991) noted that backward chaining may be particularly effective for individuals who lack recep-tive language. For example, Hagopian, Farrell, and Amari (1996) used backward chaining to treat liquid refusal by a child with severe developmental disabilities and gastrointestinal problems. They first delivered reinforcement contingent upon swallowing with no liquid in the mouth following a verbal prompt to do so. When this response was performed correctly for two consecutive trials, the next response was added to the chain, and reinforcement was provided contin-gent upon accepting and swallowing water placed in the mouth from a syringe. When the two responses were performed correctly for two consecutive trials, the next response was added to the chain, and so forth, until the individual per-formed the entire chain independently. The individual's consumption of water was also shown to generalize to novel settings.

With *total-* or *whole-task presentation,* the learner is required to attempt all of the steps from the beginning to the end of the chain in one trial, and the trial is not considered complete until the entire chain is complete. Total-task presen-tation has the advantage that steps of the chain are taught in the order in which they occur in the natural environment. However, some learners may have a dif-ficult time working through lengthy response chains in one trial without mak-ing many errors, unless most-to-least intrusive prompting is used. In an early study by Horner and Keilitz (1975), adolescents with mental retardation were taught to brush their teeth using total-task presentation. Instructors provided either no help, verbal instructions, demonstration and verbal instructions, or physical guidance and verbal instructions, which were applied using a least-to-most prompting hierarchy to the training of each step in the chain. As acqui-sition occurred, the number of training procedures applied to each step de-creased. Individuals received tokens and social praise for steps performed correctly. Similarly, Matson, Taras, Sevin, Love, and Fridley (1990) taught children diagnosed with both autism and mental retardation a number of self-help skills using total task presentation, including shoe tying, tooth brushing, hair combing, dressing, eating, and drinking. The procedure used in this study consisted of (a) the instructor modeling and verbally describing the behavior, (b) the instructor physically and verbally guiding the child through the entire chain, and (c) the child eventually performing each skill independently. Participants advanced from one phase to the next as mastery occurred. Not only did all of the children acquire all of the skills, the skills were maintained 1 year following training (Matson et al., 1990).

Self-help skills should not be taught in isolation but should rather be taught in the context in which the skill will ultimately be completed. To facilitate generalization across settings and people, instruction should occur in different settings and in the presence of different instructors. As mastery occurs, variations in the task materials should be introduced to facilitate generalization across stimuli. For example, if the individual is learning to wash his or her hands using a bar of soap, a bottle of hand soap might be substituted for the bar of soap. General-case instruction may be particularly effective in facilitating generalization of skills (Sprague & Horner, 1984). *General-case training* involves providing a range of different examples during training that systematically samples the range of stimulus and response variations that new situations might demand. In other words, a variety of stimuli and responses are strategically selected based on an analysis of what might occur in the different situations in which the task is completed, and those examples are incorporated into the teaching session. For example, Neef, Lensbower, Hockersmith, DePalma, and Gray (1990) used general-case instruction to teach laundry skills to adults with developmental disabilities. They taught participants to do laundry using a variety of actual and simulated washers and dryers. In some cases different responses were required to complete the task, and in other cases the physical features of the equipment were different. Generalization to untrained exemplars, such as novel washers or dryers that differed from those used in training, was more likely following general- versus single-case instruction.

Pictorial Cues and Schedules

A common deficit in persons with autism and related disorders is the failure to initiate self-help tasks in the absence of verbal instructions from others. For this reason, many individuals with autism depend upon ongoing supervision from parents or caregivers to complete their daily routines. Pictorial self-management packages are effective in facilitating the execution of self-help skills with minimal supervision from others. Rather than verbal prompts or instructions from others occasioning behavior, pictorial cues prompt the completion of and transition between tasks, thus promoting independence and autonomy (McClannahan & Krantz, 1999). One approach involves presenting a sequence of pictures in which each picture corresponds to a particular step in a chained task. Each picture is established as a discriminative stimulus for a specific step in the task analysis, such that the learner ultimately completes a skill with only the pictorial prompts occasioning correct responses; prompts from others are unnecessary. Another approach involves presenting a schedule of pictures in which each picture corresponds to a different task, such that each picture is established as a discriminative stimulus for the completion of the entire task. McClannahan and Krantz (1999) suggested that only manual guidance from behind be used to teach individuals to use activity schedules, thus preventing their behavior from coming under the control of the social behavior of others. The individual learns not only to complete self-care tasks in the absence of prompts from others, but independently transitions between such activities as well. A picture of a reinforcing item or activity is often shown last in the sequence of picture prompts or schedules, and the learner is often taught to deliver his or her own reinforcer upon task completion. Pictorial prompts and schedules can be presented in notebooks or binders, photo albums, computer-aided systems (Lancioni & O'Reilly, 2001), and, for some learners, written lists (see Figure 4.1). Pictorial prompts have the advantage that they can be easily transported from one setting to the next. An additional advantage for learners with autism is that their behavior may be more likely to come under control of visual rather than physical or verbal antecedent stimuli. Many individuals with autism enjoy visual stimulation; using picture cues may be a more enjoyable way to learn. For these reasons, pictorial cues and schedules have been widely used in domestic and vocational settings for children and adults with autism.

Individuals with autism should possess several prerequisite skills before a pictorial self-management system is introduced. McClannahan and Krantz (1999) advised that the individual should discriminate pictures from the surrounding backgrounds, match identical three-dimensional objects, match two-dimensional pictures to the corresponding three-dimensional objects, and tolerate manual guidance. Thus, pictorial management systems are not for individuals who have not yet received behavior analytic instruction on basic preacademic skills (see Chapter 2 for a discussion of teaching these discrimination skills.)

Activity schedules consist of a sequence of pictures that facilitate an individual's completion of lengthy response chains and transitions between tasks (McClannahan & Krantz, 1999; MacDuff, Krantz, & McClannahan, 1993). Pictures included in a learner's first schedule typically correspond to activities

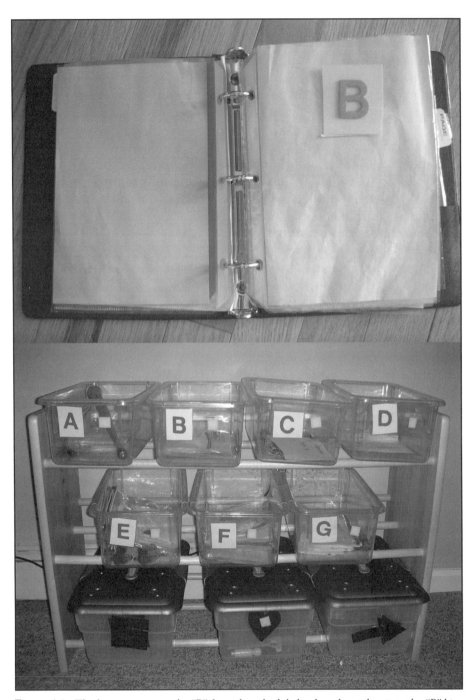

Figure 4.1. The learner removes the "B" from the schedule book and matches it to the "B" bin, which contains the materials to complete the activity.

that have clear endings and that the individual is already capable of performing. McClannahan and Krantz (1999) suggested using manual guidance from behind to teach the individual to turn the pages of his or her schedule, obtain the materials needed for each task, complete the task, return the materials, and so forth, until the schedule is complete. Thus, picture schedules may be appropriate for individuals who have already mastered self-care skills but require ongoing supervision from others to complete a sequence of tasks, such as that constituting an individual's bedtime routine, or that necessary to prepare for work in the morning. A considerable body of research has confirmed the utility of activity schedules in establishing autonomy and independence in persons with autism (MacDuff et al., 1993; Krantz, MacDuff, & McClannahan, 1993). Moreover, parents and teachers of children with autism have easily acquired the skills necessary for schedule teaching (Hall, McClannahan, & Krantz, 1995; Krantz et al., 1993.)

There are also other approaches to using visual prompts. Some of these should be distinguished from activity schedules. If the procedure involving use of visual stimuli does not explicitly emphasize bringing the behavior of the child under the stimulus control of the visual stimuli because of social prompts or consequences, then the learning process that accounts for the observed behavior change is a very different one from that involved in activity schedules.

Pierce and Schreibman (1994) demonstrated the effectiveness of pictorial self-management on the acquisition of daily living skills in children with severe autism. Picture prompts consisted of color photographs corresponding to selected steps in a task analysis, such as a picture of a child with the pajama top raised overhead corresponded to removing one's pajama top in the task analysis for getting dressed. The children were first taught to discriminate between the pictures depicting the steps in the particular chained tasks. Next, the children were taught to choose their own reinforcers, turn pages in a picture book, perform the responses depicted on the pictures, and deliver their own reinforcers. The instructors used modeling, prompting, and verbal praise during training, and the instructor's presence was eventually faded as the children achieved independence. Thus, all of the children acquired and maintained several skills. Importantly, supervision was not necessary for the maintenance of those skills, and using pictorial cues to complete the self-care tasks was shown to generalize across settings and tasks. Martin, Rusch, James, Decker, and Trtol (1982) reported similar results using picture prompts to teach adults with mental retardation to prepare complex meals. Pictures consisted of recipe cards, which included black-and-white line drawings depicting the step in the task, a number indicating the order of the step in the task, and a typed statement describing each step. Training included verbal and physical prompts as well as verbal praise for correct responses and error correction for incorrect responses.

Observational Learning and Video Modeling

An economic and efficient means for individuals with autism to acquire self-help skills is by observational learning. As discussed in Chapter 3, after acquiring generalized imitation, an individual may be more attentive to and interested in the behavior of other people. This may permit for the acquisition of untrained skills over the course of observing others who are proficient in performing the particular skill or task. Typically used to facilitate the acquisition of chained tasks, interventions that arrange for observational learning usually require the learner to observe the model perform the skill and then practice the skill until the skill is mastered. In some cases reinforcement is provided contingent upon correct responses during the practice trial. Thus, observing the behavior of a model is often a component of a treatment package that includes positive reinforcement. In variations of this procedure, the model is an individual who has not mastered the task, but who receives systematic instruction on the task while the learner observes.

Presenting the modeled task via video is a popular strategy for promoting learning in persons with developmental disabilities (Sturmey, 2003). Video modeling is defined as the viewing of a videotape of a peer or instructor successfully performing a chained task (LeGrice & Blampied, 1994). The typical protocol is similar to that described above: The learner is required to view the videotape at the beginning of an instructional session and to then attempt the task independently. As with in vivo modeling, reinforcement may be provided contingent upon correct responses during the practice trial, such that video modeling is one component of a treatment package including positive reinforcement. What is critical about both approaches is that the instructor never prompts the learner to perform particular steps in the task correctly; rather, the live or videotaped model serves as the prompt.

A number of studies have shown that children with autism and other disabilities may acquire self-help skills via the observation of in vivo models. Werts, Caldwell, and Wolery (1996) found that children with developmental delays displayed such skills as playing an audiotape, using a calculator, and sharpening a pencil after observing peer models without disabilities perform the tasks. The peer models were proficient in completing the tasks and described the steps aloud as they performed them. In a similar study, Griffen, Wolery, and Schuster (1992) showed that children with moderate mental retardation acquired most of the steps of several chained snack preparation tasks after observing other children with disabilities being directly taught the tasks. Instruction consisted of teaching all of the children to use pictorial recipe books and providing frequent praise contingent upon accuracy. Although not explicitly addressing self-help skills, Egel, Richman, and Koegel (1981) found that accuracy on discrimination tasks increased for children with autism after observing typically developing peers model the correct responses. Moreover, the skills were maintained after the peer models were removed (Egel et al., 1981).

These results suggest that video modeling may be effective not only in arranging for observational learning, but it may be cost-efficient as well: Less instructional time is necessary if learning can occur from observing one's peers. Small-group instruction, where group members observe one another being taught a particular skill or task, may be advantageous in settings where staff–student ratios are low (see also Taubman et al., 2001). Recruiting the participation of siblings of children with autism to serve as peer models in the instruction of self-help skills may encourage interaction between the two siblings and provide the sibling without autism a meaningful role in his or her sibling's treatment. However, further research is necessary to establish whether or not observing one's peers increases social interactions between the learner and other children.

Several studies have demonstrated the acquisition, generalization, and maintenance of self-help and daily living skills using video modeling. Norman, Collins, and Schuster (2001) showed that children with developmental disabilities acquired such self-help skills as cleaning their sunglasses, putting on a wristwatch, and zipping a jacket following the implementation of video modeling; moreover, the skills generalized across novel stimuli and people. In addition, Lasater and Brady (1995) showed that video modeling was effective in establishing lunch-making and laundry skills in individuals with developmental disabilities. These skills were also shown to generalize across settings. Finally, video modeling was also effective in teaching sandwich-making and coffee-making skills, with the skills generalizing across settings (Rehfeldt, Dahman, Young, Cherry, & Davis, 2003), stimuli, and people (Bidwell & Rehfeldt, 2004). Because positive reinforcement is also often used in such procedures, it may be difficult to attribute skill acquisition to the video, positive reinforcement, or both. Nonetheless, there are a number of advantages to incorporating video modeling into an instructional program. First, skill acquisition may be much more rapid using video rather than in vivo modeling (Charlop-Christy, Le, & Freeman, 2000). Second, several individuals may view a video at one time, thus reducing staff training time. Third, many individuals with autism enjoy visual stimulation such as that obtained from watching videos, so watching a video may be more enjoyable than watching a live model (Charlop-Christy et al., 2000).

Some research suggests that observational learning, whether using in vivo or video modeling, may be more effective the more similar the model is to the learner (Sherer et al., 2001). Thus, if arranging for observational learning to take place, it may be important for the model to be close in age to the learner. Self-modeling, in which the learner views an edited video of himself or herself performing accurately (Lasater & Brady, 1995), may be an optimal procedure for ensuring maximal similarity between the learner and the model. Other individuals with disabilities who are proficient in performing the task may also serve as effective models. For these procedures to be effective, it is imperative that the learner has mastered generalized imitation as well as the other readiness skills previously discussed. Video and in vivo modeling are likely to be maximally effective if the learner is interested in and attentive to other people. For recommendations on the creation of videos, the reader is referred to Dowrick (1991).

Self-Instructions

Self-management techniques are popular strategies for promoting independence in persons with disabilities. An individual self-manages when he or she emits one behavior to control the occurrence of another behavior (Skinner, 1953). In other words, a target behavior is brought under discriminative control of some other behavior that is emitted for the purposes of influencing the occurrence of the target behavior (Miltenberger, 2001, p. 385). For example, a person might place a packed gym bag next to the front door at night to make it more probable that he or she will go to the gym the next day. One self-management approach for facilitating the acquisition and maintenance of self-help skills is for the individual to state aloud brief rules or instructions prior to the completion of each step of the chained task. Appropriate for individuals with fairly well-developed verbal skills, a self-rule can be defined as a verbal response that directs other responses of the speaker (Duarte & Baer, 1994). For example, an individual's completion of the chained task of getting dressed in a work uniform may be enhanced if he or she emits simple self-statements prior to the completion of each step (i.e., "left arm through the sleeve," "right arm through the sleeve," "tie the apron in back"). Prior to training, however, it is necessary that the individual first be taught to emit the self-rules in their correct sequence in the chained task. The learner thus must state the self-rules at the appropriate time and follow them correctly (Miltenberger, 2001, p. 204). Modeling and praise for correct self-rules are typically used to establish this repertoire.

To date, not a great deal of research has been conducted on the role of self-rules in the acquisition and maintenance of self-help skills, nor have the reported studies focused exclusively on individuals with autism. Jay, Grote, and Baer (1999) taught four adults with mild mental retardation to emit and follow self-instructions, in order to improve their performance on a sorting task. They taught the participants to sort pictures and name the common features in each pair of pictures. Prior to the self-instructions intervention, participants routinely failed at the task. Jay et al. (1999) used modeling of self-instructions, approval of correct answers, and correction of incorrect answers to teach the participants to self-instruct. When participants were prompted to self-instruct, Jay et al. observed near-perfect sorting and correct self-instruction for all of the participants. Vintere, Hemmes, Brown, and Poulson (2004) showed that self-instructions facilitated gross-motor skill acquisition by typically developing pre-school children. They taught participants chained dance moves. To reduce the need for continued prompting, the instructors taught the children to voice a self-rule aloud prior to each step while simultaneously performing the step. The instructor also modeled self-rules and simultaneous completion of each step and delivered praise for steps performed correctly. The number of trials with correct responses was higher in self-instruction versus no self-instruction conditions (Vintere et al., 2004).

These studies suggest that self-instructions facilitate the acquisition of self-help skills in individuals with autism who can verbalize simple phrases. Moreover, generalization of skills to new settings is likely, as the learner's verbal repertoire can be transported easily from one setting to the next (Taylor & O'Reilly, 1997), as the learner need not rely upon verbal prompts from others in each new setting. Because it may be more socially appropriate for an individual to learn to emit self-rules silently, future research should examine the degree to which self-rules emitted at the covert level also facilitate skill acquisition and maintenance. Taylor and O'Reilly (1997) evaluated the effectiveness of covert self-rules on the acquisition of shopping skills in adults with mild intellectual disabilities. In their procedure, individuals were first taught, using modeling and verbal praise, to emit self-rules overtly prior to each step in the chained task and were then taught to emit those same rules covertly. Training was carried out in the context of completing the shopping task first in a classroom setting and then in a super-market. The self-instructions were successful in establishing proficiency in the task. When the emission of self-instructions was blocked by having the participants complete a distractor task (repeating random numbers spoken by the experimenter), accuracy in completing the chained shopping task decreased. Thus, a functional relationship between task proficiency and the emission of covert self-rules was demonstrated. They did not observe generalization of shopping to other settings or the control over nonverbal behavior by the emission of each individual self-rule. These latter issues await further programmatic study.

Although the investigation of self-instruction interventions for self-help deficits is in its infancy, results from the studies published to date appear promising. The intervention may be particularly appropriate for individuals who are verbally advanced, such as students with high-functioning autism or Asperger syndrome, whose skills are not under strong or appropriate stimulus control. It is important for practitioners to consider the large amount of training that must occur prior to the intervention, for not only must the individual learn the self-rule, but he or she must learn to emit the self-rule prior to the appropriate step in the task. During the actual training of the chained task, it may be desirable for the instructor to provide reinforcement contingent upon steps performed correctly, but eventually this should be faded, as the purpose of the intervention is for the individual to emit self-rules in the absence of assistance from others.

Contemporary Strategies for Teaching Integrated Community Living Skills

To experience the rich and diverse opportunities that integrated community living affords, individuals with autism must be proficient in completing a number of self-help skills in their respective communities. Educational efforts in recent years have focused more and more on teaching skills that will prepare individuals with autism to become enduring, contributing members of their community (Belfiore & Mace, 1994). Although not all adults with autism will achieve complete independence, each person should develop to his or her fullest potential so as to experience the richest quality of life possible. The interest in community integration and inclusion of adults with developmental disabilities has set the stage for a variety of intriguing approaches for establishing community self-help skills. We highlight several distinctive approaches to enhancing an individual's success in day-to-day community living.

Peer Tutoring

In peer tutoring, a typically developing peer without a disability teaches a student with a disability. This approach holds promise as a unique and enjoyable way to teach community skills to students with autism. In a study by Blew et al. (1985), task analysis was combined with peer tutors to teach such skills as checking out a library book, buying an item at a convenience store, purchasing a snack, and crossing a street. The peer tutors were taught how to conduct instruction using a task analysis, which included following the task analysis, modeling correct responses with and without verbal instructions, and reinforcing correct responses. After the peers had become acquainted with the children with autism, they trained the children to perform the particular tasks, with training consisting of explaining the steps in the chained tasks, modeling the target behavior, and providing feedback on performance. This strategy was effective in teaching the children the skills. Although considerable effort must be granted toward the initial training and ongoing supervision of peers, students with autism may enjoy the instruction more than if it were provided by an adult, and the instruction may produce more informal social interactions with the peer tutors.

Learning To Be Safe

An important skill for an individual to be successful in community living is recognizing and responding appropriately in potentially unsafe situations such as separation from a staff person or caregiver. In an admirable study, Taylor, Hughes, Richard, Hoch, and Coello (2004) evaluated a procedure to teach adolescents with autism to seek assistance in community settings when physically separated from parents or teachers. Three adolescents wore vibrating pagers when in community settings. Training was first conducted in the school setting. When an individual was separated from his or her teacher, he or she was paged. The individual was then taught to respond to the page by handing a card indicating that he or she was lost to a familiar adult. Prompts consisted of verbally prompting the student to say, "Excuse me," and physical guidance to approach a nearby familiar adult and produce the communication card. Verbal praise for responding to the pager was provided. Once prompts were faded and the participants were successful in giving the card to a familiar person, training was implemented in two community settings. This procedure was successful in teaching the teenagers to seek assistance when lost. Importantly, skills generalized to untrained community settings and were maintained when the pagers were activated by a parent instead of a teacher.

Providing Assistance to Others

An additional community skill that may contribute to successful social relationships in employment settings is the ability to provide assistance to others. Harris, Handleman, and Alessandri (1990) taught three adolescents with autism to offer assistance to a person stating the inability to complete such tasks as opening a cabinet door and picking up a cup. Participants verbalized the phrase, "Can I help you?" and had the motor skills necessary to provide assistance intact prior to the study. Training consisted of verbally prompting the individuals to say, "Can I help you?" in response to a confederate's indication of an inability to accomplish the task, after which time the students performed the skill necessary to complete the task. Verbal praise was provided for correct responses. Unfortunately, this study did not test for generalization across multiple settings, people, or tasks. In a recent study, Reeve (2001) expanded upon Harris et al. (1990) by using multiple exemplar training to establish stimulus and response generalization of helping responses in 5- to 6-year-old children with autism. A variety of helping responses were directly trained in the presence of a variety of different discriminative stimuli for offering assistance. Nonverbal discriminative stimuli included an adult's engagement in such activities as putting away items, locating objects, and setting up activities, while verbal discriminative stimuli included comments such as, "Time to clean up the blackboard" and "Wow, this table is messy." An instructional package consisting of live and video modeling, verbal and motor prompting, and token reinforcement plus verbal praise for correct responses was used. Helping behavior was shown to generalize to a variety of novel circumstances in which an adult needed assistance. Helping responses were maintained at 2-month follow-up. In addition, others rated the children as being more prosocial following the intervention.

Conclusion

Some of the strategies for teaching self-help skills, such as task analysis and response chaining, are the result of several decades of research in applied behavior analysis. Other strategies, such as video modeling and self-instructions, are relatively newer research endeavors that hold great promise in promoting independence. It is important for practitioners to remember that a number of readiness skills must be established prior to the teaching of self-help skills (see Chapter 3). Practitioners will also find a number of helpful resources commercially available to assist with the many techniques discussed, such as McClannahan and Krantz's (1999) thorough discussion of activity schedule teaching and Dowrick's (1991) helpful guide for using video in behavior analytic instruction.

Practitioner Recommendations

1. Toileting
    a. Ensure that the child consumes plenty of liquids.
    b. Seat the child on the toilet and provide reinforcement contingent upon appropriate sitting and eliminating.
    c. Seat the child in a chair next to toilet and provide reinforcement for staying dry (not eliminating) for a 5-minute period.

    d.   Gradually distance the chair from the toilet as the child learns to go to the toilet, remove clothing, and eliminate.

    e.   Check the child's pants every 15 to 30 minutes:

- Ask if child is dry.
- If the child is dry provide verbal praise (or tangible reinforcement if necessary).

    f.   Provide reinforcement contingent upon child asking to go to the bathroom.

2.   Creating a task analysis

    a.   Break skills down into a detailed listing of component subskills in sequential order.

    b.   State each subskill in observable and measurable terms.

    c.   Ensure that each step in the task analysis requires only one response.

    d.   Determine which chaining procedure will be used to teach the skill. Use backward chaining for those who have difficulties tolerating lengthy delays to reinforcement or those who lack receptive language skills.

    e.   Teach skills in the context that they will eventually occur.

    f.   Provide reinforcement contingent upon accurate performance of each step.

    g.   Gradually fade prompts.

    h.   Promote generalization by:

- conducting training sessions with different task materials and
- conducting training sessions in different settings and with different people.

3.   Teaching with activity schedules and pictorial cues

    a.   Establish pictures as discriminative stimuli for specific steps in a chained task or for the completion of a series of tasks.

    b.   For easy transportation, present pictorial prompts in binders, photo albums, or on portable computer systems.

    c.   Determine that the learner has the following prerequisites (McClannahan & Krantz, 1999):

- ability to discriminate pictures from surrounding backgrounds,

- ability to match identical three-dimensional shapes,
- ability to match two-dimensional pictures to corresponding 3-dimensional objects, and
- tolerates manual guidance.

d. Use manual guidance to teach schedule following.

e. Use pictorial schedules with individuals who have acquired skills but require prompts from others to initiate, complete, and transition between tasks.

4. Video modeling

a. Learner should demonstrate generalized imitation and other readiness skills before beginning instruction using video modeling.

b. Learner should view video model and imitate skill.

- Refrain from using verbal, physical, or gestural prompts during practice trials.
- Continue until mastered.

c. Deliver reinforcement contingent upon correct responses during practice trials.

d. Select models that are as similar to the learner as possible. Recruit siblings or other familiar peers.

References

Azrin, N. H., & Foxx, R. M. (1971). A rapid method of toilet training the institutionalized retarded. *Journal of Applied Behavior Analysis, 4,* 89–99.

Belfiore, P. J., & Mace, F. C. (1994). Self-help and community skills. In J. L. Matson (Ed.), *Autism in children and adults: Etiology, assessment, and intervention* (pp. 193–211). Belmont, CA: Brooks/Cole.

Bidwell, M. A., & Rehfeldt, R. A. (2004). Using video modeling to teach a domestic skill with an embedded social skill to adults with severe mental retardation. *Behavioral Interventions, 19,* 263–274.

Blew, P. A., Schwartz, I. S., & Luce, S. C. (1985). Teaching functional community skills to autistic children using nonhandicapped peer tutors. *Journal of Applied Behavior Analysis, 18,* 337–342.

Charlop-Christy, M. H., Le, L., & Freeman, K. A. (2000). A comparison of video modeling with in vivo modeling for teaching children with autism. *Journal of Autism and Developmental Disabilities, 30,* 537–552.

Christian, W. P., & Luce, S. C. (1985). Behavioral self-training for developmentally disabled individuals. *School Psychology Review, 14,* 177–181.

Cuvo, A. J. (1978). Validating task analyses of community living skills. *Vocational Evaluation and Work Adjustment Bulletin, 11,* 13–21.

Dowrick, P. W. (1991). *Practical guide to using video in the behavioral sciences.* New York: Wiley Interscience.

Duarte, A. M. M., & Baer, D. M. (1994). The effects of self-instruction on preschool children's sorting of generalized in-common tasks. *Journal of Experimental Child Psychology, 57,* 1–25.

Egel, A. L., Richman, G. S., & Koegel, R. L. (1981). Normal peer models and autistic children's learning. *Journal of Applied Behavior Analysis, 14,* 3–12.

Griffen, A. K., Wolery, M., & Schuster, J. W. (1992). Triadic instruction of chained food preparation responses: Acquisition and observational learning. *Journal of Applied Behavior Analysis, 25,* 193–204.

Hagopian, L. P., Farrell, D. A., & Amari, A. (1996). Treating total liquid refusal with backward chaining and fading. *Journal of Applied Behavior Analysis, 29,* 573–575.

Hall, L. J., McClannahan, L. E., & Krantz, P. J. (1995). Promoting independence in integrated classrooms by teaching aides to use activity schedules and decreased prompts. *Education and Training in Mental Retardation and Developmental Disabilities, 30,* 208–217.

Harris, S. L., Handleman, J. S., & Alessandri, M. (1990). Teaching youths with autism to offer assistance. *Journal of Applied Behavior Analysis, 23,* 297–305.

Horner, R. D., & Keilitz, I. (1975). Training mentally retarded adolescents to brush their teeth. *Journal of Applied Behavior Analysis, 8,* 301–309.

Jay, A. S., Grote, I., & Baer, D. (1999). Teaching participants with developmental disabilities to comply with self-instructions. *American Journal on Mental Retardation, 104,* 509–522.

Krantz, P. J., MacDuff, M. T., & McClannahan, L. E. (1993). Programming participation in family activities for children with autism: Parents' use of photographic activity schedules. *Journal of Applied Behavior Analysis, 26,* 137–138.

Lancioni, G. E., & O'Reilly, M. F. (2001). Self-management of instruction cues for occupation: Review of studies with people with severe and profound developmental disabilities. *Research in Developmental Disabilities, 22,* 41–65.

Lasater, M. W., & Brady, M. P. (1995). Effects of video self-modeling and feedback on task fluency: A home-based intervention. *Education and Treatment of Children, 18,* 389–407.

LeGrice, B., & Blampied, N. M. (1994). Training pupils with intellectual disability to operate educational technology using video prompting. *Education and Training in Mental Retardation and Developmental Disabilities, 29,* 321–330.

Lovaas, O. I. (1981). *Teaching developmentally disabled children: The me book.* Austin, TX: PRO-ED.

MacDuff, G. S., Krantz, P. J., & McClannahan, L. E. (1993). Teaching children with autism to use photographic activity schedules: Maintenance and generalization of complex response chains. *Journal of Applied Behavior Analysis, 26,* 89–97.

McClannahan, L. E., & Krantz, P. J. (1999). *Activity schedules for children with autism: Teaching independent behavior.* Bethesda, MD: Woodbine House.

Martin, J. E., Rusch, F. R., James, V. L., Decker, P. J., & Trtol, K. A. (1982). The use of picture cues to establish self-control in the preparation of complex meals by mentally retarded adults. *Applied Research in Mental Retardation, 3,* 105–119.

Matson, J. L., Benavidez, D. A., Compton, L. S., Paclawskyj, T., & Baglio, C. (1996). Behavioral treatment of autistic persons: A review of research from 1980 to present. *Research in Developmental Disabilities, 17,* 433–465.

Matson, J. L., Taras, M. E., Sevin, J. A., Love, S. R., & Fridley, D. (1990). Teaching self-help skills to autistic and mentally retarded children. *Research in Developmental Disabilities, 11,* 361–378.

Miltenberger, R. G. (2001). *Behavior modification: Principles and procedures.* Belmont, CA: Thomson Learning.

Neef, N. A., Lensbower, J., Hockersmith, I., DePalma, V., & Gray, K. (1990). In vivo versus simulation training: An interactional analysis of range and type of training exemplars. *Journal of Applied Behavior Analysis, 23,* 447–458.

Norman, J. M., Collins, B. C., & Schuster, J. W. (2001). Using an instructional package including video technology to teach self-help skills to elementary students with mental disabilities. *Journal of Special Education, 16,* 5–18.

Pierce, K. L., & Schreibman, L. (1994). Teaching daily living skills to children with autism in unsupervised settings through pictorial self-management. *Journal of Applied Behavior Analysis, 27,* 471–481.

Reeve, S. A. (2001). Effects of modeling, video modeling, prompting, and reinforcement strategies on increasing helping behavior in children with autism. *Dissertation Abstracts International: Section B: The Sciences & Engineering, 62*(3-B), 1561.

Rehfeldt, R. A. (2002). Chaining. In M. Hersen & W. Sledge (Eds.), *Encyclopedia of Psychotherapy* (pp. 365–369). New York: Academic Press.

Rehfeldt, R. A., Dahman, D., Young, A., Cherry, H., & Davis, P. (2003). Teaching a simple meal preparation skill to adults with moderate and severe mental retardation using video modeling. *Behavioral Interventions, 18,* 209–218.

Richman, G. S., Reiss, M. L., Bauman, K. E., & Bailey, J. S. (1984). Teaching menstrual care to mentally retarded women: Acquisition, generalization, and maintenance. *Journal of Applied Behavior Analysis, 17,* 441–451.

Sherer, M., Pierce, K. L., Paredes, S., Kisacky, K. L., Ingersoll, B., & Schreibman, L. (2001). Enhancing conversation skills in children with autism via video technology: Which is better, "self" or "other" as a model? *Behavior Modification, 25,* 140–158.

Skinner, B. F. (1953). *Science and human behavior.* New York: Free Press.

Smith, M. D., & Belcher, R. (1985). Teaching life skills to adults disabled by autism. *Journal of Autism and Developmental Disorders, 15,* 163–175.

Sprague, J. R., & Horner, R. H. (1984). The effects of single instance, multiple instance, and general case training on generalized vending machine use by moderately and severely handicapped students. *Journal of Applied Behavior Analysis, 17,* 273–278.

Sturmey, P. (Ed.). (2003). Special section on use of video technology. *Journal of Positive Behavior Interventions, 5,* 3–34.

Sulzer-Azaroff, B., & Mayer, G. R. (Eds.). (1991). *Behavior analysis for lasting change.* Orlando, FL: Holt, Rinehart, & Winston.

Taras, M. E., & Matese, M. (1990). Acquisition of self-help skills. In J. L. Matson (Ed.), *Handbook of behavior modification with the mentally retarded* (2nd ed., pp. 272–303). New York: Plenum.

Taubman, M., Brierley, S., Wishner, J., Baker, D., McEachin, J., & Leaf, R. F. (2001). The effectiveness of a group discrete trial instructional approach for preschoolers with developmental disabilities. *Research in Developmental Disabilities, 22,* 205–219.

Taylor, B. A., Hughes, C. E., Richard, E., Hoch, H., & Coello, A. R. (2004). Teaching teenagers with autism to seek assistance when lost. *Journal of Applied Behavior Analysis, 37,* 70–82.

Taylor, I., & O'Reilly, M. F. (1997). Toward a functional analysis of private verbal self regulation. *Journal of Applied Behavior Analysis, 30,* 43–58.

Vintere, P., Hemmes, N. S., Brown, B. L., & Poulson, C. L. (2004). Gross-motor skill acquisition by preschool dance students under self-instruction procedures. *Journal of Applied Behavior Analysis, 37,* 305–322.

Werts, M. G., Caldwell, N. K., & Wolery, M. (1996). Peer modeling of response chains: Observational learning by students with disabilities. *Journal of Applied Behavior Analysis, 29,* 53–66.

CHAPTER

Social Behavior

Dorothea C. Lerman
University of Houston, Clear Lake

Valerie M. Volkert
Louisiana State University

Linda LeBlanc
Western Michigan University

T he term *social behavior* typically refers to responses that occur within the context of reciprocal interactions, including responses required to effectively initiate, sustain, and terminate verbal and nonverbal exchanges with others. Skinner (1953) defined social behavior as "the behavior of two or more people with respect to one another or in concert with respect to a common environment" (p. 297). He pointed out that social behavior, like any other form of behavior, is subject to the same analyses, modification, and control as other forms of behavior using a natural science approach.

As discussed by Smith, McAdam, and Napolitano in Chapter 1, deficits in social behavior are a defining characteristic of autism. However, the quantity, duration, and quality of social exchanges between children with autism and adults or peers vary widely across individuals, depending on such factors as the child's age, degree of cognitive impairment, and the setting or context in which behavior is observed (Matson & Swiezy, 1994), and may vary for an individual across settings. As a group, children and adolescents with autism are less likely to respond to initiations from peers, to approach and imitate peers, to share toys with others, to offer assistance to others, and to seek or respond to adult attention (National Research Council, 2001). Even among children who readily initiate play or conversation with peers, social responses may seem atypical because they are repetitive, one-sided, or unusual in other ways. For example, subtle but important aspects of interaction, such as appropriate eye contact, facial expressions, and gestures, may be lacking. Children with autism also have difficulty interpreting or reacting appropriately to others' emotional responses and do not easily learn to take the perspective of others, an ability that is considered an important precursor for a variety of social skills such as empathy, turn taking, and sharing (Ozonoff & Miller, 1995). Thus, it is not surprising that children and adolescents with autism form fewer friendships with peers than do those without autism.

Social behavior is closely related to skills in other key developmental areas, such as communication and play. In fact, a small group of studies have identified some social responses that appear to be a determinant of success in other areas. The extent to which a child exhibits spontaneous social initiations, engages in nonverbal aspects of joint attention such as pointing at objects and making eye contact with others, and tolerates peer proximity has been found to be correlated with progress in early intervention programs and inclusive classrooms (Ingersoll, Schreibman, & Stahmer, 2001; Koegel, Koegel, & McNerney, 2001; Koegel, Koegel, Shoshan, & McNerney, 1999; Mundy, Sigman, & Kasari, 1990). Although the nature of these relationships is unclear, these types of social responses likely increase the number of opportunities that a child has to learn from others (Ingersoll et al., 2001). For example, McDonald and Hemmes (2003) found that staff began to interact more with a child who had been taught to spontaneously initiate interactions with adults.

Despite the importance of social behavior, it is frequently overlooked or relatively neglected compared to other targets in educational programs for children and adolescents with autism. In this chapter, we provide an overview of best practices for teaching social skills by summarizing current research findings on behavioral interventions for social behavior and generating detailed guidelines for practitioners and caregivers on the basis of this research.

Selecting Social Behaviors

Research has shown that children and teens with autism can learn a variety of social skills. In a vast majority of studies, multiple responses such as approaching or smiling at others, directing comments or requests to others, and sharing with others were taught as part of programs designed to increase spontaneous social initiations or to increase the quantity and duration of verbal and non-verbal social exchanges with typical peers or adults (Goldstein, Kaczmarek, Pennington, & Shafer, 1992; Kamps et al., 1992; Thiemann & Goldstein, 2001; Zanolli & Daggett, 1998). Responses intended to improve qualitative aspects of interaction, such as the appropriate use of eye contact, facial expressions, and gestures, also have been successfully taught (Buffington, Krantz, McClannahan, & Poulson, 1998; Charlop & Trasowech, 1991; Gena, Krantz, McClannahan, & Poulson, 1996; Klinger & Dawson, 1992; Taras, Matson, & Leary, 1988; Tiegerman & Primavera, 1984). Most recently, a growing number of studies have targeted complex social skills such as conversational speech, perspective taking, and joint attention (Charlop-Christy & Daneshvar, 2003; Charlop-Christy & Kelso, 2003; LeBlanc et al., 2003; Pierce & Schreibman, 1995; Stevenson, Krantz, & McClannahan, 2000).

One of the most difficult tasks facing teachers and caregivers is to select among the myriad social responses that could be incorporated into a child's educational program. A learner's current social skills should be assessed to identify appropriate targets for instruction and to obtain a baseline by which to evaluate the effects of the intervention. A number of published curricula include extensive sections on social behavior, making this task much easier (Freeman, Drake, & Tamir, 1997; Maurice, Green, & Foxx, 2001; McAfee, 2001; Weiss & Harris, 2001). Table 5.1 shows examples of beginning, intermediate, and advanced social skills that are commonly targeted. However, selecting responses for instruction should be guided by a host of considerations, including (a) the child's communication skills, (b) the norms and conditions in the child's home or school environment (e.g., number of opportunities to engage in the behavior), (c) the availability of natural reinforcers for the target response (e.g., likelihood that it will lead to reinforcing interactions with peers; Gaylord-Ross, Haring, Breen, & Pitts-Conway, 1984; Strain & Fox, 1981), and (d) the presence of behavior or reinforcers that may compete with targeted social skills (e.g., social avoidance, disruptive behavior, or perseverative speech). The social behavior of typically developing peers is an important benchmark for determining which skills to select and the terminal level of performance (e.g., duration of eye contact, number of social initiations; Shabani et al., 2002; Strain, 1983). An emphasis should be placed on social responses that are likely to be relevant across multiple social contexts (e.g., proximity or eye contact versus specific statements). Initiating social interactions and responding to the initiations of others are separate skills that must be taught directly (Oke & Schriebman, 1990).

Important prerequisite skills for some types of social behavior are readily evident. For example, shaping interactions with adults rather than with peers is a logical place to start if a child is not yet attending to or imitating adults. It may be very difficult to teach more advanced social skills such as offering assistance

TABLE 5.1

Examples of Beginning, Intermediate, and Advanced Social Skills
Commonly Targeted in Educational Programs

1. Beginning

- Establishes eye contact (Dawson & Galpert, 1990; Harris, Handleman, & Fong, 1987; Klinger & Dawson, 1992; Koegel & Frea, 1993)
- Initiates greetings (Gaylord-Ross, Haring, Breen, & Pitts-Conway, 1984; Matson, Sevin, Box, Francis, & Sevin, 1993)
- Follows instructions to play with peer (McGrath, Bosch, Sullivan, & Fuqua, 2003)
- Requests preferred items (Charlop & Trasowech, 1991; Wert & Neisworth, 2003)
- Follows eye gaze and point of another with respect to a specific object (Whalen & Schreibman, 2003)
- Requests information (Taylor & Harris, 1995)
- Reciprocates comments about objects (Thiemann & Goldstein, 2001)
- Takes turns or shares with others (McGrath et al., 2003; Oke & Schreibman, 1990)

2. Intermediate

- Requests attention or acknowledgment of adults or peers (Krantz & McClannahan, 1998; Taylor & Levin, 1998; Thiemann & Goldstein, 2001; Zanolli & Daggett, 1998)
- Initiates bids for joint attention (Whalen & Schreibman, 2003)
- Asks questions during reciprocal interactions (Charlop-Christy & Kelso, 2003; Stevenson, Krantz, & McClannahan, 2000)
- Offers assistance to adult or peer (Harris, Handleman, & Alessandri, 1990)
- Invites adult or peer to join play activity (Gaylord-Ross et al., 1984; Nikopoulos & Keenan, 2004; Shabani et al., 2002)
- Responds to peer's requests (Pierce & Schreibman, 1997)
- Comments about play activities (Krantz & McClannahan, 1993; Thiemann & Goldstein, 2001)

3. Advanced

- Uses appropriate gestures (Buffington, 1998; Thiemann & Goldstein, 2001)
- Uses statements and gestures to express emotion (Gena, Krantz, McClannahan, & Poulson, 1996)
- Responds correctly to questions about the perspective of others (Charlop-Christy & Daneshvar, 2003; LeBlanc et al., 2003)
- Asks questions to gain information (Williams, Donley, & Keller, 2000)
- Reciprocates social information (Charlop-Christy & Kelso, 2003)
- Recognizes and labels emotions (Solomon, Goodlin-Jones, & Anders, 2004; Silver & Oakes, 2001)
- Demonstrates conversational skills (e.g., topic-based turn-taking, appropriate tone of voice, and volume control; Koegel & Frea, 1993)
- Resolves conflicts (Solomon et al., 2004)
- Demonstrates sportsmanship skills (Keeling, Myles, Gagnon, & Simpson, 2003)

to peers until a child has learned how to approach peers. On the other hand, few empirical guidelines are available to indicate when it might be best to teach such social skills as perspective taking, joint attention, and the appropriate use of facial expressions or gestures. As such, a child's individual program must be guided by a combination of logic, published curricula, and consideration of typical developmental sequences.

For many children, responses that lead to powerful reinforcers from others, such as requesting desired objects, should be an early priority to increase the reinforcing value of social interactions (Koegel, Dyer, & Bell, 1987). It also may be advantageous to prioritize and target problem behavior that is incompatible with effective social interaction, such as social avoidance, aggression, or disruption, and skills that may produce collateral increases in other social behavior, such as self-initiations, peer imitation, and gestures (Garfinkle & Schwartz, 2002; Koegel & Frea, 1993; Oke & Schreibman, 1990). Improving social interactions with peers rather than with adults will be the long-term goal in most cases, because peer relations are especially problematic for people with autism (Koegel, Koegel, Frea, & Fredeen, 2001). Finally, targeted social responses should complement skills taught in the closely related areas of communication and play. Guidelines for selecting social skills are summarized in the practitioner recommendations at the end of this chapter.

Interventions for Social Behavior

Research on social behavior has identified a variety of effective instructional strategies for children and adolescents with autism. Further research is needed, however, to determine how to best match or tailor these strategies to individual children and types of social behavior. Overall, the current literature suggests that similar procedures can be used to teach a variety of different social responses. Nonetheless, certain strategies may seem better suited to teaching certain social skills than others.

Commonly used interventions for social behavior can be roughly divided into two types: adult-mediated interventions implemented by a teacher or caregiver and peer-mediated interventions implemented by peers who have been taught how to prompt and reinforce social interactions in children with autism. If peer interaction is targeted for change, peer-mediated interventions are appealing for a number of reasons. In particular, social skills training may be more effective when peers receive some training as well (Odom & Strain, 1986). Adult-delivered prompts and reinforcement also have been found to disrupt ongoing social exchanges between children and their peers, which might impede efforts to increase the duration and quality of reciprocal interactions (Strain & Kohler, 1999).

Nonetheless, some studies indicate that peer training alone may not be adequate to increase social initiations in children with autism, especially those who have few social skills or engage in high levels of problem behavior (Oke & Schreibman, 1990; Zanolli, Daggett, & Adams, 1996). Peer training also is relatively time consuming and may not be practical if peers are unavailable to participate. Finally, as discussed in more detail below, direct adult intervention may be critical for ensuring that social skills taught by peers will generalize to other settings and peers and maintain over the long run. In short, the ideal program for social behavior contains elements of both adult- and peer-mediated interventions. However, for organizational purposes, these interventions will be discussed in separate sections on the following pages.

Adult-Mediated Strategies

Adult-mediated interventions have a number of effective antecedents and consequences for social behavior in children and adolescents with autism. Commonly, a therapist, teacher, or parent will prompt and reinforce certain types of social behavior after arranging the context in which the target response(s) should occur (e.g., interactive play, conversational exchange). Social behavior may be directed toward the therapist, another adult, or a peer during training. Even when peer interactions are targeted, the adult may initially serve as the recipient of interaction, for example, the child will role-play with the adult, if the child does not have prerequisites for learning to interact with peers (Coe, Matson, Fee, Manikam, & Linarello, 1990) or if peers are not readily available to participate in training. However, peers are typically included at some point in the training to ensure that social behavior will generalize from the adult to peers.

Antecedents for Social Behavior

To enhance learning, social skills training is often conducted during relatively structured situations, yet within the context of naturalistic activities such as interactive play with peers (Sarokoff, Taylor, & Poulson, 2001; Zanolli, Daggett, & Adams, 1996) or regularly scheduled tasks (Krantz & McClannahan, 1998). Typically, the adult will establish the relevant antecedent for the social behavior, perhaps asking the child a question or sitting across from the child with a preferred toy, and provide some type of prompt to increase the likelihood of the behavior. Prompts are then gradually faded to transfer control from the prompt to the natural antecedent. Generalization of the social response from the controlled teaching situation to the natural environment also is evaluated, particularly if training is conducted in a location that is separate from the home, school, or community setting (Gena et al., 1996; Koegel, Koegel, Hurley, & Frea, 1992).

Verbal, gestural, model, and physical prompts are highly effective for teaching a variety of social skills. For example, to teach a child to greet an adult who enters the room, a verbal model (e.g., adult says "hello") may be provided if the child does not say "hello" within 2 s after the adult's entrance. The interval between the adult's entrance and the prompt is lengthened gradually (e.g., increased by 2 s every two consecutive sessions) until the child begins to respond before the model is provided (Charlop, Schreibman, & Thibodeau, 1985; Ingenmey & Van Houten, 1991; Matson, Sevin, Box, Francis, & Sevin, 1993; Taylor & Harris, 1995).

More recently, other types of prompts have been developed to teach social skills. These prompts require less adult interference while the child or adolescent is interacting with others and may be easier to fade than response prompts. For example, tactile prompts delivered via a vibrating device worn by the child can be established as an antecedent for verbal initiations in children with autism (Shabani et al., 2002; Taylor & Levin, 1998). During initial teaching sessions, participants were verbally prompted to direct social initiations toward the therapist when the device vibrated. Verbal prompts were faded until the vibration alone occasioned the behavior. After placement of the device was faded from the child's hand to the child's pocket, the vibration was effective in prompting the child to direct verbal initiations toward peers or adults during free-play activities. However, future research will need to examine strategies to transfer control from the tactile prompt to the natural antecedent.

Textual prompts in the form of scripts or cue cards also have been increasingly employed to teach verbal interactions between children with autism and adults or peers (Charlop-Christy & Kelso, 2003; Krantz & McClannahan, 1993, 1998; Sarokoff et al., 2001; Thiemann & Goldstein, 2001). A script has consisted of just one or two words such as "look" or "watch me" printed on a card that was placed in a child's daily activity schedule to prompt initiations (Krantz & McClannahan, 1998), as well as a more extensive series of six or seven conversational statements to prompt responses during reciprocal interactions (Krantz & McClannahan, 1993). Training with scripts increased both scripted and unscripted interactions. For instance, Charlop-Christy and Kelso (2003) taught children to engage in seven-line conversations about a variety of topics. During training, the child sat across from the therapist. The therapist began the conversation by asking a question such as, "What did you do today?" and handing the child a cue card with the answer to the question and a reciprocal question (e.g., "I went to school. What did you do today?"). The child was verbally instructed to read the script. In turn, the therapist responded to the prompted question with an answer and another question ("I went to school, too.

What did you do at school?"), and training continued in this manner for the remainder of the scripted exchange. Acquisition of the scripted conversations maintained when the cue cards were withdrawn, and the results generalized across settings, people, and new conversational topics. A more systematic approach for fading textual prompts has been demonstrated in other studies. For example, Krantz and McClannahan (1998) faded the scripts and cue cards by cutting away portions of the cards before withdrawing them completely, and Krantz and McClannahan (1993) gradually eliminated portions of the scripted text from the cards until nothing but single quotation marks remained. Finally, Sarokoff et al. (2001) modified the script procedure by embedding stimuli related to the topics of conversational exchanges, such as a candy package, within the textual prompts (i.e., statements about the candy). They then faded the textual scripts as described by Krantz and McClannahan (1993) until only the stimuli remained.

Textual prompts are particularly useful because they can be available throughout an activity (Thiemann & Goldstein, 2001), do not necessarily depend on the behavior of someone else, and can be transported across different locations and conversational partners (Krantz & McClannahan, 1993). However, scripts may be most effective for children whose behavior is especially sensitive to pictorial or written prompts or children who already have a history of receiving reinforcement for using written activity schedules (Krantz & McClannahan, 1993). Interestingly, in one study, audiotaped scripts successfully increased social interactions among children who could not read (Stevenson et al., 2000).

Video modeling alone and in combination with other prompts such as verbal instruction has been used to teach verbal and nonverbal social initiations, perspective-taking, and play in children with autism (Charlop-Christy & Daneshvar, 2003; Charlop & Milstein, 1989; LeBlanc et al., 2003; Nikopoulos & Keenan, 2004; Oke & Schreibman, 1990). In most studies, the child was shown videotaped segments depicting an adult or peer engaging in appropriate social behavior and then was given the opportunity to exhibit the modeled response(s) immediately after viewing the video. Training continued in this manner until the participant met a prespecified acquisition criterion during the postviewing sessions. In other studies, children observed and evaluated their own social behavior (Oke & Schreibman, 1990; Wert & Neisworth, 2003) or social exchanges of peers (Thiemann & Goldstein, 2001). At least one study indicated that video modeling may be especially useful for promoting maintenance and generalization of social behavior (Charlop-Christy, Le, & Freeman, 2000).

Teaching children to self-monitor may effectively increase a variety of social responses, including appropriate facial expressions, voice volume, social initiations, and responses to others' initiations (Koegel et al., 1992; Koegel & Frea, 1993; Shearer, Kohler, Buchan, & McCullough, 1996; Strain, Kohler, Storey, &

Danko, 1994). For example, children were first taught to discriminate between correct and incorrect social responses and then to self-monitor by clicking a wrist counter or placing a mark on a data sheet each time they engaged in the behavior (Koegel et al., 1992; Koegel & Frea, 1993).

Two other antecedent strategies that may reduce the frequency of adult-delivered prompts during naturally occurring situations are behavioral momentum (Davis, Brady, Hamilton, McEvoy, & Williams, 1994) and priming (Zanolli & Daggett, 1998; Zanolli et al., 1996). Behavioral momentum procedures, or "high-probability instructional sequences," increase the likelihood that a child will respond when instructed to interact with others. Typically, the instructor presents two or three requests associated with a high probability of compliance (e.g., "Pick up the toy") immediately before a request to engage with a peer (e.g., "Roll the toy to [peer]"). In contrast, priming is conducted prior to an activity in which unprompted targeted responses are expected to occur. Zanolli et al. (1996) used priming sessions that consisted of 10 to 14 trials during which they prompted the child to initiate social interactions toward a peer, who had been taught to deliver social and tangible reinforcers contingent on each initiation. Participants interacted more with peers during play activities that immediately followed these priming sessions. Subsequently, Zanolli and Dagget (1998) found that the rate of reinforcement for interactions during the priming sessions was positively related to the rate of spontaneous initiations during the activity sessions.

Despite the voluminous research on antecedents for social behavior, practitioners have few empirical guidelines for determining which instructional technique to select, such as live versus video modeling or tactile versus textual prompts, when developing programs for social skills training. Selections could be made on the basis of a number of factors. Children often have a previous history of responding to certain prompts more readily than others or have already shown success with certain instructional strategies. The clinician should take advantage of any known history of effective prompts or briefly assess the effectiveness of different types of prompts with a simple behavior to determine which would be promising for use with more complex behavior. Textual prompts can be used only with children who have good sight-reading skills. Video modeling may be particularly effective for children with poor attending skills who demonstrate a strong preference for television viewing. In addition, certain antecedents seem uniquely suited for teaching specific types of social skills (e.g., video-taped modeling for perspective taking and conversational scripts for reciprocal interactions). Depending on the child's skill level and the social context, approaches that require less adult intervention during ongoing social exchanges also may be preferable (e.g., priming, self-monitoring, tactile prompts). Complex or multiple social skills may be easier to teach via a combination of antecedent strategies (Matson et al., 1993; Thiemann & Goldstein, 2001) For example, Thiemann and Goldstein (2001) employed social stories, written text cues, and video feedback to teach social communication to five children with autism.

A plan for eliminating artificial prompts and programming for generalization should be incorporated from the beginning of social skills interventions (Stokes & Baer, 1977; Stokes & Osnes, 1989). Although systematic fading strategies have been demonstrated in some studies, further research is needed. Transfer of stimulus control from prompts to natural antecedents for social interaction may be easier to arrange when training is conducted in naturalistic settings, such as in the home or classroom (McGee et al., 1992). However, for some children, it may be difficult or impractical to conduct training in naturalistic contexts. One possible solution is to initially modify the setting to minimize distractions and then slowly reintroduce stimuli that are likely to be present in the natural environment (e.g., Zanolli et al., 1996). For example, training could be conducted in the child's classroom when the majority of children are out of the room. After the child has acquired the social response, the number of children who are present in the social situation should be gradually increased over time. To further promote generalization, social skills training should be conducted with multiple interactive partners and across multiple settings and situations that closely resemble those present in the child's everyday life. It also may be helpful to teach children and adolescents multiple variations of each targeted social response, such as different ways to offer assistance or to solicit attention, and how to record and evaluate their own social behavior (see Stokes & Baer, 1977; Stokes & Osnes, 1989, for further discussion). Teaching the child responses that are likely to be reinforced by others, such as sharing toys with peers or smiling at and greeting adults, also may ensure that social behavior generalizes and maintains. Finally, generalization may be more likely to occur when tests for generalization, often called "probe sessions," during which all instructional components are removed, are interspersed frequently with training sessions (Buffington et al., 1998). Strategies to promote generalization are summarized in Table 5.2, along with illustrative examples of each technique.

Consequences for Social Behavior

The naturalistic consequences of social interaction such as attention and conversation are not potent enough to maintain a social repertoire in many children and adolescents with autism. This may be especially true if verbal or physical contact or close proximity function as conditioned or unconditioned aversive stimuli for the individual. For these reasons, adults or peers often deliver strong tangible reinforcers such as tokens and food contingent on appropriate social behavior as part of social skills interventions. The resulting increase in social

TABLE 5.2
Strategies to Promote Generalization with Illustrative Examples

Strategy	Example
1. Use multiple stimulus and response exemplars.	When teaching a child to respond to a social greeting, include multiple settings, greeters, types of greetings, and ways to respond to the greeter.
2. Incorporate common salient physical and social stimuli.	When teaching a child to offer assistance, include materials, situations, and people from the child's natural environment.
3. Draw upon natural contingencies.	Teach social initiations that are likely to be reinforced by others (e.g., sharing toys with peers and smiling at or greeting others).
4. Use indiscriminable stimulus conditions.	When teaching a child to request preferred items, prompt and reinforce the response across a variety of naturally occurring activities (e.g., meals, play).
5. Use indiscriminable contingencies.	Gradually thin the schedule of reinforcement after the response is initially acquired.
6. Incorporate mediators of generalization.	Teach a child to use and transport self-recording materials or activity schedules that include prompts for social responses.
7. Reinforce instances of generalization.	Teach siblings and other caregivers to reinforce the social response when it occurs in the generalization setting or context.

Note. Adapted from "An Implicit Technology of Generalization," by T. F. Stokes and D. M. Baer, 1997, *Journal of Applied Behavior Analysis, 10,* pp. 349–367, and "An Operant Pursuit of Generalization," by T. F. Stokes and P. G. Osne, 1989, *Behavior Therapy, 20,* pp. 337–355.

behavior ensures that responding will contact the natural consequences of interaction, which may acquire reinforcing properties or at least diminished aversive properties due to the pairing of these natural consequences with tangible reinforcers.

A number of other strategies have been employed to increase the reinforcing value of social interactions, although the precise contribution of these components to the effectiveness of social skills training has not been directly evaluated. For example, social exchanges such as conversing and sharing frequently have been taught within the context of the child's preferred activities and topics. Baker, Koegel, and Koegel (1998) prompted children and their peers to play interactive games that incorporated obsessive themes of the children with autism. Social interactions of the children with autism increased during the interactive play, maintained in the absence of the teacher, and generalized to other games without those themes. The authors concluded that the use of highly preferred themes increased the children's motivation to engage in and maintain social interactions with peers.

In other studies, access to or consumption of preferred stimuli was arranged to occur as a natural consequence of social exchanges. This strategy is an integral component of naturalistic teaching techniques such as incidental teaching and pivotal response training (McGee, Almeida, Sulzer-Azaroff, & Feldman, 1992; Pierce & Schreibman, 1995). In one commonly used approach, the instructor teaches the child to request or ask questions about objects that are known to be reinforcing to the child (McGee et al., 1992; Williams, Donley, & Keller, 2000). Similarly Sarokoff et al. (2001) taught scripted conversational exchanges to children with autism, which included statements about preferred items such as food that was consumed as part of the script (e.g., the children were taught to say, "Let's eat this now"). Gaylord-Ross et al. (1984) described a similar approach in which they taught children with autism to initiate, maintain, and terminate interactions with peers. However, they selected objects that appealed to typically developing peers (e.g., video games, Walkman) for the scripted exchanges to increase the likelihood that untrained peers would respond to the participants' initiations. Programs for social behavior have been tailored to a child's interests in other ways by using textual prompts with children who showed a preference for letters and words (Charlop-Christy & Kelso, 2003) and using video modeling for children who reportedly enjoyed watching videos (Charlop-Christy et al., 2000).

Finally, some authors have suggested that pairing physical contact or proximity with highly preferred activities and conversations may reduce the aversive properties of peer interaction (Koegel et al., 1987; McEvoy et al., 1988). McEvoy et al. (1988), for example, prompted participants to physically interact with peers by hugging them and patting them on the back while engaging in highly preferred games, songs, and dances as part of group "affection activities." This intervention was associated with an increase in the frequency and duration of spontaneous interactions between the children and peers. Koegel et al. (1987) measured the frequency of social avoidance behavior (e.g., moving away from an adult, closing eyes) when children were prompted to play or converse with an adult. Fewer avoidance responses occurred when child-preferred activities were incorporated into the interactions than when activities were chosen by the adult. The authors hypothesized that the inclusion of child-preferred activities increased the reinforcing value and/or reduced the aversive properties of the interactions.

Tactics to increase the reinforcing value of the natural consequences of social interaction also should be incorporated into educational programs. A variety of highly preferred tangible reinforcers should be identified using systematic preference assessments (Fisher et al., 1992; Pace, Ivancic, Edwards, Iwata, & Page, 1985) and embedded within social skills training as described above (see Chapter 2 for more on preference assessments). Preference for these items should be reassessed on a frequent basis—at least weekly for some clients and daily for others—and reinforcers should be varied to prevent rapid satiation. Identifying and incorporating items that are highly preferred by typically developing peers may improve peer receptiveness to social interactions with the child with autism and increase the likelihood of long-term maintenance (Gaylord-Ross et al., 1984). Whenever possible, access to potent reinforcers should be arranged to occur as a direct consequence of social initiations such as requesting highly preferred items. Frequent opportunities to prompt and reinforce social interactions with adults and peers should be scheduled to occur throughout the child's day. As responding increases and contacts the natural consequences of social interaction, arbitrary reinforcers for correct social behavior should be gradually faded by systematically thinning the reinforcement schedule or delaying reinforcer delivery when appropriate. Guidelines for designing and implementing adult-mediated interventions are summarized in the practitioner recommendations at the end of this chapter.

Peer-Mediated Strategies

In peer-mediated intervention, typically developing peers are taught to prompt and reinforce social interactions with children with autism. It is the most prevalent approach to social skills training in the literature (McConnell, 2002). Peer-mediated strategies offer a number of benefits whether implemented alone or combined with adult intervention. In fact, peers should receive some type of training whenever possible because they generally fail to respond to the social initiations of children and adolescents with autism in a manner that will maintain the behavior (Pierce & Schreibman, 1995). Peer training also may ensure that peers become discriminative stimuli for interactions, increasing the likelihood of long-term maintenance and generalization (Odom, Chandler, Ostrosky, McConnell, & Reaney, 1992). Finally, as previously noted, the involvement of typically developing peers may reduce the necessity for adult-delivered prompts and reinforcement, which can disrupt ongoing social exchanges between children.

The voluminous research in this area indicates that classmates and siblings can learn effective strategies for occasioning and reinforcing the social initiations and reciprocal responses of children with autism (Coe, Matson, Craigie, & Gossen, 1991; Goldstein et al., 1992; Lee & Odom, 1996; McGee et al., 1992; Pierce & Schreibman, 1997; Shafer, Egel, & Neef, 1984; Strain & Danko,

1995; Strain, Kerr, & Ragland, 1979). The efficacy of this approach has been demonstrated for children with a variety of skill levels and across a broad range of social responses. Nevertheless, further research is needed on ways to ensure that the social behavior of both the typically developing peer and the child with autism will generalize to other settings, contexts, and people, as well as maintain over the long run.

Antecedents for Peer Social Behavior

Peer behavior can greatly influence both the quality and quantity of reciprocal interactions exhibited by children with autism (Kohler, Strain, & Shearer, 1992). Peers have been taught to prompt social responses by organizing play, sharing, obtaining the child's attention, commenting on activities and objects, offering assistance to the child, and asking the child to share, among other things (Goldstein et al., 1992; Odom et al., 1992). Peers also have been taught to implement specific instructional techniques that have been shown to be effective with children with autism, such as incidental teaching, pivotal response training, and discrete trial instruction (Blew, Schwartz, & Luce, 1985; McGee et al., 1992; Pierce & Schreibman, 1997).

In most studies, the peer initially participated in instructional sessions with an adult, who taught the selected skills using verbal instruction, modeling, and role play. While role-playing as the child with autism, the adult provided multiple opportunities for the peer to learn how to occasion and respond to the child's behavior and how to persist if the child failed to reciprocate peer social initiations (Oke & Schreibman, 1990; Sainato, Goldstein, & Strain, 1992). In other studies, teaching occurred with peers initially interacting with typically developing peers (Goldstein et al., 1992) or with children with autism (McGee et al., 1992; Shafer et al., 1984). Instruction continued for a predetermined number of sessions or until the peer's behavior met a training criterion (Goldstein et al., 1992; Hoyson, Jamieson, & Strain, 1984; McGee et al., 1992; McGrath, Bosch, Sullivan, & Fuqua, 2003; Odom et al., 1992). The experimenters typically assessed peer social behavior within the context of group play activities either concurrently with or immediately following initial training with the adult. One or more trained peers and a single child with autism generally participated in these activities, during which the adult prompted the peer to interact with the target child. As described in the next section, they delivered some type of reinforcer to the peer for exhibiting the correct social responses. For example, in Sainato et al. (1992), teachers provided a verbal prompt if no interactions had occurred for more than 20 s. Zanolli et al. (1996) used a constant time-delay procedure to increase peers' responses to social initiations. If the child with autism directed an initiation to the peer and the peer did not respond to this initiation within 1 s, the teacher delivered a verbal prompt, "[Name] talked to you, what do you do?" If the peer did not respond within 1 s of the first prompt, the teacher delivered another verbal prompt: "Say something, and give him a treat."

Other antecedents have been used to occasion the behavior of peers during reciprocal interactions with children and teens with autism. For example, prior to each interaction session, Oke and Schreibman (1990) conducted a 5-min review with the peer, during which the relevant skills were described and the peer answered questions about the interactions (e.g., "How are you going to get [Name] to play with you?"). Sainato et al. (1992) asked peers to review the targeted social responses by flipping through a self-evaluation book prior to play activities. In addition, prior to each session, the teacher introduced the play activity, presented a few ideas on how to play, and pointed to posters displayed in the play area that illustrated the strategies taught to the peers. A variety of other prompts such as gestures, pictures, and checklists also have been combined with verbal prompts to increase peer social behavior (Goldstein et al., 1992; McGee et al., 1992; Thiemann & Goldstein, 2001).

Several studies have evaluated strategies to reduce the frequency of adult-delivered prompts, but attempts to completely eliminate them while maintaining peer behavior often have failed. Prompts may be successfully faded by carefully arranging for the transfer of control from these prompts to stimuli in the natural environment (McGee et al., 1992; Odom et al., 1992). For example, Odom et al. (1992) faded teacher prompts by combining verbal prompts with a visual feedback system and then gradually faded both instructional components. Initially, the teacher delivered verbal prompts whenever social interactions had not occurred for 30 s and filled in a happy face on a clipboard each time the peer initiated an interaction. Verbal prompts were faded first by changing the content of the statements delivered to the peers from specific instructions to general reminders about the targeted social behaviors and by reducing the frequency of the prompts. The teacher gradually faded the visual feedback by making the happy faces visible to the peers only at the end of the session and then asking the peers to simply visualize the happy faces "in their heads" while she provided more general feedback about their performance. Peer initiations maintained during the play activities after the prompts and feedback were completely withdrawn. Other strategies may be useful when attempting to reduce or eliminate adult-delivered prompts. For example, peers have been taught to prompt each other to interact with children with autism (Kohler et al., 1995; Kohler, Strain, Maretsky, & DeCesare, 1990).

Consequences for Peer Social Behavior

Reciprocal interactions among children with autism and their typically developing peers are more likely to persist when the interactions are reinforcing for all of the children. Thus, peers are often taught to reinforce the social responses of children with autism using the same strategies used by adults (i.e., delivering potent tangible reinforcers for appropriate requests and arranging for social interactions to occur within the context of preferred activities). In turn, adults typically reinforce the correct social behavior of peers during and after initial peer training to increase and maintain their social interactions. For example, in Oke and Schreibman (1990), peers earned a star for each successful initiation and for each 30-s interval during which social interaction continued uninterrupted. The experimenter indicated when each star was earned using a light tap on the one-way window of the session room, and the peers could exchange the stars for preferred items at the end of each session. Sainato et al. (1992) taught peers to evaluate whether each of four targeted social skills strategies had successfully occasioned a social response from the child with autism by marking a "yes" or a "no" next to four small pictures that illustrated each strategy. Peers self-evaluated their performance after each play session and then compared their ratings to those collected by the experimenter. Each strategy on the experimenter's rating sheet was marked with a star if the peer and experimenter agreed that the strategy had been implemented successfully. The peer was allowed to choose a small tangible reward for receiving at least three of the possible four stars.

Adult-delivered feedback during or immediately following play activities also has been used as a consequence for peer social behavior (Odom et al., 1992; Thiemann & Goldstein, 2001). Performance feedback alone may have reinforcing properties, discriminative functions, or a combination of both. For example, in Odom et al. (1992), the teacher filled in a happy face on a clipboard each time the peer initiated an interaction and showed the peer the number of happy faces earned at the end of each play session. Although the authors noted that reinforcement was not delivered for peer performance, it is possible that the happy faces also functioned as conditioned reinforcers for the peers. Thiemann and Goldstein (2001) used videotapes to provide feedback about peer social initiations immediately following 10-min play activities. The experimenter paused the videotape after correct peer initiations, and the peer and target child evaluated the performance by circling a "yes" or "no" next to written descriptions of the correct social responses. The peer and child also evaluated videotaped segments of the child's behavior, which, if incorrect, set the occasion for further instruction via modeling and discussion. The checks were exchanged for tickets that could be exchanged for a variety of rewards.

Peer training is an important and effective component of social skills programs for children and teens with autism. Research is only beginning to identify factors that may directly influence the effectiveness of peer-mediated interventions for the child with autism (see Strain & Kohler, 1999, for further discus-

sion). However, two variables that are likely to be important are the types of social behavior taught to the peers and the fidelity with which the peers prompt
and reinforce social initiations and responses of the child with autism. Thus, it
may be particularly useful to teach peers how to persist if a social initiation fails
to be reciprocated or if social interaction occasions inappropriate behavior. At
least one study indicated that inappropriate behavior with peers may decrease if
the child with autism also receives some adult-directed social skills training
(Oke & Schreibman, 1990). When a child's problem behavior is particularly severe, clinicians should implement an intervention to decrease the behavior prior
to or simultaneously with the peer-mediated social behavior program (Strain &
Kohler, 1999). (See Smith, Vollmer, and St. Peter Pipkin, Chapter 7, this volume, for a review.) Peers also should be taught to deliver potent tangible reinforcers for appropriate social responses during reciprocal interactions. Finally,
children who enjoy interacting with others, have good attending skills, and are
socially competent may be more successful as peer trainers than children without these characteristics (see Taylor, 2001, for further discussion).

Peer-mediated programs are relatively labor intensive and may require up
to several months of training when peers are taught complex interventions for
social behavior such as pivotal response training (Pierce & Schreibman, 1997).
Nevertheless, some type of peer training should be incorporated into social
skills programs for children and adolescents with autism. Group peer-training
procedures, which have been shown to be effective, may increase the feasibility
of peer-mediated interventions (Goldstein et al., 1992; Haring & Breen, 1992;
Odom et al., 1992; Shafer et al., 1984). Providing some adult-directed training
to the child with autism in addition to peers also may enhance the efficacy and
practicality of the peer-training approach.

Although the literature is replete with examples of successful training models, few strategies have been identified for ensuring that peer behavior will maintain and generalize across children, settings, and other contexts in the absence
of adult prompts and reinforcement. More important, social behavior of the
child with autism has rarely been shown to generalize spontaneously across untrained typically developing peers. Generalization may be more likely to occur if
(a) the child is exposed to multiple trained peers (Pierce & Schriebman, 1997);
(b) training is conducted across multiple settings, contexts, and stimuli, such as
different conversational topics or toys; (c) the child with autism receives some
training from an adult in addition to peers (Oke & Schreibman, 1990); and
(d) peers are taught to fade their use of prompts and reinforcement when interacting with the child with autism. Guidelines for designing and implementing
peer-mediated interventions are summarized in the practitioner recommendations at the end of this chapter.

Conclusion

Procedures based on the principles of applied behavior analysis have been shown to be highly effective for teaching a wide range of social responses to children and adolescents with autism, including such complex social behavior as perspective taking and joint attention. The growing literature in this area has identified a number of effective approaches for occasioning and reinforcing the social initiations and reciprocal responses of children with autism. Research also has begun to identify strategies to promote the long-term maintenance and generalization of these skills, although further work is needed. Additional research also is needed to address the problem of defining and teaching more advanced interpersonal behavior such as resolving conflicts, expressing forgiveness, and showing empathy toward others. Nonetheless, on the basis of current research, relatively comprehensive social skills curricula and guidelines for best practices are now available to assist practitioners and caregivers (Freeman et al., 1997; McAfee, 2001; Taylor, 2001; Weiss & Harris, 2001).

 ## PRACTITIONER RECOMMENDATIONS

SELECTING TARGETS

1. Assess the child's current social repertoire and consider important prerequisites for the selected targets.
2. Consider the child's communication skills, the norms and conditions in the child's natural environment, and the availability of natural reinforcers for the response.
3. Evaluate behavior of peers to obtain benchmarks for the terminal forms and levels of the social responses.
4. Target problem responses that compete with problem social behavior (e.g., aggression). Target responses should
    a. result in powerful reinforcers from others (e.g., requesting desired objects) and
    b. be relevant across multiple social contexts (e.g., using gestures).
5. Teach the child how to initiate interactions with others as well as how to respond appropriately to others' initiations.
6. Target interactions with peers whenever possible.
7. Teach social responses that complement current targets in the areas of communication and play.

DEVELOPING AND IMPLEMENTING ADULT-MEDIATED INTERVENTIONS

1. Use the least intrusive prompts that are effective, as indicated by past performance on educational programs and the results of brief pretreatment assessments.
2. Consider the child's current behavioral repertoire and the targeted social response when selecting prompts (e.g., textual prompts for good readers; videotaped modeling for perspective taking).
3. Develop a plan for fading prompts quickly and systematically.
4. Program for generalization from the outset of treatment (see Table 5.2).
5. Pair the natural consequences of social interaction with tangible and activity reinforcers that are highly preferred by the child and peers.
6. Frequently reassess preference for tangible and activity reinforcers, and vary reinforcers to prevent satiation.
7. Arrange for potent reinforcers to be delivered as a direct consequence of social interaction (e.g., requesting or sharing highly preferred items).
8. Schedule opportunities to prompt and reinforce social interactions throughout the child's day.
9. Gradually fade arbitrary reinforcers as social behavior increases and contacts natural reinforcing consequences.

DEVELOPING AND IMPLEMENTING PEER-MEDIATED INTERVENTIONS

1. Include peer training whenever possible.
2. Select socially competent peers who enjoy interacting with others and have good attending skills.
3. Teach peers responses that have been shown to occasion the social behavior of children with autism (e.g., organizing play, sharing).
4. Using verbal instruction, modeling, and role play, provide multiple opportunities for peers to learn how to prompt and reinforce the child's behavior and how to persist if a social initiation fails to be reciprocated by the child.
5. Prompt and reinforce the correct social behavior of peers during and after initial peer training to increase and maintain their social interactions.
6. Systematically fade prompts delivered to peers.
7. Program for generalization from the outset of treatment (see Table 5.2).
8. Teach peers how to respond if social interaction occasions inappropriate behavior from the child. If necessary, directly target severe problem behavior.
9. Provide some adult-directed training to the child with autism.

References

Baker, M. J., Koegel, R. L., & Koegel, L. K. (1998). Increasing the social behavior of young children with autism using their obsessive behaviors. *Journal of the Association for Persons with Severe Handicaps, 23,* 300–308.

Blew, S. H., Schwartz, L. S., & Luce, S. C. (1985). Teaching functional community skills to autistic children using non-handicapped peer tutors. *Journal of Applied Behavior Analysis, 18,* 337–342.

Buffington, D. M., Krantz, P. J., McClannahan, L. E., & Poulson, C. L. (1998). Procedures for teaching appropriate gestural communication skills to children with autism. *Journal of Autism and Developmental Disorders, 28,* 535–545.

Charlop, M. H., & Milstein, J. P. (1989). Teaching autistic children conversational speech using video modeling. *Journal of Applied Behavior Analysis, 22,* 275–285.

Charlop, M. H., Schreibman, L., & Thibodeau, M. G. (1985). Increasing spontaneous verbal responding in autistic children using a time delay procedure. *Journal of Applied Behavior Analysis, 18,* 155–166.

Charlop, M. H., & Trasowech, J. E. (1991). Increasing autistic children's daily spontaneous speech. *Journal of Applied Behavior Analysis, 24,* 747–761.

Charlop-Christy, M. H., & Daneshvar, S. (2003). Using video modeling to teach perspective taking to children with autism. *Journal of Positive Behavior Interventions, 5,* 12–21.

Charlop-Christy, M. H., & Kelso, S. E. (2003). Teaching children with autism conversational speech using a cue card/written script program. *Education and Treatment of Children, 26,* 108–127.

Charlop-Christy, M. H., Le, L., & Freeman, K. (2000). A comparison of video modeling with in vivo modeling for teaching children with autism. *Journal of Autism and Developmental Disorders, 30,* 537–552.

Coe, D. A., Matson, J. L., Craigie, C. L., & Gossen, M. A. (1991). Play skills of autistic children: Assessment and instruction. *Child & Family Behavior Therapy, 13,* 13–40.

Coe, D. A., Matson, J. L., Fee, V., Manikam, R., & Linarello, C. (1990). Training nonverbal and verbal play skills to mentally retarded and autistic children. *Journal of Autism and Developmental Disorders, 20,* 177–187.

Davis, C. A., Brady, M. P., Hamilton, R., McEvoy, M. A., & Williams, R. E. (1994). Effects of high-probability requests on the social interactions of young children with severe disabilities. *Journal of Applied Behavior Analysis, 27,* 619–637.

Dawson, G., & Galpert, L. (1990). Mothers' use of imitative play for facilitating social responsiveness and toy play in young autistic children. *Development and Psychopathology, 2,* 151–162.

Fisher, W. W., Piazza, C. C., Bowman, L. G., Hagopian, L. P., Owens, J. C., & Slevin, I. (1992). A comparison of two approaches for identifying reinforcers for persons with severe and profound disabilities. *Journal of Applied Behavior Analysis, 25,* 491–498.

Freeman, S., Drake, L., & Tamir, I. (1997). *Teach me language: A language manual for children with autism, Asperger's syndrome and related developmental disorders.* Langley, British Columbia: SKF Books.

Garfinkle, A., & Schwartz, I. S. (2002). Peer imitation: Increasing social interactions in children with autism and other developmental disabilities in inclusive preschool classrooms. *Topics in Early Childhood Special Education, 22,* 26–38.

Gaylord-Ross, R. J., Haring, T. G., Breen, C., & Pitts-Conway, V. (1984). The training and generalization of social interaction skills with autistic children. *Journal of Applied Behavior Analysis, 17,* 229–247.

Gena, A., Krantz, P. J., McClannahan, L. E., & Poulson, C. L. (1996). Training and generalization of affective behavior displayed by youth with autism. *Journal of Applied Behavior Analysis, 29,* 291–304.

Goldstein, H., Kaczmarek, L., Pennington, R., & Shafer, K. (1992). Peer-mediated intervention: Attending to, commenting on, and acknowledging the behavior of preschoolers. *Journal of Applied Behavior Analysis, 25,* 289–305.

Haring, T. G., & Breen, C. G. (1992). A peer-mediated social network intervention to enhance the social integration of persons with moderate and severe disabilities. *Journal of Applied Behavior Analysis, 25,* 319–333.

Harris, S. L., Handleman, J. S., & Alessandri, M. (1990). Teaching youths with autism to offer assistance. *Journal of Applied Behavior Analysis, 23,* 297–306.

Harris, S. L., Handleman, J. S., & Fong, P. L. (1987). Imitation and self-stimulation: Impact on the autistic child's behavior and affect. *Child and Family Therapy, 9,* 1–21.

Hoyson, M., Jamieson, B., & Strain, P. S. (1984). Individualized group instruction of normally developing and autistic-like children: The LEAP curriculum model. *Journal of the Division of Early Childhood, 8,* 157–172.

Ingenmey, R., & Van Houten, R. (1991). Using time delay to promote spontaneous speech in an autistic child. *Journal of Applied Behavior Analysis, 24,* 591–596.

Ingersoll, B., Schreibman, L., & Stahmer, A. (2001). Differential treatment outcomes for children with autistic spectrum disorder based on level of peer social avoidance. *Journal of Autism & Developmental Disorders, 31,* 343–349.

Kamps, D. M., Leonard, B. R., Vernon, S., Dugan, E. P., Delquadri, J. C., Gershon, B., et al. (1992). Teaching social skills to students with autism to increase peer interactions in an integrated first-grade classroom. *Journal of Applied Behavior Analysis, 25,* 281–288.

Keeling, K., Myles, B. S., Gagnon, E., & Simpson, R. L. (2003). Using the power card strategy to teach sportsmanship skills to a child with autism. *Focus on Autism and Other Developmental Disabilities, 18,* 105–111.

Klinger, L. G., & Dawson, G. (1992). Facilitating early social and communicative development in children with autism. In S. F. Warren & J. Reichle (Eds.), *Causes and effects in communication and language intervention* (Vol. 1, pp. 157–186). Baltimore: Brookes.

Koegel, L. K., Koegel, R. L., Frea, W. D., & Fredeen, R. M. (2001). Identifying early intervention targets for children with autism in inclusive school settings. *Behavior Modification, 25*, 745–761.

Koegel, L. K., Koegel, R. L., Hurley, C., & Frea, W. D. (1992). Improving social skills and disruptive behavior in children with autism through self-management. *Journal of Applied Behavior Analysis, 25*, 341–353.

Koegel, L. K., Koegel, R. L., Shoshan, Y., & McNerney, E. K. (1999). Pivotal response intervention II: Preliminary long-term outcome data on self-initiations. *Journal of the Association for Persons with Severe Handicaps, 24*, 186–198.

Koegel, R. L., Dyer, K., & Bell, L. K. (1987). The influence of child-preferred activities on autistic children's social behavior. *Journal of Applied Behavior Analysis, 20*, 243–252.

Koegel, R. L., & Frea, W. D. (1993). Treatment of social behavior in autism through the modification of pivotal social skills. *Journal of Applied Behavior Analysis, 25*, 369–377.

Koegel, R. L., Koegel, L. K., & McNerney, E. K. (2001). Pivotal areas in intervention for autism. *Journal of Clinical Child Psychology, 30*, 19–32.

Kohler, F. W., Strain, P. S., Hoyson, M., Davis, L., Donina, W. M., & Rapp, N. (1995). Using a group-oriented contingency to increase social interactions between children with autism and their peers: A preliminary analysis of corollary supportive behaviors. *Behavior Modification, 19*, 10–32.

Kohler, F. W., Strain, P. S., Maretsky, S., & DeCesare, L. (1990). Promoting positive and supportive interactions between preschoolers: An analysis of group-oriented contingencies. *Journal of Early Intervention, 14*, 327–341.

Kohler, F. W., Strain, P. S., & Shearer, D. D. (1992). The overtures of preschool social skill intervention agents: Differential rates, forms, and functions. *Behavior Modification, 16*, 525–542.

Krantz, P. J., & McClannahan, L. E. (1993). Teaching children with autism to initiate to peers: Effects of a script-fading procedure. *Journal of Applied Behavior Analysis, 26*, 121–132.

Krantz, P. J., & McClannahan, L. E. (1998). Social interaction skills for children with autism: A script-fading procedure for beginning readers. *Journal of Applied Behavior Analysis, 31*, 191–202.

LeBlanc, L. A., Coates, A. M., Daneshvar, S., Charlop-Christy, M. H., Morris, C., & Lancaster, B. M. (2003). Using video modeling and reinforcement to teach perspective-taking skills to children with autism. *Journal of Applied Behavior Analysis, 36,* 253–257.

Lee, S., & Odom, S. L. (1996). The relationship between stereotypic behavior and peer social interaction for children with severe disabilities. *Journal of the Association for Persons with Severe Handicaps, 21,* 88–95.

Matson, J. L., Sevin, J. A., Box, M. L., Francis, K. L., & Sevin, B. M. (1993). An evaluation of two methods for increasing self-initiated verbalizations in autistic children. *Journal of Applied Behavior Analysis, 26,* 389–398.

Matson, J. L., & Swiezy, N. (1994). Social skills training with autistic children. In J. L. Matson (Ed.), *Autism in children and adults: Etiology, assessment and intervention* (pp. 241–260). Pacific Grove, CA: Brooks/Cole.

Maurice, C., Green, M., & Foxx, R. (Eds.). (2001). *Making a difference: Behavioral intervention for autism.* Austin, Texas: PRO-ED.

McAfee, J. (2001). *Navigating the social world: A curriculum for individuals with Asperger's syndrome, high functioning autism and related disorders.* Arlington, TX: Future Horizons.

McConnell, S. R. (2002). Interventions to facilitate social interaction for young children with autism: Review of available research and recommendations for educational intervention and future research. *Journal of Autism and Developmental Disorders, 32,* 351–372.

McDonald, M. E., & Hemmes, N. S. (2003). Increases in social initiation toward an adolescent with autism: Reciprocity effects. *Research in Developmental Disabilities, 24,* 453–465.

McEvoy, M. A., Nordquist, V. M., Twardosz, S., Heckman, K. A., Wehby, J. H., & Denny, R. K. (1988). Promoting autistic children's peer interaction in an integrated early childhood setting using affection activities. *Journal of Applied Behavior Analysis, 21,* 193–200.

McGee, G. G., Almeida, M. C., Sulzer-Azaroff, B., & Feldman, R. S. (1992). Promoting reciprocal interactions via peer incidental teaching. *Journal of Applied Behavior Analysis, 25,* 117–126.

McGrath, A. M., Bosch, S., Sullivan, C. L., & Fuqua, R. W. (2003). Training reciprocal social interactions between preschoolers and a child with autism. *Journal of Positive Behavior Interventions, 5,* 47–54.

Mundy, P., Sigman, M., & Kasari, C. (1990). A longitudinal study of joint attention and language development in autistic children. *Journal of Autism and Developmental Disorders, 20,* 115–128.

National Research Council. (2001). *Educating children with autism.* Committee on educational interventions for children with autism. C. Lord & J. P. McGee (Eds.), Division of Behavioral and Social Sciences and Education. Washington, DC: National Academy Press.

Nikopoulos, C. K., & Keenan, M. (2004). Effects of video modeling on social initiations by children with autism. *Journal of Applied Behavior Analysis, 37,* 93–96.

Odom, S. L., Chandler, L. K., Ostrosky, M., McConnell, S. R., & Reaney, S. R. (1992). Fading teacher prompts from peer-initiation interventions for young children with disabilities. *Journal of Applied Behavior Analysis, 25,* 307–317.

Odom, S. L., & Strain, P. S. (1986). A comparison of peer-initiation and teacher-antecedent interventions for promoting reciprocal social interaction of autistic preschoolers. *Journal of Applied Behavior Analysis, 19,* 59–71.

Oke, N. J., & Schreibman, L. (1990). Training social initiations to a high-functioning autistic child: Assessment of a collateral behavior change and generalization in a case study. *Journal of Autism and Developmental Disorders, 20,* 479–497.

Ozonoff, S., & Miller, J. N. (1995). Teaching theory of mind: A new approach to social skills training for individuals with autism. *Journal of Autism and Developmental Disorders, 25,* 415–433.

Pace, G. M., Ivancic, M. T., Edwards, G. L., Iwata, B. A., & Page, T. J. (1985). Assessment of stimulus preference and reinforcer value with profoundly retarded individuals. *Journal of Applied Behavior Analysis, 18,* 249–255.

Pierce, K., & Schreibman, L. (1995). Increasing complex social behaviors in children with autism: Effects on peer-implemented pivotal response training. *Journal of Applied Behavior Analysis, 28,* 285–295.

Pierce, K., & Schreibman, L. (1997). Multiple peer use of pivotal response training social behaviors of classmates with autism: Results from trained and untrained peers. *Journal of Applied Behavior Analysis, 30,* 157–160.

Sainato, D. M., Goldstein, H., & Strain, P. S. (1992). Effects of self-evaluation on preschool children's use of social interaction strategies with their classmates with autism. *Journal of Applied Behavior Analysis, 25,* 127–141.

Sarokoff, R. A., Taylor, B. A., & Poulson, C. L. (2001). Teaching children with autism to engage in conversational exchanges: Script fading with embedded textual stimuli. *Journal of Applied Behavior Analysis, 34,* 81–84.

Shabani, D. B., Katz, R. C., Wilder, D. A., Beauchamp, K., Taylor, C. R., & Fischer, K. J. (2002). Increasing social initiations in children with autism: Effects of a tactile prompt. *Journal of Applied Behavior Analysis, 35,* 79–83.

Shafer, M. S., Egel, A. L., & Neef, N. A. (1984). Training mildly handicapped peers to facilitate changes in the social interaction skills of autistic children. *Journal of Applied Behavior Analysis, 17,* 461–476.

Shearer, D. D., Kohler, F. W., Buchan, K. A., & McCullough, K. M. (1996). Promoting independent interactions between preschoolers with autism and their nondisabled peers: An analysis of self-monitoring. *Early Education & Development, 7,* 205–220.

Silver, M., & Oakes, P. (2001). Evaluation of a new computer intervention to teach people with autism or Asperger's syndrome to recognize and predict emotions in others. *Autism, 5,* 299–316.

Skinner, B. F. (1953). *Science and human behavior*. New York: The Free Press.

Solomon, M., Goodlin-Jones, B. L., & Anders, T. F. (2004). A social adjustment enhancement intervention for high functioning autism, Asperger's syndrome, and pervasive developmental disorder NOS. *Journal of Autism and Developmental Disorders, 34*, 649–668.

Stevenson, C. L., Krantz, P. J., & McClannahan, L. E. (2000). Social interaction skills for children with autism: A script-fading procedure for nonreaders. *Behavioral Interventions, 15*, 1–20.

Stokes, T. F., & Baer, D. M. (1977). An implicit technology of generalization. *Journal of Applied Behavior Analysis, 10*, 349–367.

Stokes, T. F., & Osnes, P. G. (1989). An operant pursuit of generalization. *Behavior Therapy, 20*, 337–355.

Strain, P. S. (1983). Identification of social skill curriculum targets for severely handicapped children in mainstreamed preschools. *Applied Research in Mental Retardation, 4*, 369–382.

Strain, P. S., & Danko, C. D. (1995). Caregivers' encouragement of positive interaction between preschoolers with autism and their siblings. *Journal of Emotional & Behavioral Disorders, 3*, 2–12.

Strain, P. S., & Fox, J. J. (1981). Peer social initiations and the modification of social withdrawal: A review and future perspective. *Journal of Pediatric Psychiatry, 6*, 417–433.

Strain, P. S., Kerr, M. M., & Ragland, E. U. (1979). Effects of peer-mediated social initiations and prompting/reinforcement procedures on the social behavior of autistic children. *Journal of Autism and Developmental Disorders, 9*, 41–54.

Strain, P. S., & Kohler, F. W. (1999). Peer-mediated intervention for young children with autism: A 20-year retrospective. In P. M. Ghezzi, W. L. Williams, & J. E. Carr (Eds.), *Autism: Behavior Analytic Perspectives* (pp. 189–211). Reno, NV: Context Press.

Strain, P. S., Kohler, F. W., Storey, K., & Danko, C. D. (1994). Teaching preschoolers with autism to self-monitor their social interactions: An analysis of results in home and school settings. *Journal of Emotional and Behavioral Disorders, 2*, 78–88.

Taras, M. E., Matson, J. L., & Leary, C. (1988). Training interpersonal skills in two autistic children. *Journal of Behavior Therapy and Experimental Psychiatry, 19*, 275–280.

Taylor, B. A. (2001). Teaching peer social behavior to children with autism. In C. Maurice, M. Green, & R. Foxx (Eds.), *Making a difference: Behavioral intervention for autism* (pp. 83–93). Austin, TX: PRO-ED.

Taylor, B. A., & Harris, S. L. (1995). Teaching children with autism to seek information: Acquisition of novel information and generalization of responding. *Journal of Applied Behavior Analysis, 28*, 3–14.

Taylor, B. A., & Levin, L. (1998). Teaching a student with autism to make verbal initiations: Effects of a tactile prompt. *Journal of Applied Behavior Analysis, 31,* 651–654.

Thiemann, K. S., & Goldstein, H. (2001). Social stories, written text cues, and video feedback: Effects on social communication of children with autism. *Journal of Applied Behavior Analysis, 34,* 425–446.

Tiegerman, E., & Primavera, L. H. (1984). Imitating the autistic child: Facilitating communicative gaze behavior. *Journal of Autism and Developmental Disorders, 14,* 27–38.

Weiss, M. J., & Harris, S. L. (2001). *Reaching out, joining in: Teaching social skills to young children with autism.* Rockville, MD: Woodbine House.

Wert, B. Y., & Neisworth, J. T. (2003). Effects of video self-modeling on spontaneous requesting in children with autism. *Journal of Positive Behavior Interventions, 5,* 30–34.

Whalen, C., & Schreibman, L. (2003). Joint attention training for children with autism using behavior modification procedures. *Journal of Child Psychology & Psychiatry, 44,* 456–468.

Williams, G., Donley, C. R., & Keller, J. W. (2000). Teaching children with autism to ask questions about hidden objects. *Journal of Applied Behavior Analysis, 33,* 627–630.

Zanolli, K., & Daggett, J. (1998). The effects of reinforcement rate on the spontaneous social initiations of socially withdrawn preschoolers. *Journal of Applied Behavior Analysis, 31,* 117–125.

Zanolli, K., Daggett, J., & Adams, T. (1996). Teaching preschool age autistic children to make spontaneous initiations to peers using priming. *Journal of Autism and Developmental Disorders, 26,* 407–422.

CHAPTER

COMMUNICATION INTERVENTION

Jeff Sigafoos
University of Tasmania

Mark F. O'Reilly
University of Texas

Ralf W. Schlosser
Northeastern University

Giulio E. Lancioni
University of Bari

Autism Spectrum Disorders (ASD) are characterized by delayed or atypical development in a number of behavioral domains. Communication is one area of functioning in which delays and atypical development are prominent. Sturmey and Sevin (1994) noted that poor communication skills are a core feature in many definitions of autism. Indeed, a diagnosis of ASD is based in part on the degree of impairment in the speech–language–communication domain (American Psychiatric Association, 1994).

This chapter reviews the application of procedures designed specifically for developing communication skills in individuals with ASD. In addition, we consider the emerging literature on procedures for arranging supportive environments to promote the use of newly acquired communication skills in home, school, vocational, and other community settings. We begin by conceptualizing communication within a behavioral framework and then consider the range and nature of communication deficits and excesses associated with ASD. While discussing the nature of communication deficits and excesses associated with ASD, we will illustrate exemplary behavioral procedures for ameliorating these problems. This is followed by discussion of how to develop an effective communication-learning environment to address the communication deficits and excesses associated with ASD. We then describe several contemporary communication-focused curricula that are consistent with a behavioral conceptualization of communication and based on empirically validated principles of learning. Finally, we consider strategies for supporting parents, teachers, and staff as they work to enhance the communication abilities of individuals with ASD.

Conceptual Issues in Communication Intervention

Within applied behavior analysis (ABA), communication is conceptualized as operant behavior controlled by verbal and nonverbal antecedent stimuli and establishing operations and maintained by listener-mediated reinforcing consequences. From this perspective, communication is no different from other classes of operant behavior. The behavioral conceptualization of communication as operant behavior is very different from linguistic accounts where communication is often described as the production of underlying grammatical knowledge or as a process of information exchange involving shared meanings (Losee, 1999). However, while behavior analysts view communication as a class of operant behavior, they also acknowledge that communication has some unique characteristics that set it apart from other classes of operant behavior.

The major feature distinguishing communication from other behavior is that communicative acts are effective only indirectly through the mediation of a listener (Skinner, 1957). This feature distinguishes it from other forms of operant behavior that act directly on the environment. For example, a child with autism could gain access to a picture book by reaching for it. The act of reaching is not communicative because it operates directly on the physical environment to produce the reinforcing consequence (i.e., access to the book). If the book were out of reach, however, reaching would not be directly effective. In this instance, the child might be taught to say or sign, "I want book." Whether this response were effective in producing reinforcement would depend on whether there was a listener present who could mediate reinforcement for the child. To mediate reinforcement in this example, at least three conditions must be present for the listener: (a) hearing the child speak or seeing the child make the signs;

(b) being able to decipher what the child said, or being able to "read" the child's manual signs; and (c) being willing and able to retrieve the book for the child. One potential problem with communicative behavior, unlike behavior that is directly effective, is that the probability of reinforcement, therefore, depends on a present, attentive, and willing listener. Given these prerequisites, reinforcement of communicative acts is generally less consistent than reinforcement for acts that affect the environment directly. Ferster (1961) suggested that this inconsistency might help to explain some of the communicative deficits associated with autism. Specifically, because reinforcement of verbal operants is relatively less consistent, the child may fail to acquire much verbal behavior and instead engage in stereotyped responses such as body rocking and finger flicking, which are simple motor responses that act directly on the environment to produce automatic reinforcement on a consistent basis.

Skinner (1957) provided a functional analysis of communication or verbal behavior. In his functional analysis of verbal behavior, Skinner defined several classes of verbal operants (see Table 6.1). Note that in Skinner's account, the term *verbal behavior* does not apply only to speech. Likewise, not all speech is verbal behavior, as not all speech is mediated by the behavior of a listener. Echolalia, for example, is often maintained by automatic positive reinforcement. In fact, verbal behavior can take many forms, such as vocalizations, leading, gestures, manual signs, or pointing to a picture on a communication board. Any behavior that operates indirectly and requires another person to mediate reinforcement is "verbal" within Skinner's (1957) conceptualization. In this chapter, the term *verbal behavior* is used synonymously with the term *communication skills.*

Communicative intervention focuses on building a repertoire of appropriate communicative forms that will function as mands, tacts, echoics, intraverbals, and autoclitics. Sundberg and Michael (2001) argued that communication intervention for individuals with ASD should emphasize direct instruction of each of the verbal operants outlined by Skinner (1957) rather than the more traditional focus on vocabulary building. With this emphasis, they argued that the individual would be more likely to acquire the skills necessary to function effectively as a "speaker."

Curricula Based on Verbal Behavior

In developing individualized curricula based on Skinner's (1957) analysis of verbal behavior, initial learning targets are selected by considering the communication deficits and excesses of the individual. This is done by using standardized assessment tools or by conducting behavioral assessments.

TABLE 6.1
The Basic Verbal Operants

Operant	Definition and Example
Mand	The mand is controlled by deprivation or aversive stimulation and re-inforced by a characteristic consequence that matches the form of the response. The mand *food*, for example, would be controlled by hunger and reinforced by giving the person a preferred food item. Requesting and rejecting are examples of mands.
Tact	The tact is controlled by a prior nonverbal stimulus, such as some object or event in the environment. The function of the tact is to direct the listener's attention to the object or event. The tact *rain*, for example, would be controlled by water droplets falling from the sky. Reinforcement occurs when the listener thanks the speaker. Naming, labeling, and commenting are examples of tacts.
Echoic	An echoic response is controlled by the partner's prior verbal behavior, with the form of the echoic response matching the form produced by the speaker. The teacher says *truck*, for example, and the child responds by producing exactly the same word. Imitation of speech is an example of echoic responding.
Intraverbal	An intraverbal is also controlled by the partner's prior verbal behavior, but in this case the form of the response does not match the form produced by the speaker. Instead the response is contextually related to the prior verbal stimulus. If the parent asks a child what she wants for a birthday present, appropriate intraverbal responses could include *doll, bicycle,* or *pony.*
Autoclitic	An autoclitic response occurs in association with some other verbal behavior on the part of the speaker and indicates something about the speaker's motivational state. For example, a child might mand assistance with a difficult task by saying *I need help*, but the mand is more likely to be effective with some listeners by adding the autoclitic *really*, as in *I really need your help.* Thus the autoclitic can impact on the probability that the listener will mediate reinforcement.

Duker, van Driel, and van de Bercken (2002) developed a standardized instrument for assessing verbal operants—the *Verbal Behavior Assessment Scale* (VerBAS)—which provides ratings of mands, tacts, and echoics in the vocal, gesture, and graphic mode. The VerBAS is still in development, but so far it appears to have adequate reliability and validity for assessing deficits in verbal operants among individuals with a range of developmental disabilities.

With behavioral assessment, the presence or absence of specific communication skills is recorded in relation to opportunities for communication (Ogletree,

Pierce, Harn, & Fisher, 2002). One approach is to deliberately create structured opportunities in an attempt to evoke specific communication skills.

Sigafoos, Kerr, Roberts, and Couzens (1994) used this approach to first assess and then develop communicative requesting in 26 children with developmental disabilities. The children's teachers created opportunities for requesting using the missing-item format, blocked response, and delayed assistance strategies (see Table 6.2). The results showed that the children's requesting increased as the teachers used these strategies to create more opportunities for communication.

Another approach to behavioral assessment is to conduct naturalistic observations. In a naturalistic observation, an observer may simply record the number and types of communicative acts that occur in a given period of time, with no attempt made to directly evoke communicative behavior by creating opportunities to request, reject, or comment. One potential problem with naturalistic assessment is that the individual's communicative responses may depend on the number and type of opportunities that arise during the observation. Consequently, communication behavior must be assessed in relation to the number and types of opportunity provided.

TABLE 6.2
Strategies for Creating Opportunities for Communication

Strategy	Description
Time delay	Preferred items or activities are present, but access is delayed until a request occurs. For example, a toy is placed on the table, but access to it is delayed for 10 s.
Missing item	An item that is needed for a preferred activity is missing. For example, a child may be given a coloring book but not the crayons.
Blocked response	A response is blocked momentarily or an ongoing activity is interrupted. For example, the child is blocked from reaching for a toy, creating a need for the child to request it.
Incomplete presentation	An initial request is followed by incomplete presentation of the requested item. For example, after requesting a toy that has several parts, the child is given only half of the parts.
Delayed assistance	Required assistance is delayed until a request occurs. For example, if the person needs help to open a jar of ketchup, the communicative partner waits for the person to ask for help.
Wrong-item format	Individual is given a nonmatching referent. For example, the individual requests water but is given a pencil. This creates a need for the person to clarify the initial request.

Sigafoos, Roberts, Kerr, Couzens, and Baglioni (1994) assessed communication responses in relation to opportunities in 37 children with developmental disabilities. Observers entered the children's classrooms and watched the teacher and children across a number of days. Each daily session of 15 min was divided into 10-s intervals. For each interval, the observer recorded whether the teacher provided an opportunity for communication and, if so, what type of opportunity was provided. Opportunities were classified into one of four types based on Skinner's (1957) analysis of verbal behavior: (a) tact, (b) mand, (c) intraverbal, and (d) echoic. If an opportunity was provided, the child was then observed for the next 10 s to determine his or her response. Child responses were coded as (a) appropriate, (b) inappropriate, or (c) no response. The results showed that approximately 14% of intervals contained opportunity for communication. Most (55%) opportunities were related to the tact function, followed by mands (25%), intraverbals (15%), and echoics (5%). Opportunities were incorporated into a range of classroom activities including self-care (21%), leisure (20%), transition (12%), and preacademic instruction (10%). On average, children responded appropriately 38% of the time and inappropriately 9% of the time. They were prompted to respond on 22% of the opportunities, and made no response on 29% of the opportunities.

The data from this study enabled the researchers to assess communicative skills in relation to naturally arising opportunities. However, these data are limited because it is not clear whether the times selected for the observations provided a representative sample of the children's communicative skills. This is because so much depended on the number and types of opportunities provided by teachers, and these opportunities were not necessarily provided systematically or consistently across sessions.

Partington and Sundberg (1998) developed a more systematic approach to assessment, known as the *Assessment of Basic Language and Learning Skills* (ABLLS). This instrument includes task analyses of a range of verbal behaviors, including both speaker (expressive language) and listener (receptive language) skills. The ABLLS can be used for several purposes, including identifying communication deficits in the repertoires of individuals with ASD. The identified deficits might then become the focus of behavioral intervention. A unique aspect of the ABLLS is that it is grounded in Skinner's (1957) analysis of verbal behavior. The ABLLS therefore merges behavioral assessment tactics with a behavioral conceptualization of communication as verbal behavior.

While the ABLLS can be useful in identifying communication deficits in individuals with ASD and related developmental concerns, clinicians and educators will still need to consider how best to address the identified deficits. In some cases, assessment information may indicate the need to consider alternative forms of communication. This issue will be considered in more depth later in this chapter. For now, it is important to highlight the possibility that when alternative forms of communication such as manual signs or picture-based communication boards are indicated, support may also be required to develop the skills of the person's communicative partners. Parents, teachers, peers, and staff may need specific training to learn how to mediate the alternative forms of communication being taught to the individual with ASD. Development of these partner or listener skills can therefore be viewed as a type of support to complement ABA interventions focused on addressing the individual's communication deficits and excesses. Procedures for supporting listeners are considered later in this chapter.

Communication Deficits and Excesses in ASD

Individuals with ASD can present with a range of communication deficits and excesses (Schloper & Mesibov, 1985). Behavior analysts examine communication problems in terms of the specific behavior that is either deficient because it occurs infrequently, or not at all, or that is in excess because it occurs too frequently or out of context. The type and extent of communication impairments associated with ASD vary across individuals because ASD is not a homogeneous condition. Although language problems are defining characteristics of ASD (American Psychiatric Association, 1994), some deficits, such as mutism, indicate a more severe impairment. Other communicative problems, such as echolalia, may signal a higher level of functioning and better prognosis in terms of outcomes from behavioral intervention. Children who acquire some speech before the age of 5 years, for example, show better gains during behavioral intervention than children who remain nonspeaking (Lovaas, 1977).

Mutism

One of the more striking deficits associated with ASD is the failure to develop speech. Approximately 30% to 50% of individuals with autism fail to acquire any appreciable amount of spoken language (National Research Council, 2001), and many of these individuals will remain nonspeaking throughout their lives. Given this high prevalence of mutism, communication intervention to develop alternative forms of communication is a major priority for many individuals with ASD. Mirenda (2003) argued that "many individuals with autism are candidates for augmentative and alternative communication (AAC) systems, either to supplement (i.e., augment) their existing speech or to act as their primary (i.e., alternative) method of expressive communication" (p. 203).

Mutism should not be interpreted as a lack of communicative potential because, even though speech may not develop, the individual with ASD might nonetheless acquire a variety of informal or prelinguistic acts that function as verbal operants. Some of the prelinguistic forms that might be present in the repertoires of individuals with ASD and used to communicate include reaching, leading, pointing, vocalizations, and tantrums (Wetherby & Prizant, 2000). Because these prelinguistic behaviors are mediated through the behavior of a listener, they also are examples of verbal behavior. Evidence suggests that individuals with ASD will often produce these types of informal or prelinguistic responses as mands, while at the same time having little to no behavior related to more social communicative functions, such as the tact or intraverbal (Wetherby & Prizant, 1992).

Interventions for Mutism

Lovaas, Berberich, Perloff, and Schaeffer (1966) demonstrated the effectiveness of a four-step procedure for shaping speech in children with autism who initially had no functional speech. First, the instructors reinforced the children with food for any type of vocalization and for looking at the instructor's mouth. This contingency produced an increase in the frequency of vocalizations and increased attending to the instructor. Next, vocalizations were reinforced only if they followed the instructor's vocalization closely in time. For instance, the instructor would say a word such as "mama," and any vocalization that occurred within 6 s would be reinforced. When the children's vocalizations occurred consistently in response to the instructor's model, reinforcement was withheld until the vocalizations more closely matched that of the instructor. That is, the children were required to produce a vocalization that sounded increasingly similar to that of the instructor (e.g., "ma," "maa," "mama"). In this way, speech sounds and words were shaped and brought under the stimulus control of another person's behavior. Once some speech had been acquired, new words were taught to expand the children's vocabulary. Although this procedure can be effective, not all children appear to be able to acquire speech in this manner.

For children who remain nonspeaking, there has been growing recognition of the communicative potential of their existing prelinguistic acts. This recognition has led to the development of interventions focused on replacing the prelinguistic behaviors with alternative forms of communication (Tait, Sigafoos, Woodyatt, O'Reilly, & Lancioni, 2004). For example, if a child leads an adult's hand to toys, foods, and other preferred objects, a logical intervention goal would be to teach the child more appropriate mand forms, such as using manual signs to request these same objects. Teaching opportunities occur at times when the child approaches an object or person (Drasgow, Halle, & Sigafoos, 1999). By leading an adult's hand to a toy, for example, the child is probably indicating that the toy may be a reinforcer, and hence it can be used in teaching a more advanced form of communication. Carr and Kemp (1989) described an intervention procedure for replacing leading with a more appropriate pointing response. The intervention was evaluated with four children with autism, who ranged from 3 to 5 years of age. During baseline, the children would consistently lead the trainer's hand to access preferred objects. To replace leading, the children were taught to point to objects they wanted. The experimenters used verbal and physical prompts to evoke the pointing response, which was then reinforced by access to the preferred objects. As the pointing response increased, leading decreased, suggesting that pointing had come to replace leading as the more probable mand form.

Keen, Sigafoos, and Woodyatt (2001) used a similar procedure to replace prelinguistic behaviors in three children with autism. Initially, three communicative functions (e.g., requesting a snack, indicating a choice for one of two toys, and greeting a peer) were selected for each child. Next, the existing prelinguistic behaviors of reaching and looking, which appeared to currently serve these functions, were identified using a direct behavioral assessment. The assessment involved (a) offering a preferred item, (b) offering a choice of two items, and (c) having a peer approach the child and say hello. These conditions were designed to create the opportunity for requesting, choice making, and greeting, respectively. After creating the opportunity, the child was observed for the next 10 s. During this 10-s interval, the researchers recorded what, if anything, the child did, such as reaching for the item, leading the adult's hand to the item, or vocalizing as the peer approached. Replacement forms that were more recognizable and symbolic were defined to achieve these same functions. After a baseline phase, teachers prompted and reinforced the replacement forms but ignored the existing prelinguistic forms (i.e., placed these forms on extinction). With these procedures, the targeted replacement forms increased, and the children's existing prelinguistic behavior decreased. This inverse relation suggests that the procedures were effective in replacing prelinguistic behavior with more conventional forms of functional communication. Keen et al.'s results provide support for the applicability of ABA procedures for enhancing the communication skills of children with ASD who are nonspeaking and who fail to make progress during intervention to shape functional speech.

Echolalia

Echolalia refers to the persistent repetition of auditory stimuli in an apparently nonfunctional and stereotyped manner (Rhode, 1999). For example, an adult asks, "What's your name?" and the child replies by simply repeating the question.

Echolalia is a major disorder of social–communicative functioning that is highly prevalent in children with ASD (American Psychiatric Association, 1994). It is also a problem that appears highly persistent. Many of the 11 children originally described by Kanner (1943/1985) remained highly echolalic 28 years later (Kanner, 1971). In the absence of effective intervention, echolalia is likely to remain a serious and long-term problem.

Echolalia can be immediate or delayed. With *immediate echolalia*, the child imitates the auditory stimulus within a few seconds of its presentation. With *delayed echolalia*, the imitative response occurs minutes, hours, days, or even months after the child first heard the stimulus. Echolalia is further classified as unmitigated or mitigated (Roberts, 1989). *Unmitigated echolalia* refers to the exact imitation of another's speech in terms of the actual words or sentences reproduced and intonation patterns (Schreibman, Kohlenberg, & Britten, 1986). With *mitigated echolalia*, the child imitates the first few words spoken by another and then produces self-initiated speech (Hadano, Nakamura, & Toshihiko, 1998). Although imitation is often deficient in autism (Smith & Bryson, 1998), unmitigated echolalia suggests that some children's imitative skills are atypical rather than deficient, in that their imitative behavior is under inappropriate stimulus control. The phenomenon of mitigated echolalia further suggests that echolalia may facilitate self-initiated speech and perhaps even overall language development (Bebko, 1990).

Echolalia shares some of the properties of the echoic response (see Table 6.1), but as Bondy, Tincani, and Frost (2004) explained, not all instances of echolalia are necessarily verbal behavior. For some individuals with ASD, echolalia may be maintained by automatic positive reinforcement and unrelated to listener-mediated reinforcement (Lovaas, Newsom, & Hickman, 1987). Thus, although echolalia may be viewed as an operant, it is not necessarily always a verbal operant. A potentially important variable for understanding the nature of echolalia is whether the behavior is sensitive to audience control. If echolalia occurs more often in the presence of a listener, then it may have a communicative function. In contrast, if the behavior occurs more frequently in the absence of a listener, then it is perhaps better interpreted as a form of self-stimulation reinforced by automatic positive sensory consequences.

Researchers have identified several contextual factors that influence echolalia, which support its interpretation as an operant, and possibly as verbal behavior. For example, Rydell and Mirenda (1991) discovered that a more restricted adult interaction style elicited more echolalia in three boys with autism. Charlop (1986) found that familiarity influenced echolalia in five children and young adults with autism. Specifically, echolalia was more likely when unfamiliar therapists presented unfamiliar tasks as compared to when familiar persons presented familiar tasks. Paccia and Curcio (1982) demonstrated that echolalia in five children with autism varied as a function of the type of questions asked.

They also showed that echoic responses often involved a modification of the examiner's questions. Similarly, Carr, Schreibman, and Lovaas (1975) found that echolalia was more likely when the child did not seem to comprehend the verbal stimulus, as indicated by lack of response to teacher-presented instructions. Together, these data suggest that echolalia is often differentially sensitive to environmental and social variables.

In addition to signaling lack of comprehension or understanding, echolalia may have a social–communicative function. Prizant and Rydell (1984) noted that echolalia has typically been viewed as a type of rote imitation that is automatically reinforced and with no particular linguistic function. However, Prizant and Duchan (1981) and Prizant and Rydell (1984) suggested that echolalia may function as a form of conversational marker related to turn taking and self-regulation. For example, the individual might repeat what a conversational partner has just said as a way of maintaining a social communicative interaction with that person.

Interventions for Echolalia

While echolalia is often seen as behavioral excess, general strengthening of communication skills, rather than mere suppression of echolalic responding, may represent an effective behavioral treatment for echolalic individuals with ASD. This treatment suggestion is based on evidence that echolalia is related to overall receptive and expressive language ability. Roberts (1989) found echolalia was inversely related to receptive language development in 10 children with autism. Howlin (1982) showed that echolalia decreased as linguistic competence increased in 26 boys ages 3 to 12 years with ASD. These data suggest that behavioral intervention to increase the overall communication ability in both the expressive and receptive domain may lead to collateral reductions in echolalia.

In addressing echolalia, there has been some success in replacing it with functional speech using operant procedures, such as prompting and fading (Lovaas, 1977). The general approach is for the instructor to exploit the child's echolalia as a prompt for the target response. For example, the instructor might show a child a cookie and ask, "What is this?" Instead of waiting for the child to echo the question, the instructor would immediately say, "Cookie." The child is therefore likely to echo the last word, rather than the entire initial question. The echoic prompt is then faded by speaking the word "cookie" with less and less volume and emphasis over successive learning opportunities. A variation of this approach is known as the *cues-pause-point procedure* (Foxx, McMorrow, Faw, Kyle, & Bittle, 1987; McMorrow & Foxx, 1986; McMorrow, Foxx, Faw, & Bittle, 1987). The procedure involves several steps. First, the trainer holds his or her right finger to prompt the child to remain silent. If any child verbalizations occur at this point, the trainer says, "No" or "Shh." This is called the pause prompt. Next, the trainer points to the stimulus materials and asks, "What is this?" The pause prompt is then removed, signaling the child to respond. In this way, echolalia is replaced with tact (object naming) responses.

Lack of Maintenance and Generalization

Another often noted problem is that the communication responses taught to individuals with ASD are not always maintained once training has ended. In addition, newly acquired responses often fail to generalize to other trainers, settings, or materials. Stokes and Baer (1977) conceptualized maintenance and generalization in terms of a failure to establish appropriate stimulus control over responding, rather than reflecting some deficit on the part of the individual. Given this conceptualization, the solution was to incorporate additional procedures into training to promote maintenance and generalization. Along these lines, Stokes and Baer reviewed several procedures for promoting maintenance and generalization, many of which have empirical support for promoting maintenance and generalization of communication skills in individuals with ASD. Duker, Didden, and Sigafoos (2004) provided a detailed description of behavioral procedures that have been used to promote maintenance and generalization of communication responses over time and across settings, instructors, and materials. These procedures include the following: (a) teach functional responses, (b) reduce instructional control, (c) teach multiple exemplars, (d) use intermittent reinforcement, and (e) program common stimuli. Table 6.3 describes each of these procedures.

While the failure to generalize and maintain newly acquired communication skills has been viewed in terms of stimulus control, Drasgow et al. (1999) argued that generalization failures might also be related to motivational variables. During a generalization assessment, a child may fail to produce a newly acquired mand form outside of the structured training environment. Although this outcome could indicate that the training program did not establish appropriate stimulus control over responding, it could also reflect a lack of motivation to communicate. Drasgow et al. argued that clinicians should ensure that the motivation to communicate is present when generalization and maintenance are assessed.

Lack of Spontaneity

In addition to maintenance and generalization problems, researchers have also noted that newly acquired vocabulary frequently does not occur spontaneously

TABLE 6.3
Procedures for Promoting Generalization and Maintenance

Procedure	Description
Teach functional responses	The form of the communication response should provide an effective signal to a range of listeners. Manual signs, for example, may be effective only with listeners who know sign language. A voice-output communication device, in contrast, is likely to be more functional because the speech output will be understood by more listeners.
Reduce instructional control	Communication skills are often taught in structured training sessions. While a highly structured approach can facilitate acquisition, it may also bring responding under narrow stimulus control. This problem can be addressed by reducing stimulus control during training. To reduce stimulus control, training should be implemented in a variety of settings, with a variety of listeners and materials. In addition, the prompts and cues used in training should be varied.
Teach multiple exemplars	Communication response might not generalize because too few exemplars were used in training. Generalization can be improved by including multiple exemplars in training. For example, instead of teaching a child to mand for books and toys using only one book and one toy, the trainer should offer a variety of books and toys.
Use intermittent reinforcement	Acquisition is facilitated by reinforcing each communicative response, but continuous reinforcement schedules may not match the contingencies operating outside of the training environment. Maintenance can be improved by shifting to a more intermittent schedule of reinforcement, such as a variable ratio or variable interval schedule.
Program common stimuli	A common stimulus is a discriminative stimulus that is found not only in the training environment, but also in the natural environment. If the stimuli that come to control responding during training are also found outside the training environment, then generalization is more likely to occur.

Note. From "Strengthening Communicative Behaviors for Gaining Access to Desired Items and Activities," by J. Sigafoos and P. Mirenda, 2002, in J. Reichle, D. R. Beukelman, & J. C. Light (Eds.), *Exemplary Practices for Beginning Communicators: Implications for AAC*, p. 133, Baltimore: Brookes. Reprinted with permission.

(Charlop, Schreibman, & Thibodeau, 1985; Lovaas, 1977). For example, the individual might not produce newly acquired communicative forms without being verbally prompted to do so by the teacher or parent. When this occurs the individual is often said to be prompt dependent. However, as with generalization and maintenance, the lack of spontaneity is not necessarily a deficit or dependency inherent in the individual with ASD. Instead, behavior analysts view the lack of spontaneity as an instructional problem related to a failure in bringing the response under appropriate stimulus control. That is, the individual may lack spontaneity because he or she was never taught to respond in the absence of a verbal prompt by the teacher or parent or because teaching inadvertently brought the child's speech under narrow stimulus control such as an expectant look or verbal prompt from the parent or teacher.

In addition, part of the spontaneity problem appears to have stemmed from the fact that individuals were often taught to tact (i.e., to name objects or make comments), whereas spontaneous use involves the production of mands, as in requesting access to preferred objects. Tacts and mands are separate and functionally independent communication skills (Lamarre & Holland, 1985). Thus, teaching a word as an object name did not automatically enable the individual to use that word to make a request and vice versa.

Efforts to address spontaneity were advanced by Halle's (1987) influential conceptual paper, which argued that spontaneity could be viewed as controlled along a continuum of antecedents that set the occasion for communication. Responses that require physical, gestural, or verbal prompting are less spontaneous than responses controlled by the presence of an object or a particular state of deprivation (e.g., requesting a drink when thirsty). Promotion of more spontaneous communication can therefore be seen as a process of transferring stimulus control along this continuum from instructional prompts to more natural contextual cues.

Transfer of stimulus control procedures have been used with success to develop more spontaneous communication in people with ASD. In one illustrative study, Hamilton and Snell (1993) used a least-to-most prompting sequence to transfer control from modeling and verbal prompting to natural opportunities (see Chapter 2 for more on this prompting procedure). A 15-year-old boy with autism, severe mental retardation, and no speech participated. Training opportunities were conducted across four settings: classroom, school cafeteria, community, and home. In these settings, the boy carried a wallet containing 116 symbols representing a range of foods, beverages, activities, and emotions. The purpose of the intervention was to increase use of the symbols in the communication wallet to make requests. A multiple baseline across settings design was used to evaluate the procedures. Each day the child received 20 opportunities to communicate. Opportunities were those that arose naturally or were created by an adult. For example, if the child was looking around the room for his coat to go outside, this became a natural opportunity for teaching the child to request by pointing to the symbol for "coat" in his communication wallet.

During baseline, when an opportunity arose or was created, the teacher waited 5 s without approaching or looking expectantly at the child. If the child pointed to the correct symbol, he was given what he had asked for. Thus, pointing to a symbol in the communication book functioned as a mand. No prompting was given during baseline. During intervention, the teacher used a least-to-most prompting sequence to prompt a correct response if one did not occur within 5 s. The prompt levels were (a) expectant looking (EL), (b) EL plus question (e.g., "What do you want?"), (c) EL plus mand (e.g., "Show me 'coat' in your book"), and (d) EL plus mand plus model (e.g., teacher pointed to correct symbol). A 5-s constant time delay separated each prompt level. Transfer of stimulus control was accomplished by fading the prompts. Prompts were faded in four phases. In Phase 1, the experimenters gave all prompts. In Phase 2, the experimenters faded the model. In Phase 3, the mand was faded. Finally, in Phase 4, the question was faded. An expectant look continued to be used if the child did not request within 5 s. The data from baseline revealed low rates of spontaneous requesting (mean = 11% of the opportunities). Spontaneous (i.e., unprompted) requesting in the classroom gradually increased during Phases 1 through 4. During maintenance probes, spontaneous requesting occurred during more than 75% of the opportunities. Gradually increasing trends were observed during baseline in the other settings, but increased further when intervention began, eventually reaching 75% of the opportunities. This study suggested that the least-to-most prompt sequence was effective in transferring control of requests from teacher modeling and verbal prompting to the more natural context, which included the listener looking expectantly at the child.

In another relevant study, Woods (1984) created two conditions for teaching spontaneous tacting of pictures, objects, and locations. In the first condition, two boys with autism were taught to name objects portrayed in picture books. A 7-s time-delay procedure was used. If the child did not produce a correct tact within 7 s, the instructor prompted the child to tact a picture by asking, "What do you see there?" For the second condition, the boys were accompanied around the school and exposed to various objects and locations. When approaching a location, such as an office, the instructor waited 7 s and then provided a model of the correct tact if the child failed to tact within the delay interval. Unprompted tacts increased in both conditions with the introduction of the delayed prompting procedures. Responding in the absence of the verbal prompt, "What do you see there?" was greater in the second condition. There was greater spontaneity in the second condition, which may have reflected the fact that verbal instructions were not presented as part of the training procedure in the second condition, or it may reflect the fact that the stimuli in the first and second conditions were different. Despite this confound, Woods demonstrated that children with autism could be taught to emit spontaneous tacts under fairly natural conditions using the delayed prompting technique.

Communicative Phenotype in ASD

Scheuermann and Webber (2002) noted that even when a high level of speech and language has developed, the communication of individuals with ASD is often characterized by certain odd and unusual features, including (a) unusual voice tone and inflection, (b) pronoun reversals, (c) lack of variety in sentence structure, and (d) immature grammar (e.g., simple noun–verb formats). Scheuermann and Webber also noted that the extent of the individual's presenting communication problems is often used to distinguish autism from related conditions such as Asperger syndrome. This suggests that the presenting communication profile may have diagnostic relevance.

It is unclear whether the communication deficits and excesses associated with ASD represent a unique behavioral phenotype. Duker et al. (2002) compared the communication profiles of individuals with Down syndrome, Angelman syndrome, and Pervasive Developmental Disorder (PDD) using the *Verbal Behavior Assessment Scale*. There were major differences in communication profiles. Specifically, individuals with Down syndrome and PDD had less developed mands, relative to tacts and echoics. People with Angelman syndrome, in contrast, had better skills in the mand function, relative to tacts, and also had very weak echoic skills. It is also important to note that there was considerable within-syndrome variability. Still, these data suggest the possibility of distinct communicative phenotypes associated with developmental disability syndromes. Duker et al. suggested possible implications for intervention, for example that children with Down syndrome and PDD require intervention to teach mands, but individuals with Angelman syndrome should have more training in tacts. Behavioral intervention should therefore aim to create an environment that provides a better match between nervous system and environment.

Creating an Effective Communication Learning Environment

Communication occurs across activities, communication partners, and settings. Therefore, communication intervention should be embedded into every activity and setting in which the individual with ASD is expected to function, including all communication partners with whom the individual is expected to interact. To promote rapid acquisition of new communication skills, there may also be a benefit in providing intensive and more structured training during dedicated teaching sessions. The use of discrete trial teaching during highly structured sessions has been contrasted with more naturalistic approaches in which learning opportunities are embedded within a range of typical daily activities. There is much debate as to which approach is better for developing communication skills in individuals with ASD.

Delprato (2001) articulated the differences between discrete trial teaching and more naturalistic approaches for teaching communication skills to children with autism. Discrete trial teaching is characterized by highly structured training sessions during which the trainer presents stimuli to the individual, prompts correct responses as necessary, and differentially reinforces and shapes correct responses. This approach often relies on arbitrary reinforcement. For example, with the child and teacher seated at a table, the teacher initiates each trial by presenting a stimulus, such as by holding up an object and asking, "What is this?" Correct responses from the child are followed by an unrelated reinforcer, such as a bite of cookie or sip of juice. During a 20-min session, 40 to 50 such trials might be completed.

Naturalistic approaches, in contrast, are implemented during everyday activities, such as playtime, lunch, or community outings. In addition, the teacher relies on child-initiated opportunities, rather than teacher-presented stimuli. There is also reliance on natural reinforcers. For example, during recess, the child might initiate an opportunity by approaching a preferred piece of equipment. At this point, the teacher would briefly interrupt the child from playing to create the need for communication (e.g., saying, "I want _____"). Access to the item reinforces the communicative behavior.

In his review of studies comparing discrete trial teaching to more naturalistic approaches for teaching communication skills to children with autism, Delprato (2001) concluded that naturalistic approaches were more effective, but it is not clear whether this review included all relevant studies or how the relative effectiveness of these studies was compared. In addition, the distinction between discrete trial teaching and naturalistic approaches to communication intervention is somewhat arbitrary. It may be better to view the various ways of presenting learning opportunities along a continuum. Highly structured sessions with teachers presenting stimuli in discrete trials may be of considerable initial benefit in promoting rapid acquisition, especially for individuals who fail to initiate. Bambara and Warren (1993) suggested that there are indeed appropriate contexts for the use of structured training sessions that include a large number of discrete trials. They also reported the potential benefits of using massed and discrete trial training as including increased opportunities to practice difficult response and shape the topography of the response, which may be especially important when attempting to teach speech or manual signs.

Once new communication forms have been acquired during highly structured training sessions, then more naturalistic approaches can be adopted to facilitate generalization and maintenance. In addition, the two approaches are not necessarily mutually exclusive, but might be combined and implemented concurrently. The important point is that learning opportunities should be presented in ways that fit the context.

Within ABA there are many ways in which learning opportunities can be presented, ranging from a large number of discrete trials within a specific teaching context to more naturalistic approaches where one or two opportunities are embedded in the natural flow of existing daily routines. In addition, one would be mistaken to assume that discrete trial teaching requires an artificial context. There is no reason why a number of discrete trials could not be embedded in a range of typical routines, as well as, throughout the day. Requests for food, for example, could be taught at breakfast, lunch, snack times, and dinner, whereas requests for toys could be taught during all playtimes. During such times, the trainer may decide to implement 20 to 30 trials, thereby providing an increased number of learning opportunities within the natural context. The choice of either discrete trial teaching or more naturalistic approaches, or some combination of the two approaches, may also depend on the goals of teaching. For example, if rapid skills acquisition is required, then discrete trial teaching might be the method of choice; if increasing a wide variety of mands to compete with maladaptive behaviors is the goal, then naturalistic teaching might be selected.

Setting the Occasion for Communication Behavior

A critical aspect of setting the occasion for communication is to ensure that the individual is motivated to respond at each and every instructional opportunity. There is no sense in trying to teach a learner to request food and drink, for example, if the individual has just eaten and drunk until satiation. If the individual is not motivated when an opportunity is presented, then the instructor does not have a reinforcer, and no learning will occur. It is also possible that if the instructor persists at times when motivation is lacking, then the session may become aversive, and the individual may attempt to escape from the training situation.

Clinicians must therefore gain skills in exploiting opportunities for teaching communication. Sundberg (1993) explained how ABA therapists might either capture or contrive opportunities for teaching verbal behavior. To capture learning opportunities, instructors make use of environmental events that would ordinarily set the occasion for communication as these arise during typical activities. For example, while the instructor and child are walking in the park, an airplane might fly over. The instructor could capture this event by using it as an opportunity to teach spontaneous tacting. The antecedent is the airplane. A correct response would be for the child to point to the airplane and then produce the manual sign "airplane." An appropriate listener response ("Yes, I see. Look at that big airplane") completes the three-term contingency. More naturalistic teaching programs often rely almost exclusively on teaching communication skills in the context of captured learning opportunities.

To increase the number of learning opportunities available to the individual, instructors should also learn how to contrive or create effective opportunities for communication. To do so, the instructor manipulates some aspect of the environment to set the occasion or need for communication. Relying exclusively on incidental or captured learning opportunities may result in fewer opportunities than if additional opportunities for communication were also created by manipulating the communication-learning environment. Sosne, Handleman, and Harris (1979) argued that creating the need for communication was the critical first step in teaching communication skills to individuals with ASD. Table 6.2, presented earlier in this chapter, outlines several ways that trainers can manipulate the environment to create the need for communication in individuals with ASD. As illustrated in Table 6.2, contrived opportunities are often used to teach mands. For example, a preferred or needed object is placed out of reach, thereby creating the need for the individual to mand for the object. In a novel application of this approach, Sundberg, Loeb, Hale, and Eigenheer (2002) contrived opportunities to teach children with autism to ask *wh-* questions. They did this by hiding needed objects. To obtain the needed object, the children had to ask the trainer "Where?" as in "Where is the item?"

Although there are fewer examples in the literature (cf. Woods, 1984), the communication-learning environment could also be contrived to set the occasion for other verbal operants in addition to mands. To set the occasion for spontaneous tacting, for example, the trainer might arrange objects in the environment to evoke a comment, as in presenting a conversation piece. To set the occasion for conversational exchanges, the trainer may initiate a conversation by asking specific questions (e.g., "What did you do this weekend?")

Ensure the Target Response Occurs

It is important for trainers to ensure that every learning opportunity ends with the individual making the correct response and being reinforced for that response. During the initial stages of training, however, the individual is unlikely to make the correct response. Instead, the individual is likely to revert to existing prelinguistic forms, which could be socially inappropriate, such as leading or tantrums. Thus, there will often be a need for the clinician to preempt old forms and prompt the new form, at least during the initial stages of communication intervention. This means that the instructor will have to use one or more prompts to ensure a correct response is forthcoming from the individual. Once a correct response occurs, it can then be followed with the appropriate listener-mediated reinforcement.

Various prompts have been developed and shown to be effective for teaching communication skills to individuals with ASD (Duker et al., 2004). Response prompts include (a) spoken instructions (e.g., "Show me the sign for water"), (b) gestures (e.g., pointing to the correct line drawing on a communication board), (c) model or imitative prompts (e.g., demonstrating the correct manual sign while instructing the individual to "do this," or verbally modeling a response), and (d) physical assistance (e.g., moving the person's finger to touch the correct symbol on a speech-generating device). In addition, various prompting strategies or hierarchies have been empirically validated for teaching a variety of communication forms and functions to individuals with ASD. These include most-to-least prompting (i.e., physical prompt, model, gesture, verbal prompt) and least-to-most prompting (i.e., verbal prompt, gesture, model, followed by physical prompt), graduated guidance (using the least amount of physical guidance necessary), and delayed prompting (e.g., waiting 5 or 10 s before prompting). The basic principle is that the instructor must use a prompt or prompting strategy that will reliably evoke the correct response from the individual.

Once the individual has responded with prompting, the instructor must then begin the process of fading or eliminating the prompts so that the individual begins to respond independently. In most cases, prompts cannot be withdrawn suddenly but must be removed gradually, a process known as prompt fading. The basic principle is to gradually provide less and less prompting as the individual becomes more and more independent. There are numerous effective strategies for fading prompts (Duker et al., 2004). These include (a) systematically moving from more- to less-intrusive prompts, (b) inserting a time delay between the discriminative stimulus and the delivery of the prompt, and (c) decreasing the amount or magnitude of prompting over successive trials.

Listener-Mediated Reinforcement

Once the response occurs, whether prompted or not, the listener must deliver reinforcement as quickly as possible. Reinforcement of correct responses is critical for learning. There are at least two basic principles related to proper use of reinforcement. First, it is critical to ensure that the reinforcer delivered matches the function of the individual's communicative response. If the individual requests a drink of water, for example, the appropriate reinforcement is for the listener to give the person a glass of water to drink. This is an example of a positive reinforcement contingency. In contrast, if the individual signs "No thanks" when offered a drink, then the appropriate reinforcer is for the listener to withdraw the offered beverage. This is an example of a negative reinforcement contingency.

It is relatively easy to follow this rule when the individual produces a mand, because the mand specifies its reinforcement. Difficulties can arise, however, when teaching other verbal operants, such as the tact and intraverbal, because here the natural reinforcer is simply a relevant reply from the partner, rather than some more tangible outcome. The problem is that some individuals with ASD appear to be less than responsive to such social consequences. It would therefore be difficult to teach them to tact, for example, without using some sort of instructional or artificial consequence as reinforcement during teaching. This is not necessarily a problem if the schedule of reinforcement can later be thinned so that it appears as if the individual is responding to the social consequences, rather than the occasional tangible reinforcer that is really maintaining the behavior. However, Drasgow et al. (1999) suggested that when instructors rely on artificial or instructional reinforcers, such as reinforcing a child with edibles for tacting objects, they may find that the child only tacts when hungry. After training, the motivation (i.e., food deprivation) to respond may be absent at times when it would be appropriate for the child to tact. The lack of motivation may explain why communication skills often fail to generalize.

Behavioral Programs for Communication Intervention

Numerous training programs have been published for teaching communication skills to individuals with ASD (Sigafoos, 1997). Lovaas (1977) published one of the first programs for teaching communication to children with autism. His program was evidence based, comprehensive, and firmly grounded in behavioral principles. A number of contemporary programs have evolved from the pioneering work of Lovaas.

Sign Language Training Program

Carr (1982) presented evidence-based procedures for teaching sign language to children with ASD. In this program, children were initially taught several manual signs using modeling, response prompting, and reinforcement. Once several signs had been acquired, transfer-of-stimulus-control procedures were used to establish these forms as object labels and for requesting. Duker (1988) extended this work and presented step-by-step procedures for teaching gesture-mode communication skills. His teaching procedures relied on least-to-most and most-to-least prompt hierarchies. Although both of these programs focused on functional communication skills, the functions taught—for example, requesting and naming objects—were not necessarily derived from Skinner's (1957) analysis of verbal behavior. For example, in teaching requests, the individual might be offered a preferred item and prompted to make the correct sign. The presence of the object, which sets the occasion for communication, therefore, makes the requesting response part mand and part tact.

Partington and Sundberg

Partington and Sundberg (1998) suggested that this mixing of the verbal operants, as is done in many communication intervention programs, might lead to problems with respect to generalization and spontaneity. Their program therefore uses behavioral procedures to teach the verbal operants as outlined by Skinner (1957). They begin by teaching manual signs as mands and then use transfer-of-stimulus-control procedures to establish other functions for these signs, such as tacts and intraverbals. Teaching each verbal operant separately is considered necessary because simply having the sign topography in one's repertoire is no guarantee that it will be used for various functions. Thus, procedures are included in the program to ensure that each sign can be used as mand, tact, intraverbal, and echoic response. The intervention procedures used in this program are designed to establish stimulus control over manual signs. Its aim is to bring manual signs under the control of stimuli that set the occasion for communication in the natural environment. Mands should be controlled by deprivation, satiation, or aversive stimulus, whereas tacts would be controlled by the presence of an object, and intraverbals would be controlled by a prior verbal stimulus.

The Picture Exchange Communication System (PECS)

Bondy and Frost (2001) developed the Picture Exchange Communication System (PECS). In this system, the individual with ASD is taught to give an adult a picture of an object as a means of requesting that object. Training begins by identifying reinforcers. Next, pictures of reinforcers are made, and the individual is then taught to exchange the picture for the actual item. The exchange of the card therefore functions as a mand. To teach this skill, the adult physically prompts the child to give the picture to the adult in response to a gesture cue (i.e., the adult extending an open hand). When the child gives the picture to the adult, the corresponding real object is given to the child and the adult acknowledges the child's request (e.g., "Oh, you want a cookie!"). Physical prompts are faded until the child independently exchanges the picture for the real object. Next, the adult fades the gestural prompt (i.e., extending an open hand). After the child has acquired the skill of exchanging a picture to receive the corresponding real object, other pictures are introduced and discrimination training begins. Training is extended to multipicture exchanges, such as two pictures representing "I want" and "cookie," and the child is taught to exchange pictures in response to verbal cues, such as "What do you see?" and "What is it?"

According to a recent review by Odom et al. (2003), PECS is considered one of the "emerging and effective" treatments for young children with autism. The "emerging and effective" level is below the level of "well-established" treatments in the hierarchy of evidence applied in their review. This was based on the inclusion of only one controlled single-subject experimental study at the time (Charlop-Christy, Carpenter, LeBlanc, & Kellet, 2002). Since then a number of controlled single-subject experimental design studies provided additional support for the effectiveness of using PECS to promote communication in children with autism (Anderson, 2002; Ganz & Simpson, 2004; Tincani, 2004).

Selecting the Mode of Communication

An important issue that arises when designing communication intervention programs for individuals with ASD is the selection of a communicative mode. Although many individuals with developmental disabilities benefited from interventions to teach speech, others failed to make progress. To address this issue, researchers investigated communicative alternatives to speech. The two alternatives to speech are aided (e.g., PECS, voice-output devices) and unaided (e.g., manual signs, gestures) modes of communication.

Carr, Binkoff, Kologinsky, and Eddy (1978) provided the first controlled study of teaching manual signs to children with autism. In this study, four children with autism, ages 10 to 15 years, were taught to name objects by producing the corresponding manual sign when shown an object by the trainer. The training procedures consisted of prompting, fading, and reinforcement. Discriminations between objects were taught by rotating the objects presented. Using these procedures, the children acquired a set of manual signs and used these spontaneously to request access to preferred objects. Since that study, numerous studies have replicated the effectiveness of using operant procedures for teaching manual signs to individuals with developmental disabilities who failed to acquire speech (Duker & Jutten, 1997). In addition, several studies have shown that a total communication approach—involving simultaneous speech and manual sign training—results in faster acquisition of expressive and receptive language skills than speech training alone (Barrera & Sulzer-Azaroff, 1983; Remington & Clarke, 1983; Yoder & Layton, 1988).

Because manual signs are ineffective with listeners who do not know sign language (Rotholz, Berkowitz, & Burberry, 1989), investigators also showed the applicability of operant methods for teaching learners to use aided communication systems including nonelectronic communication boards, speech-generating devices, and PECS (Sigafoos & Mirenda, 2002). Only a few studies have been carried out involving selection-based systems such as communication books or wallets. One of these studies, in which a youngster with autism was taught to request across multiple contexts using a communication book (Hamilton & Snell, 1993), was reviewed earlier in this chapter. In another study, a communication book was introduced to two individuals with autism who had previously relied on manual signing to request food items (Rotholz et al., 1989). The study was conducted in community fast-food restaurants. When the individuals attempted to place orders in the restaurants using their manual signs, they were not successful because the cashiers did not understand sign language. During intervention, the communication book was introduced, in which requests were placed by pointing to line drawings of items (e.g., hamburger, Coke). Use of the picture system proved to be an effective way of ordering food in the restaurants, demonstrating that teaching the use of a communication book can be more effective than manual sign language instruction, at least in community settings where laypeople do not know manual signing.

Another form of aided communication involves the use of speech-generating devices. Research on the use of speech-generating devices by individuals with autism is still in its infancy (Mirenda, 2003; Schlosser & Blischak, 2001). A few studies, however, demonstrated that they also might be effective for some children with autism. For example, Schepis, Reid, Behrmann, and Sutton (1998) showed that the use of a naturalistic approach was effective in teaching the use of speech-generating devices in that once device use was acquired, the young children with autism who participated in the study used it to interact more frequently. In a related study, Sigafoos, Didden, and O'Reilly (2003) successfully taught three students with developmental disabilities to request access to preferred objects using a speech-generating device.

Comparative studies have the potential to inform decision making to a greater extent than studies examining the effectiveness of a single intervention (Schlosser, 2003). To date, only a few studies have been conducted comparing different modes of communication. In one study comparing PECS with manual signing, Tincani (2004) found that no consistent effectiveness pattern emerged when comparing PECS with signing. Rather, the acquisition depended on individual characteristics of the participants. Specifically, a student with weak hand-motor imitation skills performed better with PECS than with signing, whereas the student with good hand-motor imitation skills was more successful with manual signing. Anderson (2002) compared PECS with manual signing in six children with autism, ages 2 and 4 years. The two approaches were compared in terms of rates of acquisition, spontaneous use, maintenance, generalization, eye contact, vocalizations, and challenging behaviors. PECS resulted in faster acquisition across a broader range of children and better generalization to novel items. There were also some benefits associated with the manual signing modality, including higher levels of initiation, eye contact, and vocalization. A secondary purpose of Anderson's study was to identify child characteristics that may be associated with performance patterns. Acquisition rates with PECS were linked to the extent to which the child was already using prelinguistic behaviors to make requests of others (i.e., mands), whereas acquisition rates with manual signing were associated with the extent to which the child was already using prelinguistic behaviors to alert an adult to aspects of the environment (i.e., tacting). Finally, vocalization during and after treatment was associated with imitation levels and language age-equivalents before treatment. Taken together, these studies indicate that, rather than hoping to identify superior communication modalities for individuals with ASD, it may be more productive to match modalities to specific characteristics of the individuals, their communication partners, and the environments in which they are expected to communicate.

One persistent concern of many professionals and family members has to do with the impact of alternative modes of communication on natural speech production. A recent evidence-based review of studies in which alternative modes of communication were taught to individuals with ASD revealed suggestive evidence that augmentative and alternative communication (AAC) systems do enhance natural speech production (Schlosser & Blischak, 2003). Although suggestive evidence is far from convincing, it at least provides a data-based possibility. In the absence of any evidence indicating that AAC intervention may hinder natural speech, this should be reassuring to families and professionals contemplating the use of AAC systems such as manual sign and speech-generating devices as alternatives to speech for individuals with ASD.

Listener Support

An important role for clinicians working in the field of ASD involves training parents, teachers, peers, and front-line staff on how to design an effective communication-learning environment. Effective training for communication partners is important because their responsivity may affect the communication performance of individuals with ASD (Harwood, Warren, & Yoder, 2002). Implementing behavioral interventions to teach communication skills can be complicated. Parents, teachers, peers, and staff often need considerable support to learn and make use of behavioral procedures to teach communication skills to individuals with ASD and to respond to the person's communication, especially if the person is using an alternative mode of communication. In keeping with the concept of the establishing operation and the three-term contingency, listeners must learn how to (a) motivate the individual to communicate, (b) set the occasion for communication, (c) prompt, and (d) reinforce appropriate forms of communication.

Several studies have demonstrated effective procedures to train staff to be effective communicative partners to individuals with developmental disabilities. Duker and Moonen (1985) described a program for training staff and teachers to increase the use of manual signs among three students with severe or profound intellectual disability. Training was provided to one teacher and 12 residential staff, ages 21 to 32 years. The training package was multifaceted and included (a) written instructions describing the procedures, (b) live and video demonstrations of the teaching procedures, (c) cueing and feedback, and (d) group discussions. After staff received this training, they provided increased opportunities for sign use, and the students showed increased use of manual signs to make requests. Although the study demonstrated the effectiveness of this package for training staff, it remained unclear whether all components of the package were necessary.

Sigafoos, Kerr, Roberts, and Couzens (1994) evaluated a consultative approach for training teachers to provide communicative opportunities in classrooms for children with developmental disabilities. Teachers received a 1-hour in-service during which the trainer described strategies that could be used to create opportunities for requesting (e.g., missing-item format, blocked response, and delayed assistance; see Table 6.3 earlier in this chapter for examples of these and other strategies). Teachers also received a one-page description of each strategy. The innovative aspect of this training program was that the teachers then generated their own ideas on how to incorporate these strategies into classroom routines. The trainer facilitated the discussion by asking questions such as, "How might the missing-item format be used at lunch time?" and "Do you think the delayed assistance strategy could be used with Robert?" Subsequent classroom observations revealed that the teachers incorporated these strategies into a variety of typical classroom routines, resulting in more communication learning opportunities for their students.

Schepis and Reid (2003) outlined a competency-based model for training staff to enhance communication skills of individuals with developmental dis-

TABLE 6.4
Steps for Training Parents, Teachers, and Front-Line Staff

Step	Description of Step	Example
1	The consultant collaborates with staff to identify behavioral objectives that reference observable and measurable behaviors.	The client signs HELP when assistance is needed to complete daily living tasks.
2	The consultant develops a procedure for teaching the specified objective. This includes a literature search to identify empirically validated procedures (e.g., Reichle, Drager, & Davis, 2002), an adjustment of the procedure to suit individual circumstances, and a written description of the procedure.	Procedures include (a) wait 10 s for client to request help when needed, (b) if request does not occur, use least-to-most prompting, and (c) give help after request.
3	The consultant explains procedure to staff, making sure they understand each step of the procedure.	Consultant says, "At this point, wait 10 s. This will motivate the person to request help."
4	After explaining the written plan, the clinician shows the staff how to implement the plan while simultaneously describing each step of the procedure.	Consultant says, "Now I will have to use a physical prompt because the client did not respond to the model."
5	Staff practice implementing the procedure, while the consultant watches and gives feedback. This continues until staff demonstrate proficiency.	Consultant says, "Good! You waited 10 s. Now because he has not requested, you need to deliver the verbal prompt."

Note. Based on "Issues Affecting Staff Enhancement of Speech Generating Device Use Among People with Severe Cognitive Disabilities," by M. M. Schepis and D. H. Reid, 2003, *Augmentative and Alternative Communication, 19*, pp. 59–65.

abilities. Although their model was specifically geared toward staff teaching children with severe disabilities to use speech-generating devices, their approach could be applied more generally. Table 6.4 summarizes the Schepis and Reid model, and includes an illustrative example for each step.

Summary

ABA has provided effective intervention procedures for addressing the communication deficits and excesses associated with ASD. Lovaas (2002) identified a number of critical components that appear to be associated with more positive treatment outcomes for individuals with developmental disabilities. In the practitioner recommendations, we have adapted these guidelines to the design and implementation of communication intervention programs for individuals with ASD.

In closing, communication intervention is a major priority for individuals with ASD. Intervention for these individuals requires systematic instruction to address the specific deficits and excesses associated with ASD. Communication intervention for individuals with ASD must be comprehensive and ongoing, focusing on developing a wide range of communicative functions. A major role for clinicians in providing comprehensive support is to ensure that family, teachers, and staff receive adequate training in facilitating the communication development of individuals with ASD.

 ## PRACTITIONER RECOMMENDATIONS

1. Focus on measurable and observable behaviors.

   a. Behavior related to communication should be operationally defined.

   b. Definition should include a description of how the occurrence of the behavior will be measured so that progress toward goal attainment can be monitored.

2. Use evidence-based interventions. Training procedures should be based on empirically validated principles of learning, which requires an understanding of

   a. the basic operant and respondent conditioning principles that underlie effective instruction and

   b. how to capture and contrive opportunities for learning communication skills.

3. Effective instruction procedures include the use of shaping, prompting, fading, and differential reinforcement.

   a. Use goals to teach a wide range of communication skills (e.g., mands, tacts, intraverbals, echoics) using communicative modes that are appropriate for the individual (e.g., speech, gestures, speech-generating devices).

   b. Additional training procedures may be needed to ensure generalized and spontaneous use of newly acquired communication skills.

4. Parents, siblings, teachers, peers, and front-line staff should be involved in developing and maintaining the communication intervention to help ensure that the communication skills acquired by the individual will be maintained.

References

American Psychiatric Association. (1994). *Diagnostic and statistical manual of mental disorders* (4th ed.). Washington, DC: Author.

Anderson, A. E. (2002). Augmentative communication and autism: A comparison of sign language and the Picture Exchange Communication System (Doctoral dissertation, University of California at Santa Barbara, 2001). *Dissertation Abstracts International: Section B: The Sciences and Engineering, 62,* 4269.

Bambara, L. M., & Warren, S. F. (1993). Massed trials revisited: Appropriate applications in functional skill training. In R. A. Gable & S. F. Warran (Eds.), *Strategies for teaching students with mild to severe mental retardation* (pp. 165–190). Baltimore: Brookes.

Barrera, R., & Sulzer-Azaroff, B. (1983). An alternating treatment comparison of oral and total communication training programs for echolalic autistic children. *Journal of Applied Behavior Analysis, 16,* 379–394.

Bebko, J. M. (1990). Echolalia, mitigation, and autism: Indicators from child characteristics for the use of sign language and other augmentative language systems. *Sign Language Studies, 66,* 61–78.

Bondy, A., & Frost, L. (2001). The Picture Exchange Communication System. *Behavior Modification, 25,* 725–744.

Bondy, A., Tincani, M., & Frost, L. (2004). Multiply controlled verbal operants: An analysis and extension of the Picture Exchange Communication System. *The Behavior Analyst, 27,* 247–261.

Carr, E. G. (1982). Sign language. In R. Koegel, A. Rincover, & A. Egel (Eds.), *Educating and understanding autistic children* (pp. 142–157). San Diego, CA: College Hill Press.

Carr, E. G., Binkoff, J. A., Kologinsky, E., & Eddy, M. (1978). Acquisition of sign language by autistic children: I. Expressive labeling. *Journal of Applied Behavior Analysis, 11,* 489–501.

Carr, E. G., & Kemp, D. C. (1989). Functional equivalence of autistic leading and communicative pointing: Analysis and treatment. *Journal of Autism and Developmental Disorders, 19,* 561–578.

Carr, E. G., Schreibman, L., & Lovaas, O. I. (1975). Control of echolalic speech in psychotic children. *Journal of Abnormal Child Psychology, 3,* 331–351.

Charlop, M. H. (1986). Setting effects on the occurrence of autistic children's immediate echolalia. *Journal of Autism and Developmental Disorders, 16,* 473–483.

Charlop, M. H., Schreibman, L., & Thibodeau, M. G. (1985). Increasing spontaneous verbal responding in autistic children using a time delay procedure. *Journal of Applied Behavior Analysis, 18,* 155–166.

Charlop-Christy, M. H., Carpenter, M., Le, L., LeBlanc, L. A., & Kellet, K. (2002). Using the Picture Exchange Communication System (PECS) with children with autism: Assessment of PECS acquisition, speech, social–communicative behavior, and problem behavior. *Journal of Applied Behavior Analysis, 35,* 213–231.

Delprato, D. J. (2001). Comparisons of discrete-trial and normalized behavioral intervention for young children with autism. *Journal of Autism and Developmental Disorders, 31,* 315–325.

Drasgow, E., Halle, J., & Sigafoos, J. (1999). Teaching communication to learners with severe disabilities: Motivation, response competition, and generalization. *Australasian Journal of Special Education, 23,* 47–63.

Duker, P. C. (1988). *Teaching the developmentally handicapped communicative gesturing.* Berwyn, PA: Swets.

Duker, P. C., Didden, R., & Sigafoos, J. (2004). *One-to-one training: Instructional procedures for individuals with developmental disabilities.* Austin, TX: PRO-ED.

Duker, P. C., & Jutten, W. (1997). Establishing gestural yes–no responding with individuals with profound mental retardation. *Education and Training in Mental Retardation and Developmental Disabilities, 32,* 59–67.

Duker, P. C., & Moonen, X. M. (1985). A program to increase manual signs with severely/profoundly mentally retarded students in natural environments. *Applied Research in Mental Retardation, 6,* 147–158.

Duker, P. C., van Driel, S., & van de Bercken, J. (2002). Communication profiles of individuals with Down's syndrome, Angelman syndrome and pervasive developmental disorder. *Journal of Intellectual Disability Research, 46,* 35–40.

Ferster, C. B. (1961). Positive reinforcement and behavioral deficits of autistic children. *Child Development, 32,* 437–456.

Foxx, R. M., McMorrow, M. J., Faw, G. D., Kyle, M. S., & Bittle, R. G. (1987). Cues-pause-point language training: Structuring trainer statements to students with correct answers to questions. *Behavioral Residential Treatment, 2,* 103–115.

Ganz, J. B., & Simpson, R. L. (2004). Effects on communicative requesting and speech development of the Picture Exchange Communication System in children with characteristics of autism. *Journal of Autism & Developmental Disorders, 34,* 395–409.

Hadano, K., Nakamura, H., & Toshihiko, H. (1998). Effortful echolalia. *Cortex, 34,* 67–82.

Halle, J. W. (1987). Teaching language in the natural environment: An analysis of spontaneity. *Journal of the Association for Persons with Severe Handicaps, 12,* 28–37.

Hamilton, B. L., & Snell, M. E. (1993). Using the milieu approach to increase spontaneous communication book use across environments by an adolescent with autism. *Augmentative and Alternative Communication, 9,* 259–272.

Harwood, K., Warren, S., & Yoder, P. (2002). The importance of responsivity in developing contingent exchanges with beginning communicators. In J. Reichle, D. R. Beukelman, & J. C. Light (Eds.), *Exemplary practices for beginning communicators* (pp. 59–95). Baltimore: Brookes.

Howlin, P. (1982). Echolalic and spontaneous phrase speech in autistic children. *Journal of Child Psychology & Psychiatry & Allied Disciplines, 23,* 281–293.

Kanner, L. (1971). Follow-up study of eleven autistic children originally reported in 1943. *Journal of Autism and Childhood Schizophrenia, 1,* 119–145.

Kanner, L. (1985). Autistic disturbances of affective contact. In A. M. Donnellan (Ed.), *Classic readings in autism* (pp. 11–53). New York: Teachers College Press. (Original work published 1943.)

Keen, D., Sigafoos, J., & Woodyatt, G. (2001). Replacing prelinguistic behaviors with functional communication. *Journal of Autism and Developmental Disorders, 31,* 385–398.

Lamarre, J., & Holland, P. C. (1985). The functional independence of mands and tacts. *Journal of the Experimental Analysis of Behavior, 43,* 5–19.

Losee, R. (1999). Communication defined as complementary informative processes. *Journal of Information, Communication, and Library Science, 5,* 1–15.

Lovaas, O. I. (1977). *The autistic child: Language development through behavior modification.* New York: Irvington.

Lovaas, O. I. (2002). *Teaching individuals with developmental delays: Basic intervention techniques.* Austin, TX: PRO-ED.

Lovaas, O. I., Berberich, J. P., Perloff, B. F., & Schaeffer, B. (1966). Acquisition of imitative speech by schizophrenic children. *Science, 151,* 705–707.

Lovaas, O. I., Newsom, C., & Hickman, C. (1987). Self-stimulatory behavior and perceptual reinforcement. *Journal of Applied Behavior Analysis, 20,* 45–68.

McMorrow, M. J., & Foxx, R. M. (1986). Some direct and generalized effects of replacing an autistic man's echolalia with correct responses to questions. *Journal of Applied Behavior Analysis, 19,* 289–297.

McMorrow, M. J., Foxx, R. M., Faw, G. D., & Bittle, R. G. (1987). Cues-pause-point language training: Teaching echolalics functional use of their verbal labeling repertoires. *Journal of Applied Behavior Analysis, 20,* 11–22.

Mirenda, P. (2003). Toward functional augmentative and alternative communication for students with autism: Manual signs, graphic symbols, and voice output communication aids. *Language, Speech, and Hearing Services in Schools, 34,* 203–216.

National Research Council. (2001). *Educating children with autism.* Washington, DC: National Academy Press.

Odom, S. L., Brown, W. H., Frey, T., Karasu, N., Smith-Carter, L. L., & Strain, P. S. (2003). Evidence-based practices for young children with autism: Contributions for single-subject design research. *Focus on Autism and Other Developmental Disabilities, 18,* 166–175.

Ogletree, B. T., Pierce, K., Harn, W. E., & Fisher, M. A. (2002). Assessment of communication and language in classical autism: Issues and practices. *Assessment for Effective Intervention, 27,* 61–71.

Paccia, J. M., & Curcio, F. (1982). Language processing and forms of immediate echolalia in autistic children. *Journal of Speech & Hearing Research, 25,* 42–47.

Partington, J. W., & Sundberg, M. L. (1998). *The Assessment of Basic Language and Learning Skills (the ABLLS): An assessment, curriculum guide, and skills tracking system for children with autism and other developmental disabilities: The ABLLS protocol.* Pleasant Hill, CA: Behavior Analysts.

Prizant, B. M., & Duchan, J. F. (1981). The functions of immediate echolalia in autistic children. *Journal of Speech & Hearing Disorders, 46,* 241–249.

Prizant, B. M., & Rydell, P. J. (1984). Analysis of functions of delayed echolalia in autistic children. *Journal of Speech & Hearing Research, 27,* 183–192.

Reichle, J., Drager, K., & Davis, C. (2002). Using requests for assistance to obtain desired items and to gain release from nonpreferred activities: Implications for assessment and intervention. *Education and Treatment of Children, 25,* 47–66.

Remington, B., & Clarke, S. (1983). Acquisition of expressive signing by autistic children: An evaluation of the relative effects of simultaneous communication and sign-along training. *Journal of Applied Behavior Analysis, 16,* 315–327.

Rhode, M. (1999). Echo or answer? The move towards ordinary speech in three children with autism spectrum disorder. In A. Alvarez & S. Reid (Eds.), *Autism and personality: Findings from the Tavistock Autism Workshop* (pp. 79–92). London: Routledge.

Roberts, J. (1989). Echolalia and comprehension in autistic children. *Journal of Autism and Developmental Disorders, 19,* 271–281.

Rotholz, D. A., Berkowitz, S. F., & Burberry, J. (1989). Functionality of two modes of communication in the community by students with developmental disabilities. A comparison of signing and communication books. *Journal of the Association for Persons with Severe Handicaps, 14,* 227–233.

Rydell, P. J., & Mirenda, P. (1991). The effects of two levels of linguistic constraint on echolalia and generative language production in children with autism. *Journal of Autism and Developmental Disorders, 21,* 131–157.

Schepis, M. M., & Reid, D. H. (2003). Issues affecting staff enhancement of speech generating device use among people with severe cognitive disabilities. *Augmentative and Alternative Communication, 19,* 59–65.

Schepis, M. M., Reid, D. H., Behrmann, M. M., & Sutton, K. A. (1998). Increasing communicative interaction of young children with autism using a voice output communication aid and naturalistic teaching. *Journal of Applied Behavior Analysis, 31,* 561–678.

Scheuermann, B., & Webber, J. (2002). *Autism: Teaching does make a difference.* Belmont, CA: Wadsworth/Thomson Learning.

Schloper, E., & Mesibov, G. B. (Eds.). (1985). *Communication problems in autism.* New York: Plenum Press.

Schlosser, R. W. (Ed.). (2003). *The efficacy of augmentative and alternative communication: Toward evidence-based practice.* Boston: Academic Press.

Schlosser, R. W., & Blischak, D. M. (2001). Is there a role for speech output in interventions for persons with autism? A review. *Focus on Autism and Other Developmental Disabilities, 16,* 170–178.

Schlosser, R. W., & Blischak, D. M. (2003). Evidence-based practice in support of communication in autism: A process illustration. In *Proceeding of the Korean Institute of Special Education, Annual International Symposium* (pp. 97–122) (with translation into Korean (pp. 125–148). Seoul, South Korea: Korean Institute of Special Education.

Schreibman, L., Kohlenberg, B. S., & Britten, K. R. (1986). Differential responding to content and intonation components of a complex auditory stimulus by nonverbal and echolalic autistic children. *Analysis & Intervention in Developmental Disabilities, 6,* 109–125.

Sigafoos, J. (1997). A review of communication intervention programs for people with developmental disabilities. *Behaviour Change, 14,* 125–138.

Sigafoos, J., Didden, R., & O'Reilly, M. (2003). Effects of speech output on maintenance of requesting and frequency of vocalizations in three children with developmental disabilities. *Augmentative and Alternative Communication, 19,* 37–47.

Sigafoos, J., Kerr, M., Roberts, D., & Couzens, D. (1994). Increasing opportunities for requesting in classrooms serving children with developmental disabilities. *Journal of Autism and Developmental Disorders, 24,* 631–645.

Sigafoos, J., & Mirenda, P. (2002). Strengthening communicative behavior for gaining and maintaining access to desired items and activities. In J. Reichle, D. R. Beukelman, & J. C. Light (Eds.), *Exemplary practices for beginning communicators: Implication for AAC* (pp. 123–156). Baltimore: Brookes.

Sigafoos, J., Roberts, D., Kerr, M., Couzens, D., & Baglioni, A. J. (1994). Opportunities for communication in classrooms serving children with developmental disabilities. *Journal of Autism and Developmental Disorders, 24,* 259–280.

Skinner, B. F. (1957). *Verbal behavior.* Englewood Cliffs, NJ: Prentice Hall.

Smith, I. M., & Bryson, S. E. (1998). Gesture imitation in autism I: Nonsymbolic postures and sequences. *Cognitive Neuropsychology, 15,* 747–770.

Sosne, J. B., Handleman, J. S., & Harris, S. L. (1979). Teaching spontaneous-functional speech to autistic-type children. *Mental Retardation, 17,* 241–244.

Stokes, T. F., & Baer, D. M. (1977). An implicit technology of generalization. *Journal of Applied Behavior Analysis, 10,* 349–367.

Sturmey, P., & Sevin, J. A. (1994). Defining and assessing autism. In J. L. Matson (Ed.), *Autism in children and adults: Etiology, assessment, and intervention* (pp. 13–36). Pacific Grove, CA: Brooks/Cole.

Sundberg, M. L. (1993). The application of establishing operations. *The Behavior Analyst, 16,* 211–214.

Sundberg, M. L., Loeb, M., Hale, L., & Eigenheer, P. (2002). Contriving establishing operations to teach mands for information. *Analysis of Verbal Behavior, 18,* 15–29.

Sundberg, M. L., & Michael, J. (2001). The benefits of Skinner's analysis of verbal behavior for children with autism. *Behavior Modification, 25,* 698–724.

Tait, K., Sigafoos, J., Woodyatt, G., O'Reilly, M. F., & Lancioni, G. E. (2004). Evaluating parent use of functional communication training to replace and enhance prelinguistic behaviours in six children with developmental and physical disabilities. *Disability & Rehabilitation, 26,* 1241–1254.

Tincani, M. (2004). Comparing the Picture Exchange Communication System and sign language training for children with autism. *Focus on Autism and Other Developmental Disabilities, 19,* 152–163.

Wetherby, A. M., & Prizant, B. M. (1992). Profiling young children's communicative competence. In S. Warren & J. Reichle (Eds.), *Causes and effects in communication and language intervention* (Vol. 1, pp. 217–253). Baltimore: Brookes.

Wetherby, A. M., & Prizant, B. M. (2000). *Autism spectrum disorders: A transactional developmental perspective.* Baltimore: Brookes.

Woods, T. S. (1984). Generality in the verbal tacting of autistic children as a function of the "naturalness" in antecedent control. *Journal of Behavior Therapy and Experimental Psychiatry, 15,* 27–32.

Yoder, P., & Layton, T. (1988). Speech following sign language training in autistic children with minimal verbal language. *Journal of Autism and Developmental Disorders, 18,* 217–229.

CHAPTER

FUNCTIONAL APPROACHES TO ASSESSMENT AND TREATMENT OF PROBLEM BEHAVIOR IN PERSONS WITH AUTISM AND RELATED DISABILITIES

Richard G. Smith
University of North Texas

Timothy R. Vollmer and Claire St. Peter Pipkin
University of Florida

Often, persons with autism display maladaptive patterns of behavior including stereotyped (repetitive and apparently nonpurposeful) movements, self-injurious behavior (SIB), aggression, and tantrums, among others (see Table 7.1). Problem behavior exhibited by persons with autism may interfere with social and other activities, restrict opportunities for appropriate learning to occur, and, in extreme cases such as severe and chronic SIB, be life threatening.

Problem behavior associated with autism can be among the most obvious and dramatic symptoms. Whereas behavioral deficits, such as difficulties in acquiring language or other communication skills, academic underachievement, and lack of interest in imaginative activities, may not be immediately obvious to casual observers, behavioral excesses, such as SIB, aggression, and stereotypy, immediately distinguish persons with autism from their peers and can result

TABLE 7.1
Typical Forms of Problem Behavior Exhibited by Persons with Autism

Problem behavior	Definition	Examples
Aggression	Behavior that produces or has the capacity to produce tissue damage to the body of another person	Hitting, grabbing, biting, kicking, pulling hair, scratching, spitting, pinching
Stereotypy	Repetitive, apparently purposeless patterns of behavior; the individual may appear to be so deeply involved in engaging in the behavior that attempts to redirect the person are ineffective or may result in aggression, self-injury, or other maladaptive responses	Body rocking, body spinning, flapping hands in front of eyes, head movements, perseverative vocalizations or verbalizations, repetitive object manipulation (e.g., plate spinning, arranging toys in a single line), unusual preoccupation with certain toys or items
Mouthing	Placement of indigestible nonfood items in the mouth	Hand mouthing or sucking, object mouthing or sucking
Pica	Ingestion of indigestible nonfood items	Eating coins, toys, clothing items, cigarette butts, paper, or any other item not intended for human consumption
Self-injury	Behavior that produces or has the capacity to produce tissue damage to the individual's own body	Self-scratching, head or body hitting, head banging, eye poking, self-biting, self-pinching, pulling out teeth
Property destruction	Behavior that results in damage to tangible items in the environment	Striking, turning over, throwing, kicking, or otherwise destroying or producing damage to furniture, books, toys, or other items in the environment
Tantrums/ disruption	Behavior that disrupts ongoing activities and events	Screaming, crying, throwing body to the ground; may also include other forms of problem behavior such as SIB, aggression, and property destruction
Elopement	Unauthorized departure	Running away from school, home, or other settings

in stigmatization and ostracism from the community, in addition to the more direct impact on the person's quality of life. Therefore, successful assessment and treatment of behavioral excesses associated with autism are critical to the establishment of an improved quality of life for persons with autism and their families.

A Brief History of the Functional-Analytic Approach to Behavior Disorders

Over the last two decades, substantial progress has been made toward an understanding and the development of effective treatments for problem behavior. In particular, the development of a general approach known as "functional analysis" has proven particularly useful in providing a conceptual and methodological foundation for assessment and intervention (Iwata, Dorsey, Slifer, Bauman, & Richman, 1982/1994). This approach grew from Skinner's (1953) account of human behavior, which emphasizes the role of consequences in the establishment and maintenance of human behavior. The behavioral process of reinforcement is central to a functional analysis of challenging behavior observed in persons with autism and related disabilities. Prior to the late 1970s, most researchers and practitioners who were interested in behavior disorders focused on examining the effects of various treatment procedures on different types of problem behavior. Thus, clinical research and practice emphasized *structural characteristics* of both the behavior and its corresponding treatment approach, largely ignoring the underlying functional characteristics of each. For example, some practitioners might ask, "What is the best treatment for self-injury?" focusing on the topography rather than the function. Instead the practitioner should ask, "What variables control this behavior and which treatments are indicated and contraindicated by this information?" In the absence of an understanding of the *functional characteristics* of problem behavior (i.e., knowledge about the factors that contribute to the occurrence of the behavior), treatments typically incorporated the use of powerful but arbitrarily chosen reinforcers or punishers. Sometimes these efforts were successful (e.g., Bostow & Bailey, 1969); however, failures also occurred, and the prevalence of treatment failures is impossible to estimate because failures are infrequently published in the literature (Scotti, Evans, Meyer, & Walker, 1991). However, it may be instructive to consider the outcomes of a 1989 consensus conference indicating that punishment appeared to have more empirical evidence supporting its efficacy as treatment for severe behavior problems, relative to other behavioral or pharmacological treatments (National Institutes of Health, 1989). Moreover, based on the outcomes of a recent review of the literature on treatment of self-injury and aggression that showed that (a) relatively few studies were published on these topics prior to the mid-1970s and (b) a large proportion of studies published prior to the early 1980s reported the use of punishment procedures, it is reasonable to conclude that less intrusive interventions often met with limited success (Pelios, Morren, Tesch, & Axelrod, 1999).

The role of reinforcement in the development and maintenance of challenging behavior had been considered prior to the 1980s. In fact, the logic and methods of functional analysis were apparent in some of the earliest published examples of applied behavior analysis (e.g., Ayllon & Michael, 1959; Bijou, Peterson, & Ault, 1968; Lovaas, Freitag, Gold, & Kassorla, 1965). However, two pivotal publications signaled the birth of a revolutionary reformulation of how applied behavior analysts viewed and treated severe problem behaviors. Carr's (1977) conceptual review of the "motivation" of self-injury articulated three specific accounts of contingencies of reinforcement that might explain the occurrence of this type of challenging behavior: the *positive reinforcement* hypothesis, the *negative reinforcement* hypothesis, and the *self-stimulation* hypothesis. More recently, the term *automatic reinforcement* has largely replaced self-stimulation in the technical nomenclature. Carr's paper influenced the field in at least three important ways. First, it strongly indicated that much self-injury was operant in nature, maintained by either positive reinforcement, negative reinforcement, or self-stimulation (automatic reinforcement). Second, his review of the treatment literature indicated that different contingencies of reinforcement maintained problem behavior for different people. This notion carried important implications for treatment. If maladaptive behavior is maintained by different contingencies across people, then it might be important to develop treatments on an individual basis. For example, if one individual's head banging is maintained by positive reinforcement in the form of attention from caregivers, and another individual's head banging is maintained by negative reinforcement in the form of escape from task requirements, then a treatment approach that would be expected to be effective for one person's SIB (e.g., time-out for SIB maintained by positive reinforcement) might be ineffective or even deleterious for the other person's SIB (e.g., time-out might actually function as reinforcement for behavior maintained by escape from task requirements). Thus, the third general contribution of Carr's article was to emphasize the importance of knowing at the outset of treatment development what type(s) of reinforcement contingency maintained the problem behavior of the person referred for treatment.

The conceptual work of Carr, along with early applications (e.g., Ayllon & Michael, 1959), set the stage for the development of the first systematic and comprehensive approach to the identification of the reinforcement contingencies maintaining problem behavior on an individual basis. Iwata and his colleagues' (1982/1994) description of a standardized procedure to assess the operant function of self-injury was quickly recognized as a revolutionary development toward understanding the causes of SIB. This procedure allowed researchers and practitioners to conduct individualized analyses of the contingencies that maintained self-injury exhibited by different people.

Although both Carr's (1997) conceptual review and Iwata and his colleagues' (1982/1994) methodological innovation focused on self-injury, the logic and procedures of functional analysis were soon replicated and extended with other behavior disorders, including aggression (Carr, Newsom, & Binkoff, 1980), tantrums (Vollmer, Northup, Ringdahl, LeBlanc, & Chauvin, 1996), stereotypy (Mace, Browder, & Lin, 1987), bizarre vocalizations (Mace & Lalli, 1991), pica (Mace & Knight, 1986; Piazza, Hanley, & Fisher, 1996), property destruction (Bowman, Fisher, Thompson, & Piazza, 1997), mouthing (Goh et al., 1995), hair pulling (Miltenberger, Long, Rapp, Lumley, & Elliot, 1998), noncompliance (Reimers et al., 1993), running away (Piazza et al., 1997), as well as other behavior (see Hanley, Iwata, & McCord, 2003, for a comprehensive review of the functional analysis literature, including a listing of topographical variations assessed across 277 studies).

Functional analysis methods proved to be an extraordinarily fruitful research platform, yielding a body of information that allowed for broad consensus about the operant functions of problem behavior. For example, Carr's (1977) hypotheses that self-injury could be maintained by contingencies of positive reinforcement, negative reinforcement, and automatic reinforcement have received broad support across hundreds of studies (Hanley et al., 2003). In fact, further conceptual development of an operant account of problem behavior has identified four general categories of maintaining contingencies.

First, behavior disorders can be maintained by *social positive reinforcement.* This occurs when the problem behavior is followed by a change in the behavior of another person, resulting in presentation of some type of positive reinforcer into the environment. For example, self-injury may be maintained by social positive reinforcement if it produces attention in the form of statements of concern from teachers, parents, or caregivers. Alternatively, problem behavior may be maintained by *social negative reinforcement.* This occurs when the problem behavior is followed by a change in the behavior of another person such that escape from or avoidance of some aversive event or condition is enabled. For example, self-injury may be maintained by negative reinforcement if caregivers allow the person to escape from nonpreferred or aversive therapy or training routines. Problem behavior may also be maintained via contingencies of *automatic positive reinforcement.* This occurs when the problem behavior is followed by some type of positive reinforcement that is not delivered, or mediated, by another person. For example, if the visual stimulation produced by hand flapping serves as reinforcement, then hand flapping is said to be maintained by automatic positive reinforcement. Finally, problem behavior can be maintained by *automatic negative reinforcement.* This occurs when problem behavior is followed by the termination or avoidance of some aversive event or condition that is not mediated by another person. For example, if scratching one's body reduces aversive stimulation arising from an allergic skin condition, then it is said to be maintained by automatic negative reinforcement.

Since Iwata and his colleagues' (1982/1994) seminal description of an experimental method for identifying the environmental determinants of problem behavior, three general approaches to functional assessment have evolved: experimental analysis, descriptive assessment, and anecdotal assessment. Each of these approaches has a common goal: to identify the contingencies of reinforcement that maintain problem behavior. However, these approaches differ from one another in important ways, with each having relative strengths and limitations. For example, an important distinction between experimental analysis procedures and anecdotal or descriptive assessments has to do with the term *analysis*. Similar terms are used to denote functional assessment, functional analysis, and functional behavioral assessment. We use the term *functional assessment* to refer to any procedure or set of procedures designed to produce information about the events or conditions that precede or follow problem behavior. *Functional analysis* refers to a particular type of functional assessment that involves systematic manipulation of the events that precede and follow problem behavior while measuring their effects on the behavior of interest. Finally, *functional behavioral assessment* is a term that has been used in recent legislation (Individuals with Disabilities Education Act [IDEA], 2004) referring to the collection of a broad range of information (including, but not limited to, the events that precede and follow behavior) that can be used to inform the development of effective interventions for problem behavior.

Experimental procedures constitute *analyses* of operant function in that the effects of various contingencies on problem behavior are systematically demonstrated through manipulation of those contingencies. Descriptive assessment procedures involve observing target behavior in the absence of any systematic manipulation, and anecdotal assessment procedures involve gathering information about the problem behavior and its potential determinants via checklists, interviews, and other indirect methods. Thus, although each general variation assesses the operant function, only experimental methods result in a direct and systematic analysis of operant function.

Experimental Analysis

The experimental analysis, or *functional analysis*, described by Iwata and his colleagues in their seminal 1982 paper is largely recognized as the first comprehensive and "standardized" approach to assessing the functional properties of problem behavior. Although a few alternative methodologies for conducting functional analyses have been suggested (e.g., Carr & Durand, 1985), the basic procedures described by Iwata and colleagues has proven remarkably practical, durable, and general. Several methodological variations and extensions of functional analysis procedures have seen varying degrees of acceptance among researchers and practitioners (e.g., brief functional analyses [Derby et al., 1992; Vollmer, Marcus, Ringdahl, & Roane, 1995]; functional analyses of precursor behaviors [Smith & Churchill, 2002]); however, the basic format described by Iwata and his colleagues remains the foundation of most experimental analysis procedures for identifying the operant function of problem behavior.

Functional analysis usually involves exposing participants to a series of test conditions, each of which is designed to simulate a potential contingency of reinforcement for problem behavior, along with a control, or baseline condition, against which to compare the outcomes of the test conditions (functional analysis procedures are sometimes termed *analog analyses* because the test conditions are analogous to conditions thought to evoke and maintain problem behavior in the natural environment). The conditions are usually presented within a multi-element format (Sidman, 1960) in which sessions from each type of condition are rapidly alternated, either randomly or according to a prescribed sequence. However, some researchers have proposed using alternative formats such as *reversal designs* in which the presentation of test and control conditions occurs one at a time, conducting each condition until stability is observed in the outcomes (e.g., Vollmer, Iwata, Duncan, & Lerman, 1993) or *sequential test–control designs* during which presentation of test conditions occurs one at a time while interspersing control condition sessions throughout the analysis (Iwata, Duncan, Zarcone, Lerman, & Shore, 1994). When one or another of the test conditions results in increased levels of problem behavior relative to the control condition, a potential source of reinforcement for the problem behavior has been identified. Thus, a rough analogy can be drawn between functional analysis procedures and common allergy testing procedures in which patients are systematically exposed to small amounts of potential allergens in order to identify allergic sensitivities. Similarly, functional analysis arranges systematic and controlled exposure to potential maintaining contingencies in order to identify behavioral sensitivities to those contingencies.

Testing for Social Positive Reinforcement

Attention Conditions

The attention that often follows problem behavior can serve as positive reinforcement for that behavior. Statements of concern, reprimands, touching, and even guided compliance procedures have been shown to be forms of attention that can maintain problem behavior (Vollmer, Iwata, Smith, & Rodgers, 1992). In a typical test condition for attention, the participant has access to some leisure or recreational items while a therapist engages in some work or other activities that do not involve the participant. The therapist may briefly interact (e.g., for 5 to 10 s) with the participant before starting the session. If the participant displays problem behavior, the therapist stops what he or she is doing and provides brief (e.g., 5-s) attention in one or more of the forms described above. For example, while saying, "Don't do that; you're hurting me," the therapist may also gently block an aggressive participant's arm, or pat the participant's back in a "calming" motion. If more problem behavior is observed during this condition relative to a control condition, then the therapist may conclude that the participant's problem behavior is maintained because it produces attention.

Tangible Conditions

A range of items and activities that are delivered by other people as consequences, such as toys and other leisure and recreational items, food, and access to music or other activities, have been shown to reinforce problem behavior (Hanley et al., 2003). Conditions designed to test whether problem behavior is maintained by tangible reinforcement are often incorporated as standard test conditions or are added to a functional analysis if maintenance by tangible reinforcement is suspected. Typically, a tangible condition is similar to an attention condition, with the exception that the item or activity suspected of maintaining problem behavior is briefly presented as a consequence for problem behavior. The therapist may allow the participant to interact with the item or activity briefly (the time period may vary depending on the nature of the item or activity) and then withdraw it to begin the assessment. If the participant displays problem behavior, the therapist presents the item or activity briefly and then withdraws it again. These procedures are repeated throughout the session and, if more problem behavior is observed during this condition relative to a control condition, then the therapist may conclude that the participant's problem behavior is maintained because it produces access to certain items or activities.

Testing for Social Negative Reinforcement (Demand or Escape)

For some individuals, problem behavior results in the termination or avoidance of potentially aversive or nonpreferred situations or activities. A range of stimuli that are controlled by other people, such as requests to perform difficult tasks, therapeutic routines, noise, close contact, and medical examinations, have been shown to occasion problem behavior. Test conditions for negative reinforcement typically begin with the presentation of the event or condition thought to function as an aversive stimulus in the participant's natural environment. The most common events used to test for negative reinforcement are task demands. The specific tasks and presentation styles may vary, depending on the type of situation the participant normally encounters. During the task, if the participant engages in problem behavior, the therapist turns away from the participant and stops delivering task demands. If the participant continues to engage in problem behavior, other scheduled trials may be delayed. If more problem behavior is observed during this condition relative to a control condition, then the therapist may conclude that the participant's problem behavior persists because it produces escape from, or avoidance of, nonpreferred or aversive task demands.

Testing for Automatic Reinforcement (Alone, or No Interaction Condition)

Some individuals engage in problem behavior that does not seem to be affected by social consequences. In many cases, some aspects of the behavior the person is engaging in produce positively reinforcing consequences. For example, problem behavior such as eye poking may be maintained because it produces direct stimulation to the optic nerve, causing an experience of flashing light or colors (Favell, McGimsey, & Schell, 1982), or hand mouthing may be maintained because it produces stimulation to the hand or the mouth (Goh et al., 1995). On the other hand, problem behavior may be maintained via contingencies of automatic negative reinforcement, as when excessive self-scratching appears to maintain because it reduces aversive itching (Cowdery, Iwata, & Pace, 1990) or when self-injurious ear poking is maintained because it reduces stimulation arising from an ear infection (O'Reilly, 1997).

Behavior that is maintained in the absence of an identifiable source of social reinforcement presents a unique set of challenges for researchers and clinicians. In most cases, it is not possible to complete an analysis of the maintaining consequences because it is not possible to directly control those consequences (Vollmer, 1994). Consider that, in tests for both social positive reinforcement and social negative reinforcement, the presentation or removal of stimuli is directly manipulated by the therapist, and therefore conclusions about its effects can be drawn with a high degree of confidence. However, therapists often have no means to directly control potentially reinforcing events such as stimulation to the optic nerve as a consequence for eye poking or relief from an earache as a consequence for ear hitting. Therefore, inferences must often be based on indirect evidence about the maintaining contingencies. Typically, when testing for automatic reinforcement, a condition is arranged in which no cues for social reinforcement (e.g., people, potentially reinforcing items) are present in the environment, no social consequences are programmed, and no potentially aversive stimuli (e.g., task requests, therapeutic routines) are presented. If problem behavior persists in the absence of social cues or consequences, then the therapist may conclude that the participant's problem behavior is maintained because it produces some sort of automatically reinforcing consequence.

It is sometimes possible to make some inferences about the specific contingencies maintaining automatically reinforced problem behavior based on characteristics of the behavior, its patterns, or reactions to other stimuli in the environment. For example, if functional analysis outcomes show that problem behavior occurs reliably and almost exclusively during alone sessions, the therapist may suspect that a contingency of automatic positive reinforcement maintains the problem behavior. Such outcomes indicate that the behavior is most likely to occur during unstructured periods or situations that provide little stimulation, which increases the reinforcing effectiveness of self-produced stimulation. Alternatively, if problem behavior is maintained by a contingency of automatic negative reinforcement, one might expect the behavior to occur across several of the test (or even control) conditions because the aversive events that motivate the behavior (e.g., skin rashes, ear infections) would be present across conditions. Another pattern of responding suggestive of a contingency of automatic negative reinforcement would be cyclical responding, in which the behavior is observed across conditions but waxes and wanes over time. Overall increases and decreases in problem behavior that correspond with the presence and absence of potentially aversive conditions (e.g., skin rashes, ear infections) would provide further indirect evidence about the contingency of reinforcement for problem behavior. Finally, the form, or topography, of the behavior itself can suggest the type of reinforcement maintaining the behavior. Clearly, visual stimulation is a potential reinforcing consequence for eye poking, relief from discomfort associated with a dermatological problem is a potential reinforcing consequence for self-scratching, and so on.

Control or Comparison Conditions

Most functional analyses include a condition designed to function as a control or comparison condition against which measures of problem behavior derived from the test conditions are compared. Control conditions, often termed "play" conditions, are designed to reduce the likelihood of producing problem behavior maintained by the contingencies being tested. For example, to reduce the likelihood of producing problem behavior maintained by social positive reinforcement, a therapist delivers attention throughout the session, and potentially reinforcing items and activities are readily available. To reduce the likelihood of producing problem behavior maintained by social negative reinforcement, no activities or events thought to function as aversive stimuli (e.g., task demands) are presented during the session. The presence of social interaction and stimulating materials and activities reduces the likelihood of producing problem behavior maintained by automatic reinforcement. Finally, there are typically no programmed consequences for problem behavior that occurs during the control condition.

Descriptive Assessment

An alternative approach to identifying the operant function of problem behavior is the use of descriptive assessment procedures. *Descriptive assessment* involves observing and recording occurrences of the behavior in the environments in which it typically occurs (Bijou, Peterson, & Ault, 1968). Most often, potentially important antecedent and consequent events also are recorded, so that correlations between these events and problem behavior can be identified during data analysis. This type of assessment differs from functional analysis in that no environmental events are directly manipulated and, therefore, inferences about maintaining contingencies can be made only on the basis of correlations between environmental events and behavior, rather than experimental demonstrations of functional relations.

At least three general types of descriptive assessment can be found in the behavioral literature: assessments that involve only recording of the behavior and, perhaps, the time it occurred (e.g., scatter plot; Touchette, MacDonald, & Langer, 1985); assessments that involve recording the behavior when it occurs, as well as the antecedent and subsequent conditions that surround it (e.g., antecedent-behavior-consequence, or ABC, assessments; Bijou et al., 1968); and assessments that involve continuous recording of behavior and potentially relevant environmental events throughout observation intervals (e.g., Lerman & Iwata, 1993).

Scatter Plots

The *scatter plot method* for assessing problem behavior was first introduced by Touchette and his colleagues (1985). The scatter plot is a data sheet that is divided into a grid, which denotes time of day vertically and successive days horizontally (Figure 7.1). When problem behavior is observed, a mark is recorded on the location of the grid corresponding to the time and date of the occurrence.

SCATTER PLOT DATA COLLECTION FOR: _____ MONTH: _____

	1	2	3	4	5	6	7	8	9	10	11	12	13	14	15	16	17	18	19	20	21	22	23	24	25	26	27	28	29	30	31
6:00–6:15																															
6:15–6:30																															
6:30–6:45																															
6:45–7:00																															
7:00–7:15																															
7:15–7:30																															
7:30–7:45																															
7:45–8:00																															
8:00–8:15																															
8:15–8:30																															
8:30–8:45																															
8:45–9:00																															
9:00–9:15																															
9:15–9:30																															
9:30–9:45																															
9:45–10:00																															
10:00–10:15																															
10:15–10:30																															
10:30–10:45																															
10:45–11:00																															
11:00–11:15																															
11:15–11:30																															
11:30–11:45																															
11:45–12:00																															
12:00–12:15																															
12:15–12:30																															
12:30–12:45																															
12:45–1:00																															
1:00–1:15																															
1:15–1:30																															
1:30–1:45																															
1:45–2:00																															
2:00–2:15																															
2:15–2:30																															
2:30–2:45																															
2:45–3:00																															
3:00–3:15																															
3:15–3:30																															
3:30–3:45																															
3:45–4:00																															
4:00–4:15																															
4:15–4:30																															
4:30–4:45																															
4:45–5:00																															
5:00–5:15																															
5:15–5:30																															
5:30–5:45																															
5:45–6:00																															
TOTALS																															

TARGET BEHAVIORS:
1 _____
2 _____
3 _____

LEGEND:
☐: _____
☐: _____
☐: _____

NOTES:

Figure 7.1. Example of a typical scatter plot format.

As more problem behavior occurs and is recorded on the scatter plot, a visual depiction of how the behavior is distributed over time begins to emerge. Based on this information, the user can conduct more systematic observations during periods when problem behavior is most likely to occur. Alternatively, if the results of the scatter plot point to specific environmental influences on the behavior, corresponding adjustments can be made. For example, Touchette and colleagues (1985) described a case in which the outcomes of a scatter plot indicated that the self-injury of one participant occurred primarily after 3:00 P.M. This time corresponded with a number of changes in the participant's routine, including a change in afternoon activities, an increase in the number of peers present following their return from school, and the presence of a new staff member following the 3:00 P.M. shift change. Experimenters altered one of these elements—the presence of the staff member—by changing shifts so that the aide typically assigned to work in the afternoon worked in the morning and vice versa. The participant's self-injury began to occur during the morning shift. A return to the original schedule again produced a shift in self-injury to afternoon hours. Thus, the researchers were able to determine that the presence of a particular aide set the occasion for the participant's problem behavior, and subsequently a schedule was arranged so that contact between the aide and the participant was minimized. Although this resulted in elimination of the participant's self-injury, the specific reasons why it was exacerbated by the presence of the aide were never determined. This highlights a limitation of the scatter plot and of descriptive assessments more generally. Such assessments do not typically permit a definitive analysis of the specific operant contingencies controlling problem behaviors, and therefore it may be difficult or impossible to identify the reasons why interventions such as changes in schedules or personnel are effective in decreasing problem behaviors.

Another potential drawback of the scatter plot method is that, unless the participant's daily schedule is relatively constant, the scatter plot may fail to reveal orderly patterns of responding. For example, Kahng and colleagues (1998) evaluated the outcomes of 15 scatter plots to determine whether temporal patterns of responding could be discerned. These investigators were unable to identify orderly patterns in any scatter plot via visual inspection. Although the application of statistical process control procedures indicated that intervals could be identified during which problem behavior was more likely to occur for 12 of the 15 data sets, the utility of using such a procedure is not clear.

ABC Recording

The *antecedent-behavior-consequence model* is similar to the scatter plot in that data are recorded only at times when problem behavior occurs; however, ABC analyses also include recording of immediately prior and subsequent events. That is, although data are not continuously collected on the potentially relevant environmental events, this type of analysis permits an evaluation of the types of conditions and events that are typically present before occurrences of problem behavior, as well as those that are present following the behavior. If certain events or conditions are found to be consistently present before or after occurrences of problem behavior, then it may be inferred that these events play a part in evoking (for antecedent events) or maintaining (for subsequent events) the problem behavior. Although the use of ABC procedures as a primary mode of functional assessment is rarely seen in the applied behavior analytic literature, ABC assessments have become commonly used by clinicians. The prevalence of ABC assessments in schools is likely due to language in the IDEA (1997) legislation requiring the use of functional behavioral assessment in the development of positive behavior interventions and support plans. Although the legislation did not include specific guidelines to guide the process of functional behavioral assessment, several structured approaches to the assessment have been developed that incorporate the use of data generated through the ABC model (Liaupsin, Scott, & Nelson, 2000; O'Neill et al., 1997).

ABC assessments may be structured, with the observer "selecting" from predetermined categories of antecedent, behavioral, and subsequent events that are represented on the data sheet (e.g., Pyles & Bailey, 1990). Alternatively, the assessment may be open ended, in the sense that the data sheet contains blank spaces or cells into which the observer writes a freehand description of the antecedent, behavioral, and subsequent events. Each method has strengths and limitations. For example, categorizing events permits consistency and standardization in measurement with the use of operationalized definitions that may improve the validity of the assessment. On the other hand, open-ended assessments permit the observer to document potentially important events that may not be captured within narrowly defined categories. Therefore, many researchers and clinicians suggest using a combination of open-ended and structured assessments, which contain both lists of potentially important antecedent and consequential events as well as space in which to enter other potentially relevant events and conditions that are not included in the list.

A general limitation of ABC assessments is that they do not account for events that occur beyond those occurring just before and after problem behavior. By documenting only immediate antecedents and consequences, ABC assessments omit at least two potentially important pieces of information: identification of orderly relations between the problem behavior and events that occur between instances of the problem behavior and identification of the extent to which the events identified in the ABC assessment also occur at other times when the problem behavior is not occurring. The advantages of knowing about environmental events that coincide with problem behavior—whether they occur in close temporal proximity or not—are obvious. There is no reason to doubt that temporally distant events and conditions can influence behavior. The effects of events that occur outside of the immediate three-term contingency of reinforcement, such as sleep patterns (O'Reilly, 1995), recency of attention from caregivers (O'Reilly, 1999), illness (O'Reilly, 1997), and the time that one awakens in the morning (Kennedy & Itkonen, 1993), have been demonstrated in the literature. ABC assessments do not identify these potentially important influences. The importance of knowing the extent to which the stimuli identified to occur just before or after problem behavior (as identified in an ABC assessment) also occur at other times is perhaps less obvious. Briefly, to identify contingencies between events (such as behavior and its consequences), it is necessary to show that values, or measures, of one event change as a result of changes in the value of the other event. So, a contingency between behavior and a consequence is shown only when one knows that the event is more likely to be present in the environment after behavior than at other times—and it is necessary to record those events at those other times to know that. These two issues are addressed in another type of descriptive assessment, continuous recording, that will be discussed in the next section.

Continuous Recording

Continuous recording procedures involve direct observation and documentation of environmental and behavioral events as they occur in real time. A variety of specific recording methods have been used, but those used most often are *interval recording procedures,* in which observation periods are divided into equal time units (e.g., 10 s) for observation, and individual intervals are marked as containing or not containing instances of the behavior. With *partial-interval recording,* intervals are marked as containing the behavior if it is observed to occur at least once during the interval. Typically, the number of intervals are summed, divided by the total number of intervals in the observation period, and then multiplied by 100% to derive a percentage of intervals containing the behavior. Continuous recording procedures address one of the limitations of ABC recording by providing records not only of events immediately surrounding occurrences of problem behavior but also of events occurring at other times. Ongoing data are collected on environmental events and conditions that may include the presence of and interactions with other people, presentation or availability of tangible items, task presentation and withdrawal, ongoing activities, and so on. Thus, correlations may be seen between behavior and events that occur at other times during the observation period. For example, consider a case in which a mother's exit from the vicinity reliably sets the occasion for a child's problem behavior to occur 5 min later. Whereas the ABC assessment would not capture this important event, continuous recording that included measures of the coming and going of other people could reveal the correlation between the mother's exit and the subsequent problem behavior.

Another recent advance in descriptive assessment is actually a sort of hybrid method, incorporating procedures from both descriptive assessment and experimental analysis. *Structured descriptive assessment* (SDA) uses aspects of continuous recording descriptive assessments (e.g., the behavior is observed in the natural environment with people who are typically present, and data are collected on problem behavior and environmental events throughout the observation period); however, antecedent events are systematically controlled, as in experimental analyses (Anderson & Long, 2002; Freeman, Anderson, & Scotti, 2000). For example, Anderson and Long (2002) provided instructions and prompts to a teacher and a parent to conduct antecedent procedures associated with attention, task, tangible, and play conditions but asked the teacher and parent to respond to problem behavior as they normally would. Results were interpreted based on both absolute measures of problem behavior across conditions (as in experimental analysis) and conditional probabilities between environmental events and behavior. The outcomes of the SDA matched those from functional analyses, and treatments corresponding to the results were effective in decreasing problem behavior for all participants. These results tentatively suggest that the SDA may be a useful method for identifying operant functions of problem behavior in natural settings.

The practical utility of using continuous recording descriptive assessment in clinical contexts is questionable. For example, Mace and Lalli (1991) used the outcomes of a descriptive assessment to develop conditions that they later tested during experimental analysis. The results of the descriptive assessment indicated that the participant's bizarre speech was likely maintained by social reinforcement, but the type and form of reinforcement (whether positive or negative) became apparent only after conducting the experimental analysis. Furthermore, the experimental analysis test conditions used by Mace and Lalli were very similar to those used in "standard" experimental analyses (e.g., tests for social-positive reinforcement in the form of attention and social-negative reinforcement in the form of escape from demands were conducted), so the value of the contributions of the descriptive assessment in the development of the experimental analysis is questionable. Similarly, Lerman and Iwata (1993) compared the outcomes of descriptive assessments and experimental analyses for six participants and found that although the outcomes of descriptive assessments indicated when problem behavior was maintained by social versus nonsocial contingencies, they did not provide information about the types of contingencies maintaining problem behavior (positive or negative reinforcement).

A potential limitation of SDA is the sophistication required for data analysis. To develop hypotheses about the operant function of problem behavior, conditional probabilities must be calculated across a range of variables, including the probability of particular antecedents given the occurrence of behavior, the probability of the occurrence of behavior given particular antecedents, the probability of particular subsequent events given the occurrence of behavior, and the probability of the occurrence of behavior given those events. There are no specific guidelines for comparing and interpreting the resulting values, and, as noted above, even when orderly data are found, interpretations may be limited.

Practical limitations notwithstanding, descriptive assessments using continuous observation procedures have functioned as a useful research platform for investigating a wide range of variables associated with problem behavior. For example, descriptive assessments have generated information about the types of consequences that tend to follow problem behavior in residential settings (Maurice & Trudel, 1982; Thompson & Iwata, 2001) and preschool settings (McKerchar & Thompson, 2004).

Anecdotal Assessment

Anecdotal assessments involve gathering information about problem behavior through interviews, rating scales, checklists, or other secondary formats. Using one or a combination of these formats, caregivers, teachers, family members, friends, or participants themselves may provide information about characteristics of the participant, the behavior, and the environment (both immediate and general). Some methods have been developed specifically to identify the operant function of problem behavior. For example, the outcomes of the *Motivation Assessment Scale* (MAS; Durand & Crimmins, 1988) are interpreted specifically in terms of maintaining contingencies of reinforcement (e.g., attention, tangibles, escape, sensory). Other anecdotal assessments are intended to produce a more comprehensive picture of the person, behavior, and environment. For example, the *Functional Analysis Interview* (O'Neill, Horner, Albin, Storey, & Sprague, 1990) gathers information about a wide range of variables such as the topography of the behavior, medical status of the participant, sleep and eating routines, daily activities, communication skills exhibited by the participant, and more.

Although a great deal of useful information can be gained via anecdotal assessment, some question its utility to specifically identify the operant function of problem behavior (Iwata, 1994). For example, the results of several evaluations of the utility of the MAS (Durand & Crimmins, 1988) have produced inconsistent results. Whereas some research outcomes appear to support the reliability of this assessment (Durand & Crimmins, 1988; Kearney, 1994; Shogren

& Rojahn, 2003), other outcomes have been negative (Newton & Sturmey, 1991; Paclawskyj, Matson, Rush, Smalls, & Vollmer, 2001; Sigafoos, Kerr, & Roberts, 1994; Thompson & Emerson, 1995; Zarcone, Rodgers, Iwata, Rourke, & Dorsey, 1991) or inconclusive (Singh et al., 1993). Most researchers have recommended that, in light of its potential limitations, the MAS be used in conjunction with other sources of information when attempting to identify the operant function of problem behavior. Similar types of assessments, such as the *Questions About Behavioral Function* (Paclawskyj, Matson, Rush, Smalls, & Vollmer, 2000) and the *Functional Analysis Screening Tool* (Iwata, 1995), also have limited evidence in support of their utility as functional assessment tools.

A large and growing body of research showing the effectiveness of interventions corresponding to functional assessment outcomes has demonstrated its utility as a pretreatment assessment (Iwata, Pace, Cowdery, & Miltenberger, 1994). Recognition of the clinical value of a functional-analytic approach has resulted in its extension across a wide range of settings and populations, including hospitals, schools, institutions, homes, vocational programs, and outpatient clinics (Hanley et al., 2003). In fact, the IDEA amendments of 1997 included language that required the use of functional behavior assessments for a variety of situations when students with disabilities exhibit behavior problems in school settings.

Recommendations for Practitioners

The broad array of alternative functional assessment procedures presents a challenge to practitioners and consumers interested in identifying the operant function of problem behavior. Although experimental analysis clearly represents the "state-of-the-science" in terms of producing definitive information, there are several drawbacks to its use, including the need for trained therapists and observers, the time and resources needed to complete the assessment, and risks to participants and others associated with the need to evoke problem behavior in the assessment setting. How, then, should a practitioner proceed when faced with a challenging behavior whose operant function is unclear?

First, in some cases, it may be possible to identify the operant function of problem behavior through informal observations and anecdotal reports from people who know the participant. If problem behavior is observed to occur only at specific times or in a specific context, then it may be possible to infer operant function without implementing more formal assessment procedures. For example, if a student protests going to school and emits self-injury just after arrival in a school classroom (and *only* just after arrival in the classroom), it is reasonable to suspect that the behavior may be maintained by avoidance of or escape from the academic setting or routine. When an "informed guess" about the operant function of problem behavior is based on such informally gathered information, it will be very important that an intervention that corresponds only to the hypothesized maintaining contingency be systematically implemented so as to verify, or validate, the guess. For example, an intervention for problem behavior maintained by social positive reinforcement might involve withholding attention contingent on problem behavior and presenting attention as a consequence for an alternative communication response (see Function-Based Treatments later in this chapter). This procedure should be effective if and only if the behavior is actually maintained by that contingency. Thus, testing the effects of targeted intervention in this way actually becomes part of the process of identifying the maintaining contingency. If the intervention is effective, then confidence in the original account is increased; however, if the intervention is ineffective, or even deleterious, the results may point toward another account, which can then be tested by implementing an intervention corresponding to that account.

Often, the possible operant function of problem behavior is not apparent from casual observation. When no particular function is obvious, a general recommendation is to begin by accessing multiple sources of information. For example, O'Neill and colleagues (1997) have described an approach that integrates anecdotal reports with direct observation (descriptive) procedures. Using such a multidimensional approach (Sulzer-Azaroff & Mayer, 1991) can be very useful to develop hypotheses about behavioral function as well as potential intervention strategies. As with informal approaches, when multidimensional approaches suggest a particular operant function of the problem behavior, a corresponding intervention can be used to test the account.

Sometimes, the variables of which problem behavior is a function remain unclear even after conducting multidimensional anecdotal and descriptive assessments. In such cases, experimental analysis procedures may be recommended. In recent years, several extensions of experimental analysis procedures, designed to address some identified limitations of experimental analysis, have been proposed. For example, several researchers have developed abbreviated versions of experimental analyses so that the analysis can be completed in a short period of time (e.g., Northup et al., 1991; Vollmer et al., 1995), and others have proposed methods to conduct experimental analyses in ways that may reduce risks to participants (Smith & Churchill, 2002).

If it is necessary to conduct experimental analysis procedures to identify the operant function of problem behavior, it is strongly recommended that the procedures be conducted and interpreted by a qualified behavior analyst—preferably one who has been certified by the Behavior Analyst Certification Board.

Although some researchers have demonstrated that teachers and other persons without professional training in behavior analysis can rapidly acquire the skills to conduct standard functional analysis conditions (Iwata et al., 2000; Wallace, Doney, Mintz-Resudek, & Tarbox, 2004), interpretation of the outcomes of experimental analysis, as well as the development of appropriate test conditions to accommodate idiosyncratic sources of reinforcement, require the repertoire of a competent behavior analyst.

Interventions for Problem Behavior

Several strategies have been developed to intervene upon maladaptive behavior. Broadly, these interventions can be categorized as being either based on the operant function of the behavior or not based on the operant function of behavior. When based on the operant function of behavior, a manipulation is made to alter the influence of the reinforcer(s) maintaining maladaptive behavior. When not based on the operant function of behavior, a manipulation is made to in some way override the reinforcers maintaining maladaptive behavior.

Function-Based Treatments

Extinction

The most straightforward approach is to withhold the source of reinforcement maintaining the maladaptive behavior. For behavior maintained by social positive reinforcement, extinction involves ensuring that the reinforcer maintaining that maladaptive behavior no longer occurs as a consequence of the behavior. For example, if a functional analysis shows that behavior is reinforced by attention, attention is withheld following maladaptive behavior (e.g., Iwata et al., 1994). For behavior maintained by social negative reinforcement, extinction involves ensuring that escape or avoidance no longer occurs as a consequence of the behavior. For example, if a functional analysis shows that behavior is reinforced by escape from instructional demands, the maladaptive behavior no longer terminates or postpones instructional activity (Iwata, Pace, Kalsher, & Cowdery, 1990).

When behavior is automatically reinforced, extinction is far less practical than when behavior is socially reinforced. The reason is that when behavior produces its own source of reinforcement, it is difficult for a parent, teacher, or therapist to somehow remove that source of reinforcement. Given that so much of the problematic behavior displayed by individuals with autism is automatically maintained, the practical problem of extinction arises frequently. Despite the difficulties inherent in extinguishing automatically reinforced behavior, several studies have examined the approach known as sensory extinction (e.g., Luiselli, 1988; Moore, Fisher, & Pennington, 2004; Rincover & Devany, 1982). The sensory extinction approach involves making an effort to eliminate the natural and putatively reinforcing automatic consequences of behavior. For example, wearing a soft helmet may eliminate some of the sensory by-products of self-injury (Silverman, Watanabe, Marshall, & Baer, 1984). The term *sensory extinction* is actually a misnomer, insofar as it is a procedure designed to extinguish behavior (not sensory processes), but the term has been used for more than 25 years now, so we use it here for the sake of consistency.

The principal advantage of extinction as an intervention for maladaptive behavior is that it is directly prescribed by a functional analysis. When the reinforcer has been identified, it may be withheld, at least in principle. However, there are also numerous limitations to the extinction approach. First, there is a possibility of an "extinction burst": The behavior rate, intensity, or both can temporarily increase before a decrease occurs (Vollmer et al., 1998). This can be a serious limitation if the maladaptive behavior is self-injury, severe aggression, or intense tantrums in public places. To the extent that the maladaptive behavior is aversive to an adult, the adult is likely to reinforce the behavior in order to temporarily stop the behavior (Sloman et al., 2005). A second potential limitation of extinction is that variation in maladaptive behavior may be induced (Lerman, Iwata, & Wallace, 1999). For example, if self-injury is placed on extinction, it is possible that other serious behavior problems would emerge, such as aggression. A third potential limitation is that at times it is entirely impractical to withhold reinforcement. For example, if severe aggression is maintained by attention, it is not practical to withhold attention (obviously the person whom the aggression is directed toward requires protection). Similarly, if an individual displays escape behavior, it may be impractical to physically guide him or her to complete a task if he or she is extremely strong or agile. A fourth potential limitation is that even the slightest failure of treatment integrity can be hugely detrimental. For example, if a parent accidentally reinforces maladaptive behavior just 1 out of 20 times it occurs, then the maladaptive behavior is reinforced on a variable ratio (VR) 20 schedule. Such a lean and variable schedule may make behavior all the more resistant to future extinction trials (for a further discussion on the effects of using an intermittent reinforcement schedule, see Lerman, Iwata, Shore, & Kahng, 1996). As a result of these potential limitations and others, extinction is rarely recommended as an intervention in isolation. Rather, extinction is usually one component of a larger treatment package. Some of those treatment packages are described next.

Differential Reinforcement

Differential reinforcement involves providing reinforcement for some (usually alternative) behavior while minimizing reinforcement for maladaptive behavior. This definition differs from those used even in some of our own previous papers (Vollmer & Iwata, 1992). Previously, we stressed that differential reinforcement should involve an extinction component for maladaptive behavior. Although this remains true in an ideal intervention, it is not a very practical recommendation because, as discussed in the preceding section on extinction, reinforcers cannot or at least will not be withheld at all times. However, if reinforcers sometimes occur for maladaptive behavior but much more frequently occur as a consequence for alternative adaptive behavior, then the individual should begin to allocate more and more behavior toward the schedule of reinforcement maintaining adaptive behavior. Thus, a relatively simple way to think of differential reinforcement is that the presentation of reinforcers occurs at a higher rate when adaptive behavior occurs and at a lower rate when maladaptive behavior occurs.

Differential reinforcement can be divided into two general procedure types: differential reinforcement of other behavior (DRO) and differential reinforcement of alternative behavior (DRA). With DRO, reinforcers are delivered contingent on the omission of maladaptive behavior following a set period of time. Typically, the timer resets if maladaptive behavior occurs. With DRA, a specific alternative response (such as communication or compliance) is reinforced. In recent years, DRA seems to be a more prevalent approach, presumably because it involves specifically strengthening a replacement behavior. Also, DRO is probably more sensitive than DRA to failures of treatment integrity. With DRA, treatment integrity errors may be less critical because as long as the alternative behavior is reinforced on a richer schedule, more behavior should be allocated in that direction (Myerson & Hale, 1984).

Differential reinforcement procedures are usually designed to address the operant function of behavior. Specifically, the reinforcer(s) for maladaptive behavior identified via functional analysis are used to strengthen either alternative behavior (McCord, Thompson, & Iwata, 2001) or to reinforce the omission of maladaptive behavior (Lindberg, Iwata, Kahng, & DeLeon, 1999). In short, the contingencies previously maintaining maladaptive behavior are explicitly reversed during differential reinforcement. Thus, if maladaptive behavior is maintained by escape, the DRA procedure usually involves reinforcing alternative behavior with escape (Lalli, Casey, & Kates, 1995). If maladaptive behavior is reinforced by attention, the DRA procedure usually involves reinforcing alternative attention-getting behavior (Vollmer et al., 1992).

One specific type of DRA is functional communication training (FCT; Carr & Durand, 1985; Durand & Carr, 1991). Although FCT is sometimes discussed as a distinct mode of function-based treatment, it is our contention that FCT is actually a DRA treatment, in which the alternative response that is reinforced is communicative behavior. Thus, sign language, vocalizations, picture card exchanges, and so on, all represent DRA procedures that have come to be called FCT. In some literature on FCT, there has been a de-emphasis on the consequences for maladaptive behavior, and the reinforcement contingency for alternative behavior is stressed. However, there is strong evidence that the reinforcement contingency for alternative behavior is effective only in a context where it is superior to the reinforcement contingency for maladaptive behavior (Vollmer, Roane, Ringdahl, & Marcus, 1999; Worsdell, Iwata, Hanley, Thompson, & Kahng, 2000). In other words, our initial contention that reinforcement should be maximized for appropriate behavior and minimized for maladaptive behavior is equally true for FCT.

The principal advantage of differential reinforcement procedures is that they are directly derived from a functional analysis insofar as the reinforcer maintaining maladaptive behavior is used to strengthen alternative behavior. The approach is limited for reasons similar to the limitations of extinction: If behavior is automatically reinforced, it is difficult to identify and then provide stimulation similar to the automatically produced stimulation. It also might be argued that differential reinforcement procedures do not address the problem of establishing operations. For example, if maladaptive behavior occurs at a higher rate during instructional activities and the behavior has been determined to be maintained by escape, what is it about the instructional activities that makes them aversive? Perhaps there is not enough reinforcement available in the context of those instructional activities, the activities are too difficult, or the materials being used are nonpreferred. Some preliminary evidence has been presented to suggest that differential reinforcement procedures using positive reinforcement can be used to reduce escape behavior (e.g., Lalli et al., 1999). This approach is later in this chapter.

Motivational Strategies

Establishing operations are (in part) events that alter the reinforcing efficacy of stimuli (Michael, 1993). For example, deprivation from attention or food may strengthen attention or food as a reinforcer (Vollmer & Iwata, 1991). One treatment approach that is based in part on the notion of establishing operations is known as noncontingent reinforcement (NCR; Vollmer, Iwata, Zarcone, Smith, & Mazaleski, 1993). There are problems with the use of the term NCR, but those issues have been discussed elsewhere (e.g., Poling & Normand, 1999; Vollmer, 1999) and will not be revisited here.

Essentially, NCR schedules are time-based schedules in which the occurrence or nonoccurrence of maladaptive behavior does not influence reinforcer delivery. For example, if attention is shown to be a reinforcer for maladaptive behavior, then attention would be delivered at set points in time to eliminate the contingency and to reduce the motivation to engage in attention-maintained behavior. The initial studies on NCR used fixed-time (FT) schedules during which reinforcers are delivered at set points in time; however, systematic replications of the procedure have shown that variable-time (VT) schedules, during which reinforcers are delivered at varying points in time, also may be effective to decrease problem behavior (Van Camp, Lerman, Kelley, Contrucci, & Vorndran, 2000). The idea behind NCR as treatment is that the motivation to engage in maladaptive behavior should be reduced because reinforcers are delivered freely and frequently *and* because the maladaptive behavior no longer directly produces reinforcers.

As with other forms of treatment derived from a functional analysis, NCR works best when the reinforcer maintaining maladaptive behavior is used during treatment in the FT or VT schedule. Thus, the arrangement might involve noncontingent attention, noncontingent escape, or noncontingent access to tangible items. Usually, the schedule of NCR is thinned over time to make the procedure more practical. Strategies for thinning schedules are discussed later under ecological considerations.

Skills Training

An interesting approach to treatment for behavior disorders, and one that has received relatively little empirical evaluation, is *skills training*. The notion is that as new repertoires are developed and time is absorbed with various important activities (e.g., self-care, daily living skills, leisure skills), less time is available for maladaptive behavior. This general notion is supported by research on environmental enrichment (e.g., Horner, 1980) and behavioral replacement (e.g., Durand & Carr, 1987). However, very little research has been directed explicitly toward the notion that as skills develop generally, maladaptive behavior should decrease in frequency.

From a perspective of the matching law (e.g., Martens & Houk, 1989; McDowell, 1988), a skills training approach makes intuitive sense. Engaging in behavior other than the target response should be reinforced at least at some level, and therefore the more expansive the repertoire, the more that behavior should be allocated away from maladaptive behavior.

Mathematically, the quantitative interpretation can be expressed as follows:

$$R = \frac{kr}{r + r_e}$$

In this equation, commonly called the single-response matching equation, R represents the rate of responding for a targeted behavior, r is the rate of reinforcement for engaging in the target behavior, k is a free parameter typically interpreted as the maximal response rate of the target behavior, and r_e is a free parameter typically interpreted as the rate of reinforcement for all other responses. This equation shows that the rate of the target behavior should decrease as the rate of reinforcement for other responses, r_e, increases. Therefore, the matching equation predicts that increasing reinforcement for alternative behavior should necessarily decrease the rate of responding for the target (maladaptive) behavior, even if the rate of reinforcement for the maladaptive behavior remains unchanged. Skills training may increase the rate of reinforcement for other behavior, thereby competing with the maladaptive behavior.

Other Approaches to Intervention

Current research and practice emphasizes function-based interventions. However, other interventions, including those often considered intrusive, may be important for the optimal education of individuals with autism and should not be ignored. These approaches include response blocking and punishment. In addition, differential reinforcement procedures not based on a functional analysis may be used in some cases.

Response Blocking

Response blocking involves physically preventing the occurrence of the response. Blocking is typically considered an intrusive intervention because it often involves momentary manual restraint or the application of protective gear to prevent the maladaptive response from occurring. Because of its intrusive features and possible negative side effects, blocking is usually implemented as part of a larger treatment package.

Research on response blocking has typically found it to be effective across a variety of maladaptive responses (e.g., Kelley, Lerman, & Van Camp, 2002; MacDonald, Wilder, & Dempsey, 2002), but it has often been associated with serious negative side effects. For example, blocking one form of maladaptive behavior may result in increases in other equally undesirable responses, such as aggression (Hagopian & Adelinis, 2001) or stereotypy (Rapp et al., 2004). Blocking has also resulted in decreases in desirable behavior, such as appropriate interaction with leisure items (Lerman, Kelley, Vorndran, & Van Camp, 2003).

The behavioral mechanism associated with decreases in responding during response blocking remains unknown. It is possible that blocking serves as punishment for the maladaptive behavior because each attempt to engage in the maladaptive behavior results in physical blocking, a possibly aversive consequence (Lerman & Iwata, 1996). However, it is also possible that blocking decreases responding because of extinction (Smith, Russo, & Le, 1999). That is, preventing the response from occurring may be functionally similar to with-holding the reinforcer for the response. Evidence has been found for both of these hypotheses. Because response blocking is defined based on the form of the intervention, it is difficult to determine whether or when the intervention will be effective on a case-by-case basis. Even when the intervention is effective, it is difficult to determine what behavioral mechanism was responsible for the decrease in the response.

Punishment

Punishment involves either the response-contingent delivery of aversive stimu-lation or the response-contingent removal of preferred stimuli. The former type is typically called *positive punishment* or just *punishment*, and the latter type is typically called *negative punishment* or *response cost* and *time-out*. The use of punishment with any group or population is controversial (see Lerman & Vorndran, 2002). Nonetheless, a discussion of punishment as treatment for be-havior disorders displayed by individuals with autism is warranted for several reasons, including the following: (a) The term *punishment* is used not in the ev-eryday sense to imply retribution for wrongdoing, but in the technical sense of decreasing the future probability of behavior (in this case, dangerous behavior); thus it is behavior that is punished, not the individual who displays the behav-ior; (b) a great deal of research has shown that punishment can be effective in eliminating or at least decreasing dangerous behavior; (c) a functional analysis is not always feasible (e.g., when behavior is extremely low rate but high inten-sity), is not always conclusive (e.g., when the reinforcer or reinforcers for mal-adaptive behavior cannot be identified), or does not always lead to effective treatment (e.g., when behavior is automatically reinforced and those reinforcers cannot be controlled); and (d) sometimes the outcome of a functional analysis actually prescribes a punishment procedure (e.g., time-out from attention when attention is shown to be a reinforcer for maladaptive behavior).

Perhaps the most controversial applications of punishment are those that involve the contingent delivery of noxious stimulation. Over the past 40 or so years, however, various noxious stimuli have been applied as response-contingent punishment, including noxious odor (Tanner & Zeiler, 1975), nox-ious taste (Sajwaj, Libet, & Agras, 1974), shock (Linscheid, Iwata, Ricketts, Williams, & Griffin, 1990), and loud noise (Ayllon & Azrin, 1966), among oth-ers. Nevertheless, Pelios et al. (1999) found that the use of such punishment procedures has declined steadily since the development of functional analysis procedures in the field of applied behavior analysis. Thus, the current status of this type of punishment seems to be that it is reserved for the most extreme cases, such as life-threatening self-injurious behavior or aggression. There are numerous considerations in the use of punishment, including side effects such as aggression, withdrawal from or avoidance of the context in which punishment occurs, and generalization of punishment effects to unpunished responses. Moreover, punishment is largely considered to be the most intrusive of interventions for problem behavior; indeed, some practitioners and researchers have declared it unethical and universally unwarranted (e.g., Lavigna & Donnellan, 1986). Although the debate over the use of punishment to treat behavior disorders continues, it is generally accepted that if and when such procedures are deemed necessary, they should be implemented only under the supervision of properly credentialed behavior analysts in collaboration with a group of professional peers such as a behavior analysis review committee or a human rights committee.

The primary advantage of punishment is that if it is used correctly, it can produce immediate and sustained reductions in target behavior (Lerman & Vorndran, 2002). Secondary desirable effects may include (a) an increased opportunity for positive reinforcement because maladaptive behavior episodes are reduced in magnitude, duration, or frequency; (b) increased opportunity for learning new skills because maladaptive behavior episodes are reduced in magnitude, duration, or frequency; and (c) long-term negative side effects of dangerous behavior may be minimized. For example, if head banging is eliminated, medical sequela such as retinal detachment may be avoided.

Disadvantages of punishment include the fact that the context of punishment (including the punishing agent) may become a conditioned aversive stimulus that is subsequently escaped or avoided. This potential negative side effect is quite serious if the punishing agent is a parent or a teacher who hopes to use positive reinforcement as a teaching tool, because the aversive properties of stimulation may compete with the reinforcing properties. Another disadvantage is the potential for abuse; for example, someone may use the punishing stimulus contingent on nontargeted behavior. Also, there have been reports of emotional behavior, such as crying, following the use of punishment applications (Lerman & Vorndran, 2002; Sidman, 1989). It is interesting that much controversy surrounds the use of punishment, even though positive reinforcement could be equally misused (Vollmer, 2002). Also, it appears that research on punishment has virtually stopped, in part because of functional analysis approaches (Pelios et al., 1999) but also presumably because of its controversial nature. In any case, until highly acceptable and effective procedures are universally available, it seems clear that much more could be learned about the safe and appropriate application of punishment (Lerman & Vorndran, 2002).

Time-out is a form of punishment that involves the response-contingent (usually temporary) termination of the opportunity to obtain reinforcers. Like other forms of punishment, time-out can be controversial if it involves isolation, long time intervals, or both. However, exclusion or isolation (removal of the individual from a reinforcing environment) is not necessarily a defining characteristic of time-out. For example, time-out can occur if an adult stops providing any attention or other reinforcers for a period of time following a target response. The efficacy of time-out does not depend on either a long time interval or on a resetting feature (in which the time-out interval restarts contingent on each instance of problem behavior) if maladaptive behavior occurs during the time-out interval. For example, Mace, Page, Ivancic, and O'Brien (1986) showed that time-out was equally effective whether or not problematic behavior extended the time-out interval. Thus, there does not appear to be strong evidence for extended time-out intervals.

Response cost is a form of punishment that involves the response-contingent withdrawal of reinforcers. This definition sounds similar to time-out, but the difference is that reinforcers are actually taken away during a response-cost procedure. Response-cost procedures are commonly used with token reinforcement systems in classrooms (Conyers et al., 2004) or residential living facilities. The procedure can be combined with positive reinforcement (e.g., earning points for desired behavior but losing points for maladaptive behavior) or noncontingent reinforcement (e.g., providing free, or noncontingent, access to preferred stimuli, but removing those stimuli when maladaptive behavior occurs).

Although time-out and response cost are often arbitrary in relation to the function of maladaptive behavior, these procedures can be designed to address the function. For example, if maladaptive behavior is reinforced by attention, a time-out can be arranged such that attention becomes unavailable for a period of time following occurrences of maladaptive behavior. Similarly, if maladaptive behavior is reinforced by access to preferred toys, a response-cost contingency can be arranged such that maladaptive behavior produces a response-contingent loss of toys. Thus, from a standpoint of treatment logic, there are benefits to both time-out and response cost. Disadvantages of time-out and response cost include all of those associated with punishment (discussed earlier). In addition, time-out is sometimes misapplied. For example, if the putative time-out environment actually has reinforcers available (e.g., if the student is placed within hearing distance of a TV), it might not be an actual time-out. Thus, special attention must be paid to the relative value of the time-in and time-out environments (Solnick, Rincover, & Peterson, 1977).

Differential Reinforcement

If the reinforcers maintaining maladaptive behavior are unknown or not readily controlled, such as in the case of automatic reinforcement, differential reinforcement may be applied with reinforcers that are thought to possibly compete with maladaptive behavior. For example, Corte, Wolf, and Locke (1971) showed that food reinforcers could be used in a DRO arrangement to compete with SIB. Because the reinforcers for SIB were unknown (no functional analysis had been conducted), the procedure was only minimally effective.

A series of studies by Repp and Deitz and colleagues (e.g., Repp & Deitz, 1974; Repp, Deitz, & Deitz, 1976; Repp, Deitz, & Speir, 1974) elegantly demonstrated the range of formal variations of DRO and DRA using reinforcers that were arbitrary in relation to maladaptive behavior. Some of these variations involved changing the parameters of the reinforcement schedule. For DRO schedules, variations in the DRO interval include basing the interval on the average time between responses (known as the interresponse time, or IRT), on a variable amount of time, or incrementing the interval in an escalating fashion. Of these variations, basing the DRO interval on the IRT seems especially appealing because it may ensure contact with the reinforcement contingency. A second formal variation of DRO schedules involves the inclusion or exclusion of a resetting feature. When a resetting feature is included, instances of the maladaptive response reset the DRO interval. If a resetting feature is not included, reinforcers are programmed to occur at set points in time, and instances of the maladaptive behavior simply cancel the upcoming reinforcer.

Formal variations of DRA have also been used to decrease maladaptive behavior. In one such variation, reinforcement is provided for the occurrence of a response incompatible with the maladaptive behavior. For example, appropriately answering questions would be incompatible with repetitive, nonsensical vocalizations. This variation has been labeled *differential reinforcement of incompatible behavior* (DRI).

Antecedent-Based Interventions

The focus of most of the previous discussion of treatment and intervention has centered on consequent events (i.e., reinforcement or punishment). However, other treatment strategies have focused on the manipulation of antecedent events (those that come before behavior). In our view, antecedent interventions influence behavior because they in some way alter the effects of consequences. Some examples of antecedent-based interventions include manipulation of establishing operations, prompting, manipulation of stimulus control, environmental modification, and exercise.

Establishing Operations

As discussed previously, establishing operations influence behavior (in part) by altering the efficacy of events as reinforcement. For example, deprivation from attention is an establishing operation because presumably attention becomes a more potent form of reinforcement. For negatively reinforced behavior, difficult task demands may serve as establishing operations increasing the value of escape as reinforcement. In the case of attention deprivation, enriching the schedule of attention via NCR may alter the establishing operation and thus make attention-maintained maladaptive behavior less likely to occur. In the case of instructional demands, the frequency or degree of difficulty of demands can be modified such that escape is less likely to function as reinforcement (Smith & Iwata, 1997).

To illustrate interventions based on manipulation of establishing operations, consider the approach known as instructional demand fading (Zarcone, Iwata, Smith, Mazaleski, & Lerman, 1994). In this approach, instructional demands are first eliminated entirely. If there are no instructional demands, there is no reason that escape behavior should occur (assuming the escape behavior is limited to escape from instructional demands). Instructional demands are then gradually introduced, but rates of problem behavior typically remain low.

Stimulus Control

Stimulus control involves a change in the probability of behavior in the presence of particular stimuli. This relationship typically develops when a particular form of behavior is frequently followed by a predictable consequence (e.g., reinforcement, punishment, or extinction) in the presence of a certain stimulus. Stimulus control can either increase or decrease the probability of the response, depending on the consequence associated with the presence of the stimulus. Behavior is less likely to occur during stimulus conditions associated with punishment or extinction and more likely to occur during stimulus conditions associated with reinforcement.

An example of stimulus control is the increase in the probability of maladaptive behavior in the presence of someone who typically reinforces that behavior. Similarly, people who have a history with a child may exert stimulus control over maladaptive behavior. Progar et al. (2001) showed that for one child higher rates of aggression occurred in sessions that were conducted by a therapist who had a history with the child than in sessions with a novel therapist. In other words, the familiar therapist may have exerted stimulus control over the behavior. Stimulus control can be used to the benefit of treatments designed for behavior that is acceptable in one context but unacceptable in another. For example, some forms of stereotypy may be acceptable in private situations such as the home, but unacceptable in public places such as the grocery store. A treatment could be designed in which the response is placed on extinction while in public places but is reinforced in the home. Consistent implementation of such a treatment should result in lower rates of the behavior in public places but sustained rates within the home.

Environmental Enrichment

Environmental enrichment (EE) involves increasing the reinforcing qualities of the environment. In home and school settings, EE procedures usually entail adding toys, music, food, or other preferred stimuli to the environment. Because the stimuli are not delivered contingent upon behavior, EE shares features with NCR and may operate through similar mechanisms. One difference between EE and NCR is that NCR typically (although not necessarily) involves the delivery of a reinforcer maintaining the response, whereas EE does not typically use a maintaining reinforcer. Instead, EE is designed to provide alternative reinforcers that may compete with the reinforcement for the undesired response.

EE has been effective at reducing rates of stereotypy (Rapp, 2004) and self-injury (Ringdahl, Vollmer, Marcus, & Roane, 1997). A limited amount of research has tested the parameters influencing the effects of EE. However, EE may be more effective when implemented with a DRA procedure in which appropriate behavior results in reinforcement (Horner, 1980).

Exercise

A small body of literature has examined the effects of antecedent exercise on undesirable behavior. Typically, stereotypic responses are targeted for studies on antecedent exercise. For example, Powers, Thibadieau, and Rose (1992) examined the effects of 10 min of roller skating on the rate of maladaptive responses exhibited by a boy with autism and found that maladaptive responses decreased following exercise.

The research on antecedent exercise consists primarily of case reports, with no systematic replications of the procedures or results. Therefore, more research is needed before conclusions can be drawn about the general effectiveness of antecedent exercise as an intervention for maladaptive behavior. Future research should examine the duration of the exercise effects, as well as the topographies and functions of behavior for which exercise is an effective antecedent intervention. It is possible that exercise produces a general fatigue and, therefore, all behavior rates (not just maladaptive behavior rates) are reduced following exercise.

Other Considerations

Staff and Parent Training

Most behavioral interventions require implementation by an adult caregiver. Thus, careful training is an integral step in the successful treatment of maladaptive behavior. Behavioral research has shown convincingly that caregiver training that is competency based is superior to caregiver training that is didactic only (Feldman, Case, Rincover, & Towns, 1989). Competency-based training requires that the caregiver demonstrate the skill that is taught—in this case, implementation of a behavioral treatment. At a minimum, the skill should be demonstrated during role-play (Duclos, 1987). Role-play is important because actual simulations can be evaluated, but even better is to ensure that implementation is correct in the context of actual interactions with the individual who displays the maladaptive behavior.

One approach that we have adopted and evaluated over the years involves a succession of steps in parent training (Vollmer, Marcus, & LeBlanc, 1994; Marcus, Swanson, & Vollmer, 2001). First, an expert outlines the logic of the procedure to the caregivers and answers any questions. Second, the expert models implementation of the procedure during role-play, where the caregiver plays the role of the target individual. Third, the expert plays the role of the target individual and the caregiver implements the procedure while receiving immediate corrective feedback and praise. Fourth, when corrective feedback is no longer necessary, the expert then models implementation of the procedure with the target individual. Fifth, the caregiver implements the procedure with the target individual while the expert provides immediate corrective and positive feedback. Sixth, when immediate corrective feedback is no longer needed, the caregiver implements the procedure in vivo with delayed feedback only. Finally, when delayed feedback is no longer necessary, the expert monitors the implementation periodically with booster training sessions implemented as necessary. The issues concerning relapse and the need for booster training will be addressed further in a later section.

Ecology of Intervention

The context in which an intervention is implemented is an important consideration. If a treatment recommendation is made but cannot be implemented due to ecological factors, then the procedure is moot and cannot possibly be effective. Examples of ecological invalidity include asking a teacher with 30 students to implement a 10-s DRO procedure, asking a parent with a fifth-grade education to train respite workers to implement a complex behavioral intervention for her child, and so on.

Two approaches, which are not mutually exclusive, should be considered when the context surrounding an intervention makes it challenging to implement properly. The first general approach is that the ethical practitioner should push to have systems in place that will make an intervention viable. To cite a medical analogy, a physician recognizes that a child with diabetes must receive insulin shots no matter what the environmental context. To ensure that this happens, a nurse may be assigned to a school (adjustment in person power), an insulin pump might be prescribed (adjustment in technology), or necessary training regimens are followed (adjustments in standard training resources). Similarly, if a child or adult with autism engages in dangerous or potentially dangerous behavior, a first step is to ensure that the problem has been accommodated to the fullest extent possible. This may involve identifying needs for support personnel, respite care, parent training, teacher training, additional aides in school, and so on.

The second general approach is to ensure that the intervention is suited to the environmental context as much as possible. For example, if a complex intervention package is effective, which components of the procedure are necessary and sufficient to gain similar effects? What level of treatment integrity is required to gain satisfactory outcomes? Can the DRO, DRA, or NCR schedule be thinned to an extent that makes the procedure more conducive to a complex home, school, or work environment? Each of these questions will be addressed briefly below.

Throughout the history of treatment of maladaptive behavior in autism, the tendency of professionals has been to implement treatment packages proven to be effective in suppressing dangerous or maladaptive behavior. It is important to consider the possibility that only part of that treatment package may be necessary and sufficient to obtain desired results. Thus, it is important that the expert evaluate the independent effects of components of treatment packages. If only one piece of a complex treatment package is needed, caregivers are more likely to implement the procedure successfully. In our view, the issue is sometimes skirted for political reasons, such as if the successful component of a procedure is punishment, even if it is not called or recognized as punishment, while the reinforcement component may be very cumbersome and difficult to implement and may have no effect on behavior.

Treatment integrity is an issue that should be of great concern to practitioners developing treatments for maladaptive behavior (Gresham, 1989). Treatment integrity refers to the extent that a procedure is conducted as prescribed. For example, if reinforcement is supposed to be delivered every time appropriate communication occurs, then treatment integrity can be measured as a percentage of opportunities to provide reinforcement, with the number of appropriate communication instances serving as the denominator and the number of correct responses by the individual implementing treatment as the numerator. Similarly, treatment integrity can be evaluated along dimensions of correct responses to maladaptive behavior (including immediacy of responding), false-positive implementation of reinforcement (e.g., delivering reinforcement when it should not have been delivered), or false-positive delivery of punishment (e.g., delivering a punitive consequence when it should not have been delivered). There is no standard for best practice in relation to treatment integrity, other than to say that procedures should be implemented with as much integrity as possible. However, some research has shown that treatment integrity can be far less than perfect and the procedure still can have a desired effect on behavior (e.g., Vollmer et al., 1999; Northup, Fisher, Kahng, Harrel, & Kurtz, 1997).

Although many issues can be raised about ecological validity, the final one we will discuss here relates to making reinforcement schedules more practical via schedule thinning. Schedule thinning refers to the process of moving from an extremely dense and labor-intensive schedule of delivery to a relatively thin and less labor-intensive schedule. For both DRO and NCR schedules, this has been accomplished by thinning the schedule in fixed units (Vollmer et al., 1993) or by increasing the interval based on new average interresponse times (IRTs). This IRT adjusting approach works nicely because, as behavior rates decrease, the IRTs necessarily increase (note that IRTs are the reciprocal of response rates). Thus, as treatment progresses, the DRO or NCR schedule is naturally thinned (Kahng, Iwata, DeLeon, & Wallace, 2000). With DRA schedules, thinning commonly involves increasing the response requirements either by placing the alternative response on an interval schedule that gradually increases (e.g., Marcus & Vollmer, 1996) or by reinforcing the appropriate behavior only after a certain number of responses on some other task has been accomplished (Lalli et al., 1995).

Maintenance and Relapse Prevention

Maintenance refers to the extent to which a behavioral treatment yields sustained effects over time. Typically, maintenance is measured during follow-up observations, and data are plotted graphically to compare levels of maladaptive behavior, appropriate behavior, or both, after some time period has elapsed (Kazdin, 2001). Four general factors should be considered if maintenance is poor: (a) There may be procedural drift; (b) there may be new people in the environment who are not implementing the procedures; (c) the procedures used may no longer be effective due to satiation, habituation, or maturation; and (d) there may be a change in operant function. Each of these possibilities is discussed briefly in the following paragraphs.

The problem of *procedural drift* relates to treatment integrity. Some researchers have focused not only on the target individual's behavior during follow-up observations, but on the treatment implementer's behavior as well (Noell,

Gresham, & Gansle, 2002; Vollmer et al., 1994). Such observations and data collection allow for an analysis of the possibility that degradations in behavior correlate with, and perhaps are caused by, degradations in treatment integrity. If treatment effects are not maintained *and* treatment integrity is poor, a first-level safeguard is to conduct booster training sessions. If treatment effects are not maintained, yet treatment integrity is good, other more complex possibilities must be considered.

One such possibility is that the individual is now engaged in interactions with new or previously untrained individuals. This kind of information can be gained via interview (e.g., O'Neill et al., 1990) or via direct observation. The obvious solution is to further train any individuals for whom training was not previously completed. If this has no effect, it is possible that the procedure is no longer effective.

The procedure may become ineffective over time if the individual habituates to a reinforcer or punisher (Murphy, McSweeney, Smith, & McComas, 2003). Alternatively, due to changes in the individual (such as maturation), a previously effective punisher or reinforcer may no longer be effective. For example, a toy that was preferred by a child at age 4 may no longer be of interest at age 8. The possibility of lost treatment efficacy can be established by having a highly trained professional implement the procedure repeatedly with either perfect or very high levels of treatment integrity. If the procedure is ineffective under those kinds of highly controlled conditions, it is unlikely to be effective in the more natural environment. At that point, alternative treatments should be evaluated.

A related possibility is that the operant function of the behavior has changed (Lerman, Iwata, Smith, Zarcone, & Vollmer, 1994). An illustration of this phenomenon can be found in a clinical experience of the two senior authors. A functional analysis of SIB was conducted for a young man residing at a state residential facility in Florida. The outcome of the functional analysis showed that the SIB was reinforced by escape. We developed a treatment that involved escape extinction and positive reinforcement for compliance with instructional activity (preferred treats were given contingent on compliance). Over time, the instructional sessions became highly reinforcing insofar as the young man readily came to and cooperated with instructional sessions, often smiling and placing his hands on the therapists in a friendly manner. After staff training and follow-up observation, the young man was discharged from our program and returned to his regular living routine. Some months later, it was reported that SIB had resurfaced. Observations showed that procedures were being conducted with reasonable integrity. Thus, a second functional analysis was conducted. This time, the SIB was reinforced by attention, and virtually no SIB occurred in the escape condition. Thus, the prior treatment had become ineffective because it no longer addressed the operant function of his behavior.

Summary

Over the last 25 years, extraordinary progress has been made in the behavioral assessment and treatment of behavior disorders displayed by persons with autism and related developmental disabilities. The logic and procedures of functional assessment, first applied to self-injury, have since been extended toward a better understanding of the role of environmental contingencies in the establishment and maintenance of a wide range of problem behaviors, including aggression, stereotypy, mouthing, pica, and others.

Several approaches to functional assessment have emerged, including anecdotal, descriptive, and experimental procedures. Experimental methods, in particular, have proven useful to identify contingencies of reinforcement that maintain problem behavior, produce information that can be used to develop effective treatments, and provide a basic framework for a large and important body of research. Advancement and innovation continue to occur, with the goal of developing more efficient and less intrusive methods for identifying the environmental determinants of problem behavior.

Advances in our understanding of these issues have led to improvements in our ability to treat them. Whereas punishment and other interventions unrelated to the operant function of behavior characterized previous approaches, a wide range of treatments focus on directly altering events and conditions in the environment that set the occasion for and maintain problem behavior. Consideration of the contingencies of reinforcement responsible for problem behavior permits the development of individualized interventions that address the underlying causes of the behavior. Thus, interventions can reduce the motivation to engage in problem behavior (e.g., noncontingent reinforcement), reduce or eliminate the consequences that support problem behavior (e.g., extinction), and encourage appropriate responses and skills to replace problem behavior by producing the consequences previously associated with problem behavior (e.g., differential reinforcement). These interventions reduce the need for other, less effective and often more intrusive interventions that leave the "root cause" of problem behavior untreated, such as punishment, restraint, and medication.

The utility of a function-based approach is evidenced in the widespread adoption of related assessments and interventions in schools, homes, and treatment facilities. Continuing efforts to train and educate parents, teachers, caregivers, and advocates about how environmental contingencies affect problem behavior have heightened awareness of and demand for function-based assessments and treatments, culminating in legislative action requiring the use of functional assessment toward the solution of behavior problems in public school settings. Perhaps further extension of the functional assessment model will result in the development of more proactive approaches. It is hoped that improvements in our understanding of how operant contingencies contribute to the maintenance of problem behavior can be used to design environments in which persons with autism and related disabilities acquire repertoires that reduce the likelihood that problem behavior will develop and produce reinforcing consequences.

PRACTITIONER RECOMMENDATIONS

1. Determine the function of the behavior.

    a. Conduct descriptive observations to determine which possible reinforcers tend to follow behavior in the natural environment.

    b. When possible, conduct a functional analysis.

    c. Gather anecdotal assessment measures if descriptive observations and functional analysis are impossible, or as supplemental data for other assessments.

2. Develop an intervention based on the function of the behavior.

    a. Talk to relevant caregivers to determine which interventions would be manageable during everyday routines.

    b. If social reinforcers maintain the behavior, try

       • withholding reinforcers following occurrences of the behavior (extinction),

       • using the maintaining reinforcer to reinforce the non-occurrence of the response or the occurrence of a more desirable response (differential reinforcement),

       • changing the motivation to engage in the response by frequently providing the reinforcer independent of behavior (noncontingent reinforcement), and

       • reinforcing appropriate alternative forms of behavior through skills training.

3. If function-based interventions are not feasible or are ineffective, try other approaches.

    a. Reinforce the nonoccurrence of behavior or an alternative appropriate behavior using other powerful reinforcers (differential reinforcement).

    b. Change the antecedents of the behavior by

       • providing access to alternative items (environmental enrichment) or

- altering the structure of demands if behavior tends to occur in demand contexts (instructional demand fading).

c. If other interventions are ineffective and the behavior is dangerous, consider the use of more intrusive interventions.

d. Response blocking can be effective if the behavior is overt and a high level of monitoring can be maintained. Watch for possible negative side effects such as increases in other forms of undesirable behavior.

e. Punishment procedures can be used to decrease responding.

- Present an aversive item or event following the undesired behavior or remove a desirable item or event following the behavior.

- Use with caution because of negative side effects and social concerns.

- Implement only in collaboration with a group of professional peers.

4. When an effective intervention has been developed, prepare for implementation of the intervention during daily routines.

a. Train caregivers to implement procedures.

b. Determine whether the intervention is implemented effectively during daily activities.

- Ensure that the intervention package is manageable for caregivers.

- If the intervention is less effective than previously demonstrated, consider additional caregiver training or modifying the treatment package, including schedule thinning.

c. Conduct follow-ups to ensure maintenance of intervention effects. If effects have degraded, check for procedural drift, lack of implementation, changes in reinforcer efficacy, and changes in operant function.

References

Anderson, C. M., & Long, E. S. (2002). Use of a structured descriptive assessment methodology to identify variables affecting problem behavior. *Journal of Applied Behavior Analysis, 35,* 137–154.

Ayllon, T., & Azrin, N. H. (1966). Punishment as a discriminative stimulus and conditioned reinforcer with humans. *Journal of the Experimental Analysis of Behavior, 9,* 411–419.

Ayllon, T., & Michael, J. (1959). The psychiatric nurse as a behavioral engineer. *Journal of the Experimental Analysis of Behavior, 2,* 323–334.

Bijou, S. W., Peterson, R. F., & Ault, M. H. (1968). A method to integrate descriptive and experimental field studies at the level of data and empirical concepts. *Journal of Applied Behavior Analysis, 1,* 175–191.

Bostow, D. E., & Bailey, J. (1969). Modification of severe disruptive and aggressive behavior using brief timeout and reinforcement procedures. *Journal of Applied Behavior Analysis, 2,* 31–37.

Bowman, L. G., Fisher, W. W., Thompson, R. H., & Piazza, C. C. (1997). On the relation of mands and the function of destructive behavior. *Journal of Applied Behavior Analysis, 30,* 251–265.

Carr, E. G. (1977). The motivation of self-injurious behavior: A review of some hypotheses. *Psychological Bulletin, 84,* 800–816.

Carr, E. G., & Durand, V. M. (1985). Reducing problem behavior through functional communication training. *Journal of Applied Behavior Analysis, 18,* 111–126.

Carr, E. G., Newsom, C. D., & Binkoff, J. (1980). Escape as a factor in the aggressive behavior of two retarded children. *Journal of Applied Behavior Analysis, 13,* 101–117.

Conyers, C., Miltenberger, R., Maki, A., Barenz, R., Jurgens, M., Sailer, A., et al. (2004). A comparison of response cost and differential reinforcement of other behavior to reduce disruptive behavior in a preschool classroom. *Journal of Applied Behavior Analysis, 37,* 411–415.

Corte, H. E., Wolf, M. M., & Locke, B. J. (1971). A comparison of procedures for eliminating self-injurious behavior of retarded adolescents. *Journal of Applied Behavior Analysis, 4,* 201–213.

Cowdery, G. E., Iwata, B. A., & Pace, G. M. (1990). Effects and side effects of DRO as treatment for self-injurious behavior. *Journal of Applied Behavior Analysis, 23,* 497–506.

Derby, K. M., Wacker, D. P., Sasso, G., Steege, M., Northup, J., Cigrand, K., et al. (1992). Brief functional assessments techniques to evaluate aberrant behavior in an outpatient setting: A summary of 79 cases. *Journal of Applied Behavior Analysis, 25,* 713–721.

Duclos, W. A. (1987). Clinical aspects of the training of foster parents. *Child and Adolescent Social Work Journal, 4*, 187–194.

Durand, V. M., & Carr, E. G. (1987). Social influences on "self-stimulatory" behavior and treatment implications. *Journal of Applied Behavior Analysis, 20*, 119–132.

Durand, V. M., & Carr, E. G. (1991). Functional communication training to reduce challenging behavior: Maintenance and application in new settings. *Journal of Applied Behavior Analysis, 24*, 251–264.

Durand, V. M., & Crimmins, D. B. (1988). Identifying the variables maintaining self-injurious behavior. *Journal of Autism and Developmental Disorders, 18*, 99–117.

Favell, J. E., McGimsey, J. F., & Schell, R. M. (1982). Treatment of self-injury by providing alternate sensory activities. *Analysis and Intervention in Developmental Disabilities, 2*, 83–104.

Feldman, M. A., Case, L., Rincover, A., & Towns, F. (1989). Parent Education Project III: Increasing affection and responsivity in developmentally handicapped mothers: Component analysis, generalization, and effects on child language. *Journal of Applied Behavior Analysis, 22*, 211–222.

Freeman, K. A., Anderson, C. M., & Scotti, J. R. (2000). A structured descriptive methodology: Increasing agreement between descriptive and experimental analyses. *Education and Training in Mental Retardation and Developmental Disabilities, 35*, 55–66.

Goh, H., Iwata, B. A., Shore, B. A., DeLeon, I. G., Lerman, D. C., Ulrich, S. M., et al. (1995). An analysis of the reinforcing properties of hand mouthing. *Journal of Applied Behavior Analysis, 28*, 269–283.

Gresham, F. M. (1989). Assessment of treatment integrity in school consultation and prereferral intervention. *School Psychology Review, 18*, 37–50.

Hagopian, L. P., & Adelinis, J. D. (2001). Response blocking with and without redirection for the treatment of pica. *Journal of Applied Behavior Analysis, 34*, 527–530.

Hanley, G. P., Iwata, B. A., & McCord, B. E. (2003). Functional analysis of problem behavior: A review. *Journal of Applied Behavior Analysis, 36*, 147–185.

Horner, R. D. (1980). The effects of an environmental enrichment program on the behavior of institutionalized profoundly retarded children. *Journal of Applied Behavior Analysis, 13*, 473–491.

Individuals with Disabilities Education Act Amendments of 1997, 20 U.S.C. § 1401 (26).

Individuals with Disabilities Education Improvement Act of 2004. Retrieved June 30, 2005, from http://thomas.loc.gov/cgi-bin/query/z?c108:h.1350.enr:

Iwata, B. A. (1994). Functional analysis methodology: Some closing comments. *Journal of Applied Behavior Analysis, 27*, 413–418.

Iwata, B. A. (1995). *Functional analysis screening tool*. Gainesville, FL: The Florida Center on Self-injury.

Iwata, B. A., Dorsey, M. F., Slifer, K. J., Bauman, K. E., & Richman, G. S. (1994). Toward a functional analysis of self-injury. *Journal of Applied Behavior Analysis, 27,* 97–209. (Reprinted from *Analysis and Intervention in Developmental Disabilities, 2,* 3–20, 1982)

Iwata, B. A., Duncan, B. A., Zarcone, J. R., Lerman, D. C., & Shore, B. A. (1994). A sequential, test-control methodology for conducting functional analyses of self-injurious behavior. *Behavior Modification, 18,* 289–306.

Iwata, B. A., Pace, G. M., Cowdery, G. E., & Miltenberger, R. G. (1994). What makes extinction work: An analysis of procedural form and function. *Journal of Applied Behavior Analysis, 27,* 131–144.

Iwata, B. A., Pace, G. M., Kalsher, M. J., & Cowdery, G. E. (1990). Experimental analysis and extinction of self-injurious behavior. *Journal of Applied Behavior Analysis, 23,* 11–27.

Iwata, B. A., Wallace, M. D., Kahng, S., Lindberg, J. S., Roscoe, E. M., Conners, J., et al. (2000). Skill acquisition in the implementation of functional analysis methodology. *Journal of Applied Behavior Analysis, 33,* 181–194.

Kahng, S., Iwata, B. A., DeLeon, I. G., & Wallace, M. D. (2000). A comparison of procedures for programming noncontingent reinforcement schedules. *Journal of Applied Behavior Analysis, 33,* 223–231.

Kahng, S., Iwata, B. A., Fischer, S. M., Page, T. J., Treadwell, K. R. H., Williams, D. E., et al. (1998). Temporal distributions of problem behavior based on scatter plot analysis. *Journal of Applied Behavior Analysis, 31,* 593–604.

Kazdin, A. (2001). *Behavior modification in applied settings.* Belmont, CA: Wadsworth.

Kearney, C. A. (1994). Interrater reliability of the Motivation Assessment Scale: Another, closer look. *Journal of the Association for Persons with Severe Handicaps, 19*(2), 139–142.

Kelley, M. E., Lerman, D. C., & Van Camp, C. M. (2002). The effects of competing reinforcement schedules on the acquisition of functional communication. *Journal of Applied Behavior Analysis, 35,* 59–63.

Kennedy, C. H., & Itkonen, T. (1993). Effects of setting events on the problem behavior of students with severe disabilities. *Journal of Applied Behavior Analysis, 26,* 321–327.

Lalli, J. S., Casey, S., & Kates, K. (1995). Reducing escape behavior and increasing task completion with functional communication training, extinction, and response chaining. *Journal of Applied Behavior Analysis, 28,* 261–268.

Lalli, J. S., Vollmer, T. R., Progar, P. R., Wright, C., Borrero, J., Daniel, D., et al. (1999). Competition between positive and negative reinforcement in the treatment of escape behavior. *Journal of Applied Behavior Analysis, 32,* 285–296.

Lavigna, G., & Donnellan, A. (1986). *Alternatives to punishment: Solving behavior problems with non-aversive strategies.* New York: Irvington.

Lerman, D. C., & Iwata, B. A. (1993). Descriptive and experimental analysis of variables maintaining self-injurious behavior. *Journal of Applied Behavior Analysis, 26,* 293–319.

Lerman, D. C., & Iwata, B. A. (1996). A methodology for distinguishing between extinction and punishment effects associated with response blocking. *Journal of Applied Behavior Analysis, 29,* 231–233.

Lerman, D. C., Iwata, B. A., Shore, B. A., & Kahng, S. W. (1996). Responding maintained by intermittent reinforcement: Implications for the use of extinction with problem behavior in clinical settings. *Journal of Applied Behavior Analysis, 29,* 153–172.

Lerman, D. C., Iwata, B. A., Smith, R. G., Zarcone, J. R., & Vollmer, T. R. (1994). Transfer of behavioral function as a contributing factor in treatment relapse. *Journal of Applied Behavior Analysis, 27,* 357–370.

Lerman, D. C., Iwata, B. A., & Wallace, M. D. (1999). Side effects of extinction: Prevalence of bursting and aggression during the treatment of self-injurious behavior. *Journal of Applied Behavior Analysis, 32,* 1–8.

Lerman, D. C., Kelley, M. E., Vorndran, C. M., & Van Camp, C. M. (2003). Collateral effects of response blocking during the treatment of stereotypic behavior. *Journal of Applied Behavior Analysis, 36,* 119–123.

Lerman, D. C., & Vorndran, C. M. (2002). On the status of knowledge for using punishment: Implications for treating behavior disorders. *Journal of Applied Behavior Analysis, 35,* 431–464.

Liaupsin, C. J., Scott, T. M., & Nelson, C. M. (2000). *Functional behavioral assessment: An interactive training manual* (2nd ed.). Longmont, CO: Sopris West.

Lindberg, J. S., Iwata, B. A., Kahng, S., & DeLeon, I. G. (1999). DRO contingencies: An analysis of variable-momentary schedules. *Journal of Applied Behavior Analysis, 32,* 123–136.

Linscheid, T. R., Iwata, B. A., Ricketts, R. W., Williams, D. E., & Griffin, J. C. (1990). Clinical evaluation of the self-injurious behavior inhibiting system (SIBIS). *Journal of Applied Behavior Analysis, 23,* 53–78.

Lovaas, O. I., Freitag, G., Gold, V. J., & Kassorla, I. C. (1965). Experimental studies in childhood schizophrenia: Analysis of self-destructive behavior. *Journal of Experimental Child Psychology, 2,* 67–84.

Luiselli, J. K. (1988). Comparative analysis of sensory extinction treatments for self-injury. *Education and Treatment of Children, 11,* 149–156.

MacDonald, J. E., Wilder, D. A., & Dempsey, C. (2002). Brief functional analysis and treatment of eye poking. *Behavioral Interventions, 17,* 261–270.

Mace, F. C., Browder, D. M., & Lin, Y. (1987). Analysis of demand conditions associated with stereotypy. *Journal of Behavior Therapy and Experimental Psychiatry, 18,* 25–31.

Mace, F. C., & Knight, D. (1986). Functional analysis and treatment of severe pica. *Journal of Applied Behavior Analysis, 19,* 411–416.

Mace, F. C., & Lalli, J. S. (1991). Linking descriptive and experimental analysis in the treatment of bizarre speech. *Journal of Applied Behavior Analysis, 24,* 553–562.

Mace, F. C., Page, T. J., Ivancic, M. T., & O'Brien, S. (1986). Effectiveness of brief time-out with and without contingent delay: A comparative analysis. *Journal of Applied Behavior Analysis, 19,* 79–86.

Marcus, B. A., Swanson, V., & Vollmer, T. R. (2001). Effects of parent training on parent and child behavior using procedures based on functional analyses. *Behavioral Interventions, 16,* 87–104.

Marcus, B. A., & Vollmer, T. R. (1996). Combining noncontingent reinforcement and differential reinforcement schedules as treatment for aberrant behavior. *Journal of Applied Behavior Analysis, 29,* 43–51.

Martens, B. K., & Houk, J. L. (1989). The application of Herrnstein's law of effect to disruptive and on-task behavior of a retarded adolescent girl. *Journal of the Experimental Analysis of Behavior, 51,* 17–27.

Maurice, P., & Trudel, G. (1982). Self-injurious behavior: Prevalence and relationships to environmental events. In J. H. Hollis & C. E. Meyers (Eds.), *Life-threatening behavior: Analysis and intervention* (pp. 91–103). Washington, DC: American Association on Mental Deficiency.

McCord, B. E., Thompson, R. J., & Iwata, B. A. (2001). Functional analysis and treatment of self-injury associated with transitions. *Journal of Applied Behavior Analysis, 34,* 195–210.

McDowell, J. J. (1988). Matching theory in natural human environments. *Behavior Analyst, 11,* 95–109.

McKerchar, P. M., & Thompson, R. H. (2004). A descriptive analysis of potential reinforcement contingencies in the preschool classroom. *Journal of Applied Behavior Analysis, 37,* 431–444.

Michael, J. (1993). Establishing operations. *Behavior Analyst, 16,* 191–206.

Miltenberger, R. G., Long, E. S., Rapp, J. T., Lumley, V., & Elliot, A. J. (1998). Evaluating the function of hair pulling: A preliminary investigation. *Behavior Therapy, 29,* 211–219.

Moore, J. W., Fisher, W. W., & Pennington, A. (2004). Systematic application and removal of protective equipment in the assessment of multiple topographies of self-injury. *Journal of Applied Behavior Analysis, 37,* 73–77.

Murphy, E. S., McSweeney, F. K., Smith, R. G., & McComas, J. J. (2003). Dynamic changes in reinforcer effectiveness: Theoretical, methodological, and practical implications for applied research. *Journal of Applied Behavior Analysis, 36,* 421–438.

Myerson, J., & Hale, S. (1984). Practical applications of the matching law. *Journal of Applied Behavior Analysis, 17,* 367–380.

National Institutes of Health. (1989). Treatment of destructive behaviors in persons with developmental disabilities. *NIH Consensus Statement Online 1989 Sep 11–13 [cited 2005 April 22]; 7*(9): 1–15.

Newton, J. T., & Sturmey, P. (1991). The Motivation Assessment Scale: Inter-rater reliability and internal consistency in a British sample. *Journal of Mental Deficiency Research, 35,* 472–474.

Noell, G. H., Gresham, F. M., & Gansle, K. A. (2002). Does treatment integrity matter? A preliminary investigation of instructional implementation and mathematics performance. *Journal of Behavioral Education, 11,* 51–67.

Northup, J., Fisher, W., Kahng, S., Harrel, P., & Kurtz, P. (1997). An assessment of the necessary strength of behavioral treatments for severe behavior problems. *Journal of Developmental and Physical Disabilities, 9,* 1–16.

Northup, J., Wacker, D., Sasso, G., Steege, M., Cigrand, K., Cook, J., et al. (1991). A brief functional analysis of aggressive and alternative behavior in an outclinic setting. *Journal of Applied Behavior Analysis, 24,* 509–522.

O'Neill, R. E., Horner, R. W., Albin, R. W., Sprague, J. R., Storey, K., & Newton, J. S. (1997). *Functional assessment and program development for problem behavior: A practical handbook* (2nd ed.). Pacific Grove, CA: Brooks/Cole.

O'Neill, R. E., Horner, R. H., Albin, R. W., Storey, K., & Sprague, J. R. (1990). *Functional analysis of problem behavior: A practical handbook.* Sycamore, IL: Sycamore.

O'Reilly, M. F. (1995). Functional analysis and treatment of escape-maintained aggression correlated with sleep deprivation. *Journal of Applied Behavior Analysis, 28,* 225–226.

O'Reilly, M. F. (1997). Functional analysis of episodic self-injury correlated with recurrent otitis media. *Journal of Applied Behavior Analysis, 30,* 165–167.

O'Reilly, M. F. (1999). Effects of presession attention on the frequency of attention-maintained behavior. *Journal of Applied Behavior Analysis, 32,* 371–374.

Paclawskyj, T. R., Matson, J. L., Rush, K. S., Smalls, Y., & Vollmer, T. R. (2000). Questions About Behavioral Function (QABF): A behavioral checklist for functional assessment of aberrant behavior. *Research in Developmental Disabilities, 21,* 223–229.

Paclawskyj, T. R., Matson, J. L., Rush, K. S., Smalls, Y., & Vollmer, T. R. (2001). Assessment of the convergent validity of the Questions About Behavioral Function scale with analogue functional analysis and the Motivation Assessment Scale. *Journal of Intellectual Disability Research, 45,* 484–494.

Pelios, L., Morren, J., Tesch, D., & Axelrod, S. (1999). The impact of functional analysis methodology on treatment choice for self-injurious and aggressive behavior. *Journal of Applied Behavior Analysis, 32,* 185–195.

Piazza, C. C., Hanley, G. P., Bowman, L. G., Ruyter, J. M., Lindauer, S. E., & Saiontz, D. M. (1997). Functional analysis and treatment of elopement. *Journal of Applied Behavior Analysis, 30,* 653–672.

Piazza, C. C., Hanley, G. P., & Fisher, W. W. (1996). Functional analysis and treatment of cigarette pica. *Journal of Applied Behavior Analysis, 29,* 437–449.

Poling, A., & Normand, M. (1999). Noncontingent reinforcement: An appropriate description of time-based schedules that reduce behavior. *Journal of Applied Behavior Analysis, 32,* 237–238.

Powers, S., Thibadieau, S., & Rose, K. (1992). Antecedent exercise and its effects on self-stimulation. *Behavioral Residential Treatment, 7,* 15–22.

Progar, P. R., North, S. T., Bruce, S. S., DiNovi, B. J., Nau, P. A., Eberman, E. M., et al. (2001). Putative behavioral history effects and aggression maintained by escape from therapists. *Journal of Applied Behavior Analysis, 34,* 69–72.

Pyles, D. A. M., & Bailey, J. S. (1990). Diagnosing severe behavior problems. In A. C. Repp & N. N. Singh (Eds.), *Perspectives on the use of nonaversive and aversive interventions for persons with developmental disabilities* (pp. 381–401). Sycamore, IL: Sycamore.

Rapp, J. T. (2004). Effects of prior access and environmental enrichment on stereotypy. *Behavioral Interventions, 19,* 287–295.

Rapp, J. T., Vollmer, T. R., St. Peter, C., Dozier, C. L., & Cotnoir, N. M. (2004). Analysis of response allocation in individuals with multiple forms of stereotyped behavior. *Journal of Applied Behavior Analysis, 37,* 481–501.

Reimers, T. M., Wacker, D. B., Cooper, L. J., Sasso, G. M., Berg, W. K., & Steege, M. W. (1993). Assessing the functional properties of noncompliant behavior in an outpatient setting. *Child and Family Behavior Therapy, 15,* 1–15.

Repp, A. C., & Deitz, S. M. (1974). Reducing aggressive and self-injurious behavior of institutionalized retarded children through reinforcement of other behavior. *Journal of Applied Behavior Analysis, 7,* 313–325.

Repp, A. C., Deitz, S. M., & Deitz, D. E. D. (1976). Reducing inappropriate behaviors in a classroom and individual sessions through DRO schedules of reinforcement. *Mental Retardation, 14,* 11–15.

Repp, A. C., Deitz, S. M., & Speir, N. C. (1974). Reducing stereotypic responding of retarded persons by the differential reinforcement of other behavior. *American Journal of Mental Deficiency, 79,* 279–284.

Rincover, A., & Devany, J. (1982). The application of sensory extinction procedures to self-injury. *Analysis & Intervention in Developmental Disabilities, 2,* 67–81.

Ringdahl, J. E., Vollmer, T. R., Marcus, B. A., & Roane, H. S. (1997). An analogue evaluation of environmental enrichment: The role of stimulus preference. *Journal of Applied Behavior Analysis, 30,* 203–216.

Sajwaj, T., Libet, J., & Agras, S. (1974). Lemon-juice therapy: The control of life-threatening rumination in a six-month-old infant. *Journal of Applied Behavior Analysis, 7,* 557–563.

Scotti, J. R., Evans, I. M., Meyer, I. H., & Walker, P. (1991). A meta-analysis of intervention research with problem behavior: Treatment validity and standard of practice. *American Journal of Mental Retardation, 96,* 233–256.

Shogren, K. A., & Rojahn, J. (2003). Convergent reliability and validity of the Questions About Behavioral Function and the Motivation Assessment Scale: A replication study. *Journal of Developmental and Physical Disabilities, 15,* 367–375.

Sidman, M. (1960). *Tactics of scientific research.* New York: Basic Books.

Sidman, M. (1989). *Coercion and its fallout.* Boston: Authors Cooperative.

Sigafoos, J., Kerr, M., & Roberts, D. (1994). Interrater reliability of the Motivation Assessment Scale: Failure to replicate with aggressive behavior. *Research in Developmental Disabilities, 15,* 333–342.

Silverman, K., Watanabe, K., Marshall, A. M., & Baer, D. M. (1984). Reducing self-injury and corresponding self-restraint through the strategic use of protective clothing. *Journal of Applied Behavior Analysis, 17,* 545–552.

Singh, N. N., Donatelli, L. S., Best, A., Williams, D. E., Barrera, F. J., Lenz, M. W., et al. (1993). Factor structure of the Motivation Assessment Scale. *Journal of Intellectual Disability Research, 37,* 65–74.

Skinner, B. F. (1953). *Science and human behavior.* New York: Macmillan.

Sloman, K., Vollmer, T. R., Cotnoir, N., Borrero, C. S. W., Borrero, J. C., Samaha, A. L., et al. (2005). Descriptive analysis of parent reprimands. *Journal of Applied Behavior Analysis, 38,* 373–383.

Smith, R. G., & Churchill, R. M. (2002). Identification of environmental determinants of behavior disorders through functional analysis of precursor behaviors. *Journal of Applied Behavior Analysis, 35,* 125–136.

Smith, R. G., & Iwata, B. A. (1997). Antecedent influences on behavior disorders. *Journal of Applied Behavior Analysis, 30,* 343–375.

Smith, R. G., Russo, L., & Le, D. D. (1999). Distinguishing between extinction and punishment effects of response blocking: A replication. *Journal of Applied Behavior Analysis, 32,* 367–370.

Solnick, J. V., Rincover, A., & Peterson, C. R. (1977). Some determiners of the reinforcing and punishing effects of timeout. *Journal of Applied Behavior Analysis, 10,* 415–424.

Sulzer-Azaroff, B., & Mayer, R. (1991). *Behavior analysis for lasting change.* Fort Worth, TX: Holt, Reinhart & Winston.

Symons, F. J., Hoch, J., Dahl, N. A., & McComas, J. J. (2003). Sequential and matching analyses of self-injurious behavior: A case of overmatching in the natural environment. *Journal of Applied Behavior Analysis, 36,* 267–270.

Tanner, B. A., & Zeiler, M. (1975). Punishment of self-injurious behavior using aromatic ammonia as the aversive stimulus. *Journal of Applied Behavior Analysis, 8,* 53–57.

Thompson, R. H., & Iwata, B. A. (2001). A descriptive analysis of social consequences following problem behavior. *Journal of Applied Behavior Analysis, 34,* 169–178.

Thomson, S., & Emerson E. (1995). Inter-observer agreement on the motivation assessment scale: Another failure to replicate. *Journal of Applied Research in Intellectual Disabilities, 8,* 203–208.

Touchette, P. E., MacDonald, R. F., & Langer, S. N. (1985). A scatter plot for identifying stimulus control of problem behavior. *Journal of Applied Behavior Analysis, 18,* 343–351.

Van Camp, C. M., Lerman, D. C., Kelley, M. E., Contrucci, S. A., Vorndran, C. M. (2000). Variable-time reinforcement schedules in the treatment of socially-maintained problem behavior. *Journal of Applied Behavior Analysis, 33,* 545–557.

Vollmer, T. R. (1994). The concept of automatic reinforcement: Implications for behavioral research in developmental disabilities. *Research in Developmental Disabilities, 15,* 187–207.

Vollmer, T. R. (1999). Noncontingent reinforcement: Some additional comments. *Journal of Applied Behavior Analysis, 32,* 239–240.

Vollmer, T. R. (2002). Punishment happens: Some comments on Lerman and Vorndran's review. *Journal of Applied Behavior Analysis, 35,* 469–473.

Vollmer, T. R., & Iwata, B. A. (1992). Differential reinforcement as treatment for behavior disorders: Procedural and functional variations. *Research in Developmental Disabilities, 13,* 393–417.

Vollmer, T. R., Iwata, B. A., Duncan, B. A., & Lerman, D. C. (1993). Within-session patterns of self-injury as indicators of behavioral function. *Research in Developmental Disabilities, 14,* 479–492.

Vollmer, T. R., Iwata, B. A., Smith, R. G., & Rodgers, T. A. (1992). Reduction of multiple aberrant behaviors and concurrent development of self-care skills with differential reinforcement. *Research in Developmental Disabilities, 13,* 287–299.

Vollmer, T. R., Iwata, B. A., Zarcone, J. R., Smith, R. G., & Mazaleski, J. L. (1993). The role of attention in the treatment of attention-maintained self-injurious behavior: Noncontingent reinforcement and differential reinforcement of other behavior. *Journal of Applied Behavior Analysis, 26,* 9–21.

Vollmer, T. R., Marcus, B. A., & LeBlanc, L. (1994). Treatment of self-injury and hand mouthing following inconclusive functional analysis. *Journal of Applied Behavior Analysis, 27,* 331–344.

Vollmer, T. R., Marcus, B. A., Ringdahl, J. E., & Roane, H. S. (1995). Progressing from brief assessments to extended experimental analyses in the evaluation of aberrant behavior. *Journal of Applied Behavior Analysis, 28,* 561–576.

Vollmer, T. R., Northup, J., Ringdahl, J. E., LeBlanc, L. A., & Chauvin, T. M. (1996). Functional analysis of severe tantrums displayed by children with language delays: An outclinic assessment. *Behavior Modification, 20,* 97–115.

Vollmer, T. R., Progar, P. R., Lalli, J. S., Van Camp, C. M., Sierp, B. J., Wright, C. S., et al. (1998). Fixed-time schedules attenuate extinction-induced phenomena in the treatment of severe aberrant behavior. *Journal of Applied Behavior Analysis, 31,* 529–542.

Vollmer, T. R., Roane, H. S., Ringdahl, J. E., & Marcus, B. A. (1999). Evaluating treatment challenges with differential reinforcement of alternative behavior. *Journal of Applied Behavior Analysis, 32,* 9–23.

Wallace, M. D., Doney, J. K., Mintz-Resudek, C. M., & Tarbox, R. S. F. (2004). Training educators to implement functional analyses. *Journal of Applied Behavior Analysis, 37,* 89–92.

Worsdell, A. S., Iwata, B. A., Hanley, G. P., Thompson, R. H., & Kahng, S. (2000). Effects of continuous and intermittent reinforcement for problem behavior during functional communication training. *Journal of Applied Behavior Analysis, 33,* 167–179.

Zarcone, J. R., Iwata, B. A., Smith, R. G., Mazaleski, J. L., & Lerman, D. C. (1994). Re-emergence and extinction of self-injurious escape behavior during stimulus (instructional) fading. *Journal of Applied Behavior Analysis, 27,* 307–316.

Zarcone, J. R., Rodgers, T., Iwata, B., Rourke, D., & Dorsey, M. (1991). Reliability analysis of the motivation assessment scale: A failure to replicate. *Research in Developmental Disabilities, 12,* 349–360.

CHAPTER

PROGRAMMATIC ISSUES

Sandra L. Harris, Robert H. LaRue, and Mary Jane Weiss
Rutgers, The State University of New Jersey

Providing high-quality services to children, adolescents, and adults on the autism spectrum requires more than a well-developed, effective data-based set of teaching methods and curricula. Those are essential components of a good program, but there are other essential elements in the instructional process as well, including staff and family training. On the staffing side, behavior analysts, special education teachers, assistant teachers, speech therapists, job coaches, and other service providers need to be familiar with and keep apprised of the increasingly complex technology that constitutes applied behavior analysis (ABA) teaching methods for people with autism. The need to learn about the methods is continuous, starting with the fundamentals of ABA and continuing indefinitely over time as new methods are developed. The newest assistant teacher as well as the Board Certified Behavior Analyst must be in a situation of continual learning.

On the family side, parents, family members, friends, others responsible for childcare, and in some cases siblings must have access to training in ABA. Regardless of how many hours a child is in school or in a home program, usually a child with autism will spend the majority of time with family members or primary caregivers. It is crucial that those living with the person with autism are able to help teach him or her to function as a member of the family when no teachers are available. Finding the time for training may seem difficult as family members try to cope with the exceptional demands created by the needs of the person with autism and to effectively handle their own reaction to the stress of living with a person with autism, but such training may in fact help to reduce stress and increase parent self-efficacy (Sofronoff & Farbotko, 2002).

The continued training of staff and parents is especially important given the complexity of the ABA teaching methods and the consistency with which they need to be implemented. As a result such training requires considerable effort and specialized programming (Harchik, Sherman, Sheldon, & Strouse, 1992; Noell & Witt, 1999; Page, Iwata, & Reid, 1982; Wolery, 1997). Unfortunately, there is a significant discrepancy between knowledge about ABA methods obtained in research and common practice in the applied field (Jahr, 1998; Van Houten et al., 1988). The implementation of basic behavioral principles, such as reinforcement, extinction, and punishment, appear relatively simple, but the precision and consistency required for effective use of these procedures can be quite labor-intensive. Several studies have demonstrated the importance of high levels of treatment integrity required for interventions to succeed (Albin, Lucyshyn, Horner, & Flannery, 1996; Detrich, 1999; Gresham, Gansle, & Noell, 1993; Koegel, Russo, & Rincover, 1977; Noell et al., 2000; Peterson, Homer, & Wonderlich, 1982; Witt, Noell, LaFleur, & Mortenson, 1997). In addition, inconsistent use of behavioral change procedures may not produce the desired changes in target behavior or in some cases may increase maladaptive behavior (Kazdin, 1984).

This chapter focuses on programming issues separate from the educational and behavioral goals that are most often addressed. First and foremost, because staff and parent training is crucial to the continuing success of a program designed for a person with autism, the first part of this chapter focuses solely on this area. This part of the chapter is divided into three sections: (a) traditional versus behavioral skills training, (b) quality assurance in training, and (c) differences between training staff and family members, with a special focus on sibling training.

The rest of the chapter focuses on other issues that influence the effectiveness of programs for learners with autism. The second part of this chapter is devoted to the special issues facing parents and caregivers of persons with autism, including (a) coping with stress, (b) integrating psychotropic medications for behavior management when necessary, (c) addressing comorbid behavioral and psychiatric disorders, and (d) accessing excellent services for those who may not be able to afford to pay for private services. We have chosen to cover these issues because they contribute to the overall effectiveness of a program designed for a person with autism. Finally, the last part of this chapter touches upon the special issues facing professionals working within the field of ABA and autism. More specifically, this part of the chapter focuses on (a) delivering services to individuals with autism who live in environments of poverty; in rural, cultural, or linguistic isolation; or in regions or countries where there are few people trained in the delivery of ABA; (b) disseminating what we know about ABA to those who need to use it; and (c) ensuring that we think about services in a way that meets our legal and ethical obligation to deliver services to our clients and students.

Staff and Family Training

Teaching staff members and family members to be skilled in the use of ABA teaching methods requires considerable effort and specialized programming (Harchik et al., 1992; Noell & Witt, 1999; Page et al., 1982; Wolery, 1997). This section of the chapter reviews the research on these training methods, focusing first on professional staff and then on families.

Traditional Versus Behavioral Skills Training Approaches to Training Staff

Traditional staff training has included classroom lectures, discussions, workshops, in-service training, and reading training manuals (Kazdin, 1982). Using this approach, training ends when the lecture, discussion, or workshop ends. Follow-up training and feedback are not commonly used. These training procedures are marginally effective and generally do not result in increased staff implementation of ABA procedures (Noell et al., 2000; Pommer & Streedbeck, 1974; Watson & Uzzell, 1980).

In contrast to traditional approaches, *behavioral skills training* (BST) has garnered considerable empirical support for its use in training staff and maintaining skills over time. BST represents an empirically driven approach to teaching a wide variety of skills (Reid & Parsons, 1995). BST has been used effectively to teach students interviewing skills (Iwata, Wong, Riordan, Dorsey, & Lau, 1982); to train children in skills to prevent gun play (Gatheridge et al., 2004; Himle, Miltenberger, Flessner, & Gatheridge, 2004; Miltenberger et al., 2004); to teach staff to conduct paired choice preference assessments (Lavie & Sturmey, 2002); to use incidental teaching to effectively prompt, correct, and reinforce child behavior in its natural context (Schepis, Reid, Ownbey, & Parsons, 2001); to train staff and teachers to conduct analog functional analyses (Iwata et al., 2000; Moore, 2002; Wallace, Doney, Mintz-Resudek, & Tarbox, 2004); to train nursing assistants to use graduated prompting for elderly patients with dementia

(Engelman, Altus, Mosier, & Mathews, 2003); to teach staff to implement discrete trial instruction with learners with autism (Sarokoff & Sturmey, 2004); to
train institutional staff to implement self-management programs with individuals with severe to profound mental retardation (Kissel, Whitman, & Reid, 1983);
and to train parents to implement protocols for children with pediatric feeding
disorders (Mueller et al., 2003). Training should also address stimulus generalization of staff behavior such as the use of multiple exemplar training (Ducharme
& Feldman, 1992). For example, when a staff member is taught to correctly use
incidental teaching, when a child approaches a set of objects during staff training, the staff member blocks the child's approach and prompts more elaborate
language. However, after training, the staff member should emit novel untrained
responses as the child approaches new objects or emits more elaborate language
forms.

Behavioral Skills Training Approach to Teaching Skills

The BST approach to training is a multicomponent process that generally includes instructions, modeling or role playing, and corrective feedback.

Instructional Methods

Providing instructions is the most commonly used procedure for training behavior change agents. This method represents a traditional approach to training. However, the effectiveness of instructional methods is considered minimal
without follow-up training components (Harchik, Sherman, Hopkins, Strouse,
& Sheldon, 1989; McClannahan & Krantz, 1993; Richman, Riordan, Reiss,
Pyles, & Bailey, 1988). Although instructional methods are generally considered
ineffective if used alone, they remain an important component of training. Often instructions can be reduced to a statement of the purpose and importance of
the skill to be trained, a description of the task analysis of the staff performance,
and reading a copy of the task analysis (Reid & Parsons, 1995).

Modeling and Role-Playing

Modeling refers to a procedure in which the model implements a procedure
while the trainee observes the model. Several studies have validated the usefulness of modeling procedures as a component in behavioral skills training (Neef,
1995; Selinske, Greer, & Lodhi, 1991). Video modeling is a useful variant that

may reduce the need for additional staff to provide training (Lavie & Sturmey, 2002; Winnett, Kramer, Walker, Malone, & Lane, 1988).

Role-playing is closely related to modeling in that the desired behavior or procedure is modeled in a practice situation while the roles of teacher and student are alternated. Role-playing allows the rapid practice of the target skills and may improve fluency with implementation and decrease errors while allowing trainees to practice skills in a nonthreatening environment where they can receive immediate feedback from the trainer. There is considerable research supporting the use of role playing in the training process (Ducharme & Feldman, 1992; Iwata et al., 2000; Schepis et al., 2001).

Corrective Feedback

Feedback is a particularly powerful training tool and may include providing individuals with verbal or written information regarding their performance of a particular skill or behavior in order to improve performance (Alavosius & Sulzer-Azaroff, 1986) or graphs illustrating staff performance (Selinske, Greer, & Lodhi, 1991). Not only have the use of corrective feedback procedures been validated for training caregivers (Parsonson, Baer, & Baer, 1974), these procedures may represent the most important component for training and maintaining the desired target skills (Noell et al., 2000; Witt et al., 1997). In addition, research has shown that direct corrective feedback (e.g., face-to-face verbal interaction) is superior to indirect, written feedback (Green, Rollyson, Passante, & Reid, 2002).

Most effective BST protocols involve a combination of written instructions, modeling and role playing, and corrective feedback. The literature has shown that this combination of training components generally produces the greatest impact regarding behavior change (Kazdin, 1984).

Maintaining Staff Behavior

Another challenge in training staff members to implement behavioral procedures involves maintaining the trained target skills over time. Unfortunately, initial training alone is not sufficient to maintain skills for extended periods of time. Even after extensive staff training, staff behavior often reverts to pretraining levels in the absence of continued monitoring and feedback (Ingham & Greer, 1992; Noell et al., 2000).

There are several reasons why treatment integrity may decrease over time. Allen and Warzak (2000) outlined a variety of factors that impact parental nonadherence to treatment protocols. Although their article was written specifically in regard to parental treatment integrity, the same factors are likely to influence service delivery by staff. Table 8.1 lists four of the broad categories of reasons for nonadherence. There are a number of strategies that may be useful for maintaining trained skills.

Skills are most likely to be maintained in settings where consultation, training, and feedback are provided on an ongoing basis (Noell et al., 2000). Continued feedback can be delivered in writing (e.g., progress notes) or verbally (e.g., social praise). In addition to feedback, improving the general knowledge of caregivers may improve treatment integrity and, therefore, have positive effects on maintenance. Caregivers should understand that treatments sometimes need time to work and that their implementation of procedures has a direct impact on treatment effectiveness. The collection and graphing of behavioral data may provide caregivers with an additional source of feedback that can bridge the gap between the initial stages of intervention and the terminal goal. Efforts also need to be made to improve the quality of the training itself. Training caregivers to implement procedures in novel environments and in response to novel be-

TABLE 8.1
Four Categories for Parental Nonadherence

1. Establishing operations
   - Clinicians often fail to account for establishing operations when training others to implement treatments.

2. Stimulus generalization
   - Clinicians often do not train diversely enough to account for situational variations in implementation (training sufficient exemplars) and also may train implementers to use a procedure only in a narrow range of settings.

3. Response acquisition
   - The more complicated a protocol or procedure is, the less likely it will be implemented with high levels of integrity.

4. Consequent events
   - Competing punitive and reinforcing contingencies may have pronounced effects of treatment implementation. For instance, implementation of behavior change procedures may produce an escalation in coercive behavior that punishes parental compliance with a protocol.

Note. Adapted from "The Problem of Parental Nonadherence in Clinical Behavior Analysis: Effective Treatment Is Not Enough," by K. D. Allen and W. J. Warzak, 2000, *Journal of Applied Behavior Analysis*, 33, pp. 373–391. Adapted with permission.

havior can increase preparedness and confidence in what the caregivers are implementing.

Quality Assurance in Training

Monitoring the effectiveness of training procedures is important for ensuring quality assurance in staff training. However, there are few guidelines for evaluating these procedures. The effectiveness of training strategies can be evaluated in four main content areas. The first of these involves the effectiveness of the training procedures for teaching staff to perform a behavior. BST is extremely effective for training behavior change agents to implement behavioral protocols with a high degree of integrity (Reid & Parsons, 1995). The second component is related to whether or not the training results in improvements in the behavior of the clients. Evaluation of training procedures should document changes in client performance (Kuhn, Lerman, & Vorndran, 2003; Schepis et al., 2001). Third, training programs should be evaluated for how well the trained behavior generalizes to different settings or populations (Ducharme & Feldman, 1992; Shore, Iwata, Vollmer, Lerman, & Zarcone, 1995). The usefulness of training is significantly limited if the procedures are useful only in a specific setting or with specific clients. Finally, the maintenance of the trained skills over time should be evaluated in determining the effectiveness of training protocols (Ducharme & Feldman, 1992). Without continued follow up, trained skills often revert to pretraining levels (Noell et al., 2000). For training programs to be effective, they must sustain their effects over extended periods of time.

Unfortunately, BST is not commonly used for training direct-service staff (Hersen, Bellack, & Harris, 1993; Parsons, Reid, & Green, 1993; Reid & Green, 1990). There are several reasons that may account for its lack of use. One reason may be that BST procedures are more labor intensive than traditional approaches to training. Other possible contributing factors may be that people are often uncomfortable providing and receiving feedback and that many supervisory staff members are not trained to use BST. There have, however, been procedures developed to train large groups of caregivers to effectively implement behavior change procedures.

Training Large Groups of People

Although BST has been shown to be effective for training a wide variety of skills, the question remains, How does one provide high-quality training for large groups of staff members or parents? Traditional approaches to training often involve considerable expense for agencies and involve the logistical problems of scheduling training for direct-care staff and arranging coverage for their clinical duties. Another challenge involves the quality of the training itself. In general, the larger the group being trained, the less one-to-one supervisory feedback is possible, which decreases the quality contact training time. Another complication involves the high staff turnover and absenteeism that is common for facilities serving individuals with developmental disabilities (Zaharia & Baumeister, 1979).

Pyramidal training represents a useful strategy for training large groups of individuals in a cost-efficient, less time-consuming manner than traditional approaches to training. Pyramidal training involves training a small number of staff who then train other staff members. The trainers are generally administrative or other supervisory staff members who repeatedly train small groups of staff. This approach allows training to become more efficient (a group of trainers training smaller, more manageable groups of staff) and effective (higher trainee-to-trainer ratio, which increases contact time). Pyramidal training has received overwhelming empirical support. It has been shown to be effective for training small groups of staff members (Jones, Fremouw, & Carples, 1977), large groups of institutional staff (Page et al., 1982; Shore et al., 1995), families of children with behavioral problems (Adubato, Adams, & Budd, 1981; Kuhn et al., 2003), and for training parents to train other parents to use behavioral teaching skills (Neef, 1995). It has even been applied effectively in statewide training (Reid et al., 2003). In addition to training staff and caregivers to implement the procedures themselves, providing specific training in how to give feedback has been shown to improve the training model (Fleming & Sulzer-Azaroff, 1989; McGimsey, Greene, & Lutzker, 1995; Parsons & Reid, 1995).

Pyramidal training procedures offer a number of advantages as compared to traditional forms of training. Perhaps the most salient of these advantages is cost effectiveness. Training supervisory staff or parents to train others eliminates the need for continued training or consultation from outside professionals. Pyramidal training may also increase maintenance by allowing continued supervision to occur in the context of the workplace. Supervisors remain in the clinical setting and can provide continuous feedback for staff behavior. In addition, training in the work environment reduces the need to remove direct care staff from clinical obligations for training.

Teaching ABA to Parents and Siblings

There is a substantial body of research over several decades documenting that parents, like professional staff members, can master the fundamentals of ABA (Harris, 1983; Howlin, 1981; Koegel, Schreibman, Britten, Burke, & O'Neill,

1982). Nonetheless, given the many demands in their lives, the extent and depth of parental involvement is often not as extensive as that of professionals. Parents can learn ABA skills, and their children with autism show changes in behavior as a result. This kind of learning requires continual training and education. Early research indicated that parents who did not receive ongoing support in problem solving were likely to discontinue their use of ABA when they were stymied by problems that arose (Harris, 1986). We do not expect staff members to master a set of ABA teaching methods and never seek consultation and support in the future; thus, there is little reason to expect that parents can function without this ongoing support as well. They may become increasingly good at problem solving as they apply the methods over time, but even the most skilled ABA practitioner needs to brainstorm with colleagues when a recalcitrant problem arises.

The most extensive use of ABA in the home has been in early intensive intervention programs for young children where parents may be primary therapists or coordinators of services for their preschool-age child. Starting with the work of Lovaas (1987) and continuing since then in a series of partial replications and extensions of his work, parents have been taught to implement a broad gamut of ABA programs (Jocelyn, Casiro, Beattie, Bow, & Kneisz, 1998; Smith, Groen, & Wynn, 2000). Other studies have focused on teaching one or more specific skill to parents, such as the use of the natural language paradigm to increase speech (Laski, Charlop, & Schreibman, 1998), photographic activity schedules to increase participation in family activities (Krantz, MacDuff, & McClannahan, 1993), functional communication training to reduce behavior problems (Moes & Frea, 2002), pivotal response training to increase a child's motivation (Koegel, Bimbela, & Schreibman, 1996), or joint attention (Drew et al., 2002).

Early research showed that siblings, too, can learn some fundamentals of ABA (Colletti & Harris, 1977; Schreibman, O'Neill, & Koegel, 1983). In a study with sisters of children with autism, Celiberti and Harris (1993) found that these girls could learn basic behavioral skills to engage their brothers with autism in play including giving clear directions, praising good behavior, and using physical and verbal prompts. The skills were taught over the course of several play sessions and were readily mastered. Not only did independent raters evaluate the girls as more confident after training, and more interested in their brothers with autism, they also appeared more pleased by their interactions with their siblings. A caution, however, is that one would want to be certain that children wished to learn the skills before enrolling them in such a program.

Assisting family members in the process of adaptation and ensuring competency among staff members serving individuals with autism spectrum disorders are two critically important goals in empowering family members and staff members and in ensuring maximally effective intervention. It is likely that we will continue to be more effective in these realms as research and clinical practice continue to help us hone our efforts in achieving these goals. For family members in particular, training should be coupled with sensitivity to the experience of raising a child with autism.

Special Issues: Parents and Siblings

Coping with Stress

Life in a family—any family—has times of stress. Stress arises not just from sad things like a death in the family, but also from happy events, such as when a child graduates from high school. Many stressors come from normative events that happen to most of us, like the birth of a baby, and some events become exceptional stressors, such as when the parent of a young child dies or a family contends with a devastating flood or hurricane.

When a family includes someone with autism, the vulnerability to stress is greatly increased by the demands of meeting that person's special needs and managing one's feelings about the impact of the disability on the family. These parents are subject to events of greater potential stress than are parents of children who are typically developing (Holmes & Carr, 1991; Morgan, 1988) or parents who have children with other disabilities such as mental retardation (Donovan, 1988; Weiss, 2002). Although most brothers and sisters of children with autism function as well as other youngsters, there is a somewhat greater risk for discomfort in the lives of these children, just as is true for their parents (Rivers & Stoneman, 2003). Males and siblings who are younger than the child with autism may be at greater risk than females or older siblings (Hastings, 2003), although other studies with children with mental retardation have failed to support the birth-order findings (Stoneman, Brody, Davis, Crapps, & Malone, 1991). Siblings are also at increased risk for autism spectrum disorders and related disorders such as problems with speech and language (Rutter, Bailey, Simonoff, & Pickles, 1997). The presence of these disorders may serve to heighten the sibling's vulnerability to potential stressors.

Among the factors that contribute to the higher level of stress in families of people with autism is the lack of social responsiveness of the child with autism. The presence of behavior management issues, especially externally directed challenging behavior such as aggression and sleep problems, and the consequent need for parents to master a complex set of child management skills are also related to family stress. The demands of time, energy, and money can leave a family depleted emotionally, physically, and financially (Jarbrink, Fombonne,

& Knapp, 2003). The impact of chronic stress is not trivial in terms of one's psychological or physical health (Glasberg, Martins, & Harris, in press) and can even be correlated with greater cellular aging (Epel et al., 2004).

Parental stress and methods of coping can have an impact on the experiences of the siblings of children with autism. Rivers and Stoneman (2003) found that in families with higher levels of marital stress, typically developing siblings reported less satisfaction in their relationship with their brother or sister with autism and described more negative and fewer positive interactions than did children in families with less marital stress. When marital conflict was high, support from family and friends appeared to have a beneficial impact on the positive aspects of the sibling relationship.

Coping Strategies: Parents

Although living with a child with autism is stressful, some families cope better with the demands than do others, and there are some important factors that contribute to being more resilient in the face of this or any other source of stress. *Instrumental* and *palliative* strategies are both used to cope with stressful situations (Glasberg et al., in press). A good example of an instrumental coping strategy is demonstrated when parents master the fundamentals of ABA so they can address behavior problems and skill acquisition opportunities. Consistent use of ABA methods, although initially time consuming, ultimately enhances the quality of family life as the person with autism learns self-help skills, engages in less disruptive behavior, and masters recreational skills enabling him or her to share family activities. An example of a palliative coping skill would be the parent attending cognitive behavior therapy or a parent support group to examine their feelings about their child's autism and the meaning of the disability. This reflection may result in a shift in their feelings and opinions about the impact of the disability.

Instrumental coping skills can have both palliative and instrumental benefits. For example, Sofronoff and Farbotko (2002) taught parents of children with Asperger's Disorder to use parent management training (Judge, 1997) to address their child's behavior problems. Not only did the children engage in fewer behavior problems after the parents mastered the skills, but the parents reported a greater sense of personal self-efficacy.

Developing a strong, supportive social network is another example of a coping method that involves both instrumental and palliative components (Boyd, 2002; Weiss, 2002). Families who have more friends and relatives to whom they can turn may receive tangible benefits in terms of child care as well as the palliative benefits of feeling cared about and having someone with whom one can talk and share feelings.

Although the changes that occur in family life when a child has autism are stressful and demand attention, the resultant changes need not always be negative (Rodrigue, Geffken, & Morgan, 1993; Scorgie & Sobsey, 2000; Sivberg, 2002). There are many helpful ways to cope. Religious faith (Skinner, Correa, Skinner, & Bailey, 2001) friendships (Weiss, 2002), or reorganization of value systems to make their children more central in their lives and their work outside the home less important than it may have been in the past (e.g., Tunali & Power, 2002) may all be effective coping strategies. Some people find support from others who share their experience to be especially helpful. Support groups for various family members come in many forms, including parent-managed groups with little if any professional input, as well as professionally guided support groups, organized according to that professional's theoretical framework. Some groups may involve an open forum for sharing feelings, whereas others may be more focused on problem solving (Nixon & Singer, 1993). There are few data concerning more or less effective modalities for these groups.

Coping Strategies: Siblings

Siblings, like parents, rely on a variety of coping strategies to manage their concerns about their sibling with autism (Glasberg et al., in press). The specific strategies and their benefits vary with the child's age and level of intellectual maturity. Younger children who are more cognitively immature and who have less control over their environment will typically need more parental support than will older children who have more advanced problem-solving skills and greater independence. In general, younger children use fewer of the following coping methods than older siblings use (Donaldson, Prinstein, Danovsky, & Spirito, 2000): talking to a friend, relative, or parent about their concerns; generating their own solutions, such as putting valued toys in a locked closet where they are safe from their sibling's destructive behavior; thinking positively about the situation; or saying reassuring things to themselves about how the situation will eventually improve. Unlike most adults, though, siblings may also be physically or verbally aggressive toward the child with autism.

Gamble and McHale (1989) found that children who have a sibling with a disability do not differ from other children in the kinds of coping methods they adopt, but do tend to use more cognitive strategies than do other youngsters. A heavy reliance on cognitive, as opposed to action-oriented, strategies has a downside to it. Some research suggests that children who use cognitive methods are more prone to report feelings of sadness and worry (Gamble & McHale, 1989). It may be helpful for children to learn more action-oriented approaches, like talking to their parents about their concerns. Parents should also be encouraged to support their child in solving the problems that arise so that asking parents to take action on his or her behalf or generating one's own solutions is reinforcing for children.

There is only a modest body of research on the benefits of support groups for siblings, and much of this work has addressed children whose siblings have a variety of chronic disabilities (Lobato & Kao, 2002; Meyer & Vadasay, 1994). The activities in a sibling support group will vary with the ages of the participants and can include art projects, sharing both positive and negative feelings about their brother or sister, and learning the details of their sibling's disorder (Meyer & Vadasy, 1994). At the Douglass Developmental Disabilities Center, we teach siblings problem-solving skills and encourage them, in a session with their parents, to describe the things that adults should know about having a brother or sister with autism.

Providing support to families and equipping family members with the skills to be effective in their interactions with their loved one with autism is critically important. Well-supported and proficient family members cope better, feel more efficacious in their roles, and are less vulnerable to burnout.

Pharmacological Interventions

Autism is a clinical syndrome with a neurological basis. As such, psychopharmacological interventions are common treatment components for the management of behavioral problems associated with these disorders. To date, the etiology of autism remains multifactorial and poorly understood. However, it appears that autism is the result of complex genetic and physiological factors and their interaction with the environment (Ellis, Singh, & Singh, 1997). Given the complexity of autism, a wide variety of medications have been tested to treat the behavioral problems associated with autism.

Types of Psychotropic Medications

Antipsychotic medications are among the most commonly prescribed for the treatment of autism. Conventional antipsychotic medications include haloperidol and pimozide, which are effective for reducing stereotypic behavior, hyperactivity, fidgeting, and aggression (Anderson & Campbell, 1989; Ernst et al., 1992). Side effects of conventional antipsychotics include sedation, dystonia, and severe tardive dyskinesia (Campbell et al., 1993). Atypical or second-generation antipsychotic medications, such as risperidone, have been shown to have similar reductive effects on hyperactivity, stereotypy, and aggression (McDougle et al., 1998) while having less tardive dyskinesia and extrapyramidal side effects. However, these drugs have other significant negative side effects including sedation that may impair learning and cause weight gain (Singh, Matson, Cooper, Dixon, & Sturmey, 2005).

Antidepressant medications, such as clomipramine, fluoxetine, and sertraline, are also commonly prescribed for the treatment of autism and are effective for reducing obsessional behavior, hyperactivity, and aggression (Brasic et al., 1994; Koshes, 1997; Steingard, Zimnitsky, DeMaso, Bauman, & Bucci, 1997). Common side effects of antidepressant medications include restlessness, irritability, and drowsiness.

There are a variety of other, less commonly prescribed medications used to treat behavioral problems associated with autism, including anticonvulsants (e.g., sodium valproate), psychomotor stimulants (e.g., methylphenidate), antihypertensives (e.g., clonidine), opioid antagonists (e.g., naltrexone), and gastrointestinal hormones (e.g., secretin). Supporting evidence for use of these medications is less conclusive than reported for antipsychotic and antidepressant medication (e.g., Sturmey, 2005).

Effectiveness of Pharmacological Interventions

The literature regarding the effectiveness of psychotropic medications is plagued by both methodological and ethical controversy. One consistent finding is that many classes of psychotropic medication are effective for reducing some forms of maladaptive behavior associated with autism, but few studies have shown that any of these medications consistently increase adaptive behavior or learning. Another consistent finding in the literature is that medication response varies considerably from individual to individual. In most group studies, there exist responders and nonresponders. This variability in clinical response may be related to myriad different factors such as medication dose, physiological differences, and environmental factors affecting behavior. Although many double-blind trials collect data on reductions in a target autistic symptom, they rarely evaluate the impact of psychotropic medication on learning, do not collect data on the social validity of the changes reported, do not report data on individuals, and may possibly report safety data during the short duration of the trial.

Best Practices in Evaluating the Effects of Psychotropic Medications

The effects of psychotropic medications have historically been evaluated using large-group designs. Indeed, double-blind placebo-controlled group studies represent an effective means by which to determine the effectiveness of psychoactive medications. These designs are extremely effective for identifying potentially useful medications and determining how large groups of individuals respond to different dosage levels of medication. Although group designs are extremely effective to this end, they are, by design, not sensitive to individual variability of response to medication.

Single-subject research can be a useful complement to group designs for evaluating the effects of psychotropic medication. Single-subject methodologies represent a useful strategy for evaluating individual clinical response to medication. However, relatively few single-subject methods for evaluating medication effects have been empirically validated. Reinforcer assessments (Northup, Fusilier, Swanson, Roane, & Borrero, 1997; Northup, George, Jones, & Broussard, 1996) and functional analysis procedures (Crosland et al., 2003; Northup et al., 1999) are among a number of potentially useful procedures that can be used to inform decisions regarding dose titration and general effectiveness of medications on the individual level. Treatment teams using psychotropic medications should identify specific behavioral targets for psychotropic medication and collect reliable observational and social validation data to evaluate their effectiveness. Once a reliable behavior change has been observed, the treatment team will be able to explicitly judge the costs and benefits of the psychotropic medications.

Comorbid Disorders

Comorbidity of autism and psychiatric disorders is an area of interest and debate within the field. It is clear that autism can coexist with other difficulties. What is not clear is how these disorders interact and whether the comorbidity itself might help in identifying the genesis of autism (Tsai, 1996; Volkmar, Klin, & Cohen, 1997). The question of comorbidity is complex because of the wide variety and severity of behavior exhibited by individuals with autism. It is very common for individuals with autism to be hyperactive and inattentive, exhibit motor tics, and engage in perseverative behavior. It can be very difficult to separate the presence of such common behavior from an appropriate separate diagnosis.

Volkmar, Klin, and Cohen (1997) noted that more than 80% of individuals with autism may exhibit stereotyped behavior, although there is some variability in the estimates of such behavior (Brasic et al., 1994; Fombonne, 1992; McDougle et al., 1995; Rumsey, Rapoport, & Sceery, 1985). Some authors view that type of behavior as a symptom of compulsion; however, it is not clear how similar genuine obsessions and compulsions are to the repetitive thoughts and behavior of persons with Autism Spectrum Disorders (McDougle, Kresch, & Posey, 2000). Nevertheless, there has been some suggestion that medication given for Obsessive–Compulsive Disorders can ameliorate obsessive–compulsive symptoms in individuals with autism (Gordon, Rapoport, Hamburger, State, & Mannheim, 1992; McDougle et al., 2000).

Attention-Deficit/Hyperactivity Disorder (ADHD) is another important condition that often co-occurs with autism. Although many individuals with ASD exhibit both high rates of activity and deficits in attention, these problems and the potential diagnostic overlap have not been fully explored. It was originally thought that ADHD and ASD were mutually exclusive, but they are now considered potentially comorbid (Volkmar, Klin, & Cohen, 1997). Goldstein and Schwebach (2004) examined charts of children diagnosed with a *Pervasive Developmental Disorder* (PDD) or ADHD. Seven of 27 (26%) individuals with PDD met *Diagnostic and Statistical Manual of Mental Disorders* (DSM–IV; American Psychiatric Association, 2004) criteria for the combined type of ADHD, while an additional 9 (33%) met the criteria for the inattentive type of ADHD. In addition, these authors found that those exhibiting symptoms of the combined type were much more likely to experience serious impairment in daily life. It is now recommended that ADHD be considered as an additional diagnosis for persons with autism and as a target of intervention when appropriate (Ghaziuddin, Tsai, & Ghaziuddin, 1992).

Access to Services and Cultural Issues

Access to services for the treatment of ASDs varies widely around the world. In the United States quality of care for learners with autism is affected by socioeconomic factors. It is especially prominent in early intervention services, where parental advocacy and personal affluence can make a big difference in the amount and quality of services obtained, but the effects are also felt at the school-age level where affluent communities can afford more educational resources for students with autism than can communities of poverty.

It also appears that the diagnosis of autism itself has implications for access to services. Children with a diagnosis of autism are especially vulnerable to having difficulty securing appropriate specialist care, with over one third of children with autism having difficulty obtaining appropriate care from specialty physicians (Krauss, Gulley, Sciegaj, & Wells, 2003). Diagnosis itself is affected by demographics. African American children receive a diagnosis at a statistically significant later age than White children (7.9 years vs. 6.3 years; Mandell, Listerud, Levy, & Pinto-Martin, 2002). Given the importance of early intervention, such a lag in services has grave implications.

The data on such inequities in access to services are difficult to obtain. Ruble, Helfinger, Renfrew, and Saunders (2005) found that information on access to and utilization of services is lacking. These researchers reviewed data from the state Medicaid program for low socioeconomic status children in Tennessee. They were especially interested in the extent to which available services were used. Examining trends over 5 years, the researchers found that the number of children receiving services for ASDs increased. However, the rate of service use was one 10th of what would be expected given prevalence rates.

Prevalence and Related Issues

Epidemiological surveys reveal mixed information on the prevalence of ASDs, typically ranging from 0.7 to 15 per 10,000 (Fombonne, 1998), although more recent empirical papers have reported even higher prevalence rates (Centers for Disease Control and Prevention, 2003). In addition to disputes over absolute prevalence rates, there are difficulties in ascertaining relative prevalence across different groups. In general, there are problems with how well surveys have analyzed race or immigrant status (Dyches, Wilder, Sudweeks, Obiakor, & Algozzine, 2004). The data on immigration are particularly mixed, with some studies showing a higher prevalence in immigrant families (Gillberg, Steffenburg, Borjesson, & Andersson, 1987) and others showing no significant differences (Powell et al., 2000). There is a general consensus, however, that prevalence rates are higher among immigrants (Dyches et al., 2004). Explanations include higher rates of intrauterine viral infections, higher rates of brain damage in developing countries, and homeland-specific genetic disorders (Dyches et al., 2004).

A related barrier to effective services is found in problems in language comprehension and use. When English is a second language, it may be particularly difficult for the family to access services, to understand information conveyed to them by professionals, and to advocate for their child's needs. Access to parent training programs in a family's native language has been shown to increase attendance and participation (Prieto-Bayard & Baker, 1986). See the practitioner recommendations for parents at the end of this chapter.

A Multicultural Perspective

The clinician working with diverse populations needs to be sensitive to the myriad ways in which culture, religion, race, and ethnicity affect a family's experience and relationships with staff. Although some of the variables are more obvious, as in the case of language differences, others are subtler.

Cultural factors play a role in resilience in the face of stress. Different ethnic and racial groups tend to view their child's autism or related developmental disorder in different ways, and their perspective influences how parents cope. For example, Dyches et al. (2004) pointed out that one Native American group, the Mojaves, think of mental retardation as resulting from parental misdeed, whereas another group, the Navajos, think of autism as related to witchcraft or parental fault.

Degree of acculturation into the Western scientific perspective will influence the extent to which the younger generation adheres to the values of their elders. For example, although younger Latino mothers may hold more Western views about the source of developmental disorders, their elders may still attribute mental retardation to parental sin (Skinner, Bailey, Correa, & Rodriguez, 1999). Dyches et al. (2004) noted that cultural values have an impact not only on perception of the potential stressor but also on resources for coping. For example, Boyd-Franklin (1989) pointed to the strength of the extended family in supporting members of the African American community. A similar valuing of family, although grounded in somewhat different perspectives, is found in Hispanic, Native Hawaiian, and Filipino American families (Dyches et al., 2004). The wise service provider will be familiar with the cultural background of his or her students and will work with families in a way that respects their values and draws on their strengths.

Ensuring Quality Service and Dissemination

A critical issue in the legal realm is the definition of adequate or appropriate services (Wright & Wright, 1999). Part of the difficulty is the heterogenous presentation of individuals on the autism spectrum. What is adequate and appropriate for one student with an ASD may be wholly inappropriate for another. Philosophical differences regarding intensity of intervention, instructional approach, and the benefits of inclusion further muddy the waters. With the explosion of interest in and requests for services, the need to define quality services has also increased. In reality, many individuals with ASDs will be served in programs offering fewer than optimal hours of intervention. Furthermore, the variability in the training and expertise of the staff members serving the population of individuals with autism, especially in the public sector, means there will be uneven services. A hopeful note in this regard is the development by some states of guidelines for effective educational services. These include New Jersey (New Jersey Department of Education, 2004) and New York (New York State Department of Health Early Intervention Program, 1999), as well as the National Research Council's (2001) report for the U.S. Department of Education.

A major training priority is the effective dissemination of technology to the wider educational community. This is a difficult and daunting task, mainly because of the complexity and sophistication of the instructional technology within ABA. As we note in discussing staff training, it cannot be conveyed to educators in a few brief workshops.

One hopeful change in the field is the national certification credential (Shook & Favell, 1996). The Behavior Analyst Certification Board certifies professionals at a full and an associate level (http://www.bacb.com). This makes it possible for school districts and parents to assess whether a professional has expertise in ABA. Certification requires both academic and clinical experience. Academic requirements are substantial (three courses at the associate level and five at the full level). This ensures that there is a theoretical foundation in ABA, as well as a broad understanding of its applications. The clinical experience guidelines require supervised experience in the design and implementation of behavioral technology, including instructional techniques, functional assessment and analysis, and the development of behavior intervention plans. Meeting the mentoring needs of professionals engaged in the process of becoming certified is a substantial challenge, particularly at this juncture, when the numbers of certified behavior analysts is still relatively small.

This credential will most certainly propel the ABA field forward. It provides basic guidelines for professional expertise within the field, and it empowers consumers to evaluate candidates' expertise. Additional assistance for consumers can be found in the Association for Behavior Analysis Autism Special Interest Group's (2004) *Revised Guidelines for Consumers of ABA Services to Individuals with Autism and Related Disorders.* This document provides explicit information regarding the evaluation of professional competence and is available at the organization's Web site (http://www.abainternational.org/sub/membersvcs/sig/contactinfo/Autism.asp).

Summary

We addressed a broad range of topics in this chapter. In the domain of families, the research indicates that parents can be effective collaborators with professionals in the education of their children, but for some families sensitivity to the stress they face may be essential if they are to mobilize themselves for a teaching role. We also noted that there are very effective ways to train people in ABA teaching methods and that the Board Certified Behavior Analyst credential has become a useful way to identify staff members who have solid ABA training. We touched on the area of social skills development as a domain where some innovative work is being done. The chapter also examined some of the factors that may have an impact on service delivery by the ABA professional. These include the client's need for medication and the presence of comorbid diagnoses. It also includes the social context in which the family is embedded and the meaning the diagnosis on the autism spectrum has for them.

PRACTITIONER RECOMMENDATIONS

PARENTS

1. Insist on regular parent and staff training sessions that use a behavioral skills training approach from your service provider.
2. Parents and siblings should use instrumental and pallative coping skills to reduce the effects of stress related to having a family member with autism.
3. Choose medication carefully and always monitor effects on the learner's ability to function effectively within his or her environment.

   a. Medication should be used as a component of a treatment package that includes strategies to increase adaptive behavior.

   b. Medication should not be used as a form of behavior restraint.

4. Be alert for the presence of comorbid disorders that can make intervention more complex.
5. Choose behavior analysts who are board certified by the Behavior Analyst Certification Board.

PROFESSIONALS

1. Use data-based approaches to staff and parent training and ensure maintenance of skills through continuing training.
2. Recognize that family members have complex roles and are grappling with the emotional impact of raising a child with a serious and potentially lifelong disorder. They need support as well as skills.
3. Be sensitive to the impact of contextual factors including cultural traditions and socioeconomic status as variables that influence how a family copes with the needs of a person with autism.
4. Standards of ethical conduct require us all to be in a state of continuous learning.
5. Pursue board certification in behavior analysis.

References

Adubato, S. A., Adams, M. K., & Budd, K. S. (1981). Teaching a parent to train a spouse in child management techniques. *Journal of Applied Behavior Analysis, 14,* 193–205.

Alavosius, M. P., & Sulzer-Azaroff, B. (1986). The effects of performance feedback on the safety of client lifting and transfer. *Journal of Applied Behavior Analysis, 19,* 261–267.

Albin, R. W., Lucyshyn, J. M., Horner, R. H., & Flannery, K. B. (1996). Contextual fit for behavioral support plans: A model for "goodness of fit." In L. K. Koegel, R. L. Koegel, & G. Dunlap (Eds.), *Positive behavioral support: Including people with difficult behaviors in the community* (pp. 81–98). Baltimore: Brookes.

Allen, K. D., & Warzak, W. J. (2000). The problem of parental nonadherence in clinical behavior analysis: Effective treatment is not enough. *Journal of Applied Behavior Analysis, 33,* 373–391.

American Psychiatric Association. (1994). *Diagnostic and statistical manual of mental disorders* (4th ed.). Washington, DC: Author.

Anderson, L., & Campbell, M. (1989). The effects of haloperidol on discrimination learning and behavioral symptoms in autistic children. *Journal of Autism and Developmental Disorders, 19,* 227–239.

Autism Special Interest Group: Association for Behavior Analysis. 2004. Revised guidelines for consumers of ABA services to individuals with autism and related disorders. Retrieved April 24, 2006, from http://www.abainternational.org/sub/membersvcs/sig/contactinfo/Autism.asp

Boyd, B. A. (2002). Examining the relationship between stress and lack of social support in mothers of children with autism. *Focus on Autism and Other Developmental Disabilities, 17,* 208–215.

Boyd-Franklin, N. (1989). *Black families in therapy: A multisystems approach.* New York: Guilford Press.

Brasic, J. R., Barnett, J. Y., Kaplan, D., Sheitman, B. B., Aisemberg, P., Lafargue, R. T., et al. (1994). Clomipramine ameliorates adventitious movements and compulsions in prepubertal boys with autistic disorder and severe mental retardation. *Neurology, 44,* 1309–1312.

Campbell, M., Armenteros, J. L., Malone, R. P., Adams, P. B., Eisenberg, Z. W., & Overall, J. E. (1993). Neuroleptic-related dyskinesias in autistic children: A prospective, longitudinal study. *Journal of the American Academy of Child and Adolescent Psychiatry, 46,* 672.

Celiberti, D. A., & Harris, S. L. (1993). Behavioral intervention for siblings of children with autism: A focus on skills to enhance play. *Behavior Therapy, 24,* 573–599.

Centers for Disease Control and Prevention. (2003). How common is autism spectrum disorder (ASDs)? Retrieved April 24, 2006, from http://www.cdc.gov/ncbddd/autism/asd_common.htm

Colletti, G., & Harris, S. L. (1977). Behavior modification in the home: Siblings as behavior modifiers, parents as observers. *Journal of Abnormal Child Psychology, 1,* 21–30.

Crosland K. A., Zarcone, J. R., Lindauer, S. E., Valdovinos, M. G., Zarcone, T. J., Hellings, J. A., et al. (2003). Use of functional analysis methodology in the evaluation of medication effects. *Journal of Autism and Developmental Disorders, 33,* 271–279.

Detrich, R. (1999). Increasing treatment fidelity by matching interventions to contextual variables within the educational setting. *School Psychology Review, 28,* 608–620.

Donaldson, D., Prinstein, M. J., Danovsky, M., & Spirito, A. (2000). Patterns of children's coping with life stress: Implications for clinicians. *American Journal of Orthopsychiatry, 70,* 351–359.

Donovan, A. M. (1988). Family stress and ways of coping with adolescents who have handicaps: Maternal perceptions. *American Journal on Mental Retardation, 92,* 502–509.

Drew, A., Baird, G., Baron-Cohen, S., Cox, A., Slonims, V., Wheelwright, S., et al. (2002). A pilot randomized control trial of a parent training intervention for pre-school children with autism. *European Child and Adolescent Psychiatry, 11,* 266–272.

Ducharme, J. M., & Feldman, M. A. (1992). Comparison of staff training strategies to promote generalized teaching skills. *Journal of Applied Behavior Analysis, 25,* 165–179.

Dyches, T. T., Wilder, L. K., Sudweeks, R. R., Obiakor, F. E., & Algozzine, B. (2004). Multicultural issues in autism. *Journal of Autism and Developmental Disorders, 34,* 211–222.

Ellis, C. R., Singh, Y. N., & Singh, N. N. (1997). Use of behavior modifying drugs. In N. Singh (Ed.), *Prevention and treatment of severe behavior problems: Methods and models in developmental disabilities* (pp. 150–176). Pacific Grove, CA: Brooks/Cole.

Engelman, K. K., Altus, D. E., Mosier, M. C., & Mathews, R. M. (2003). Brief training to promote the use of less intrusive prompts by nursing assistants in a dementia care unit. *Journal of Applied Behavior Analysis, 36,* 129–132.

Epel, E. S., Blackburn, E. H., Lin, J., Dhabhar, F. S., Adler, N. E., Morrow, J. D., et al. (2004). Accelerated telomere shortening in response to life stress. *Proceedings of the National Academy of Science, 101,* 17312–17315.

Ernst, M., Magee, H. G., Gonzalez, N. M., Locascio, J. J., Rosenberg, C. R., & Campbell, M. (1992). Pimozide in autistic children. *Psychopharmacology Bulletin, 28,* 87–92.

Fleming, R. K., & Sulzer-Azaroff, B. (1989). Enhancing quality of teaching by direct care staff through performance feedback on the job. *Behavioral Residential Treatment, 4*, 377–395.

Fombonne, E. (1992). Diagnostic assessment in a sample of autistic and developmentally impaired adolescents: Classification and diagnosis. *Journal of Autism and Developmental Disorders, 22*, 563–581.

Fombonne, E. (1998). Epidemiological surveys of autism. In F. R. Volkmar (Ed.), *Autism and pervasive developmental disorders* (pp. 32–63). Cambridge, England: Cambridge University Press.

Gamble, W. C., & McHale, S. M. (1989). Coping with stress in sibling relationships: A comparison of children with disabled and nondisabled siblings. *Journal of Applied Developmental Psychology, 10*, 353–373.

Gatheridge, B. J., Miltenberger, R. G., Huneke, D. F., Satterlund, M. J., Mattern, A. R., Johnson, B. M., et al. (2004). Comparison of two programs to teach firearm injury prevention skills to 6- and 7-year-old children. *Pediatrics, 114*, 94–99.

Ghaziuddin, M., Tsai, L., & Ghaziuddin, N. (1992). Comorbidity of autistic disorder in children and adolescents. *European Child and Adolescent Psychiatry, 1*, 209–213.

Gillberg, C., Steffenburg, G., Borjesson, B., & Andersson, L. (1987). Infantile autism in children with immigrant parents: A population based study from Goteburg, Sweden. *British Journal of Psychiatry, 150*, 856–858.

Glasberg, B., Martins, M., & Harris, S. L. (in press). Stress and coping among family members of individuals with autism. In M. G. Baron, J. Groden, G. Groden, & L. P. Lipsett (Eds.), *Stress and coping in autism.* New York: Oxford University Press.

Goldstein, S., & Schwebach, A. (2004). The comorbidity of pervasive developmental disorder and attention deficit hyperactivity disorder: Result of a retrospective chart review. *Journal of Autism and Developmental Disorders, 34*, 329–339.

Gordon, C. T., Rapoport, J. L., Hamburger, S. D., State, R. C., & Mannheim, G. B. (1992). Differential response of seven subjects with autistic disorder to chlomipramine and desipramine. *American Journal of Psychiatry, 149*, 363–366.

Green, C. W., Rollyson, J. H., Passante, S. C., & Reid, D. H. (2002). Maintaining proficient supervisor performance with direct support personnel: An analysis of two management approaches. *Journal of Applied Behavior Analysis, 35*, 205–208.

Gresham, F. M., Gansle, K. A., & Noell, G. H. (1993). Treatment integrity in applied behavior analysis with children. *Journal of Applied Behavior Analysis, 26*, 257–263.

Harchik, A. E., Sherman, J. A., Hopkins, B. L., Strouse, M. C., & Sheldon, J. B. (1989). Use of behavioral techniques by paraprofessional staff: A review and proposal. *Behavioral Residential Treatment, 4*, 331–357.

Harchik, A. E., Sherman, J. A., Sheldon, J. B., & Strouse, M. C. (1992). Ongoing consultation as a method of improving staff performance of staff members in a group home. *Journal of Applied Behavior Analysis, 25*, 599–610.

Harris, S. L. (1983). *Families of the developmentally disabled: A guide to behavioral intervention.* Elmsford, NY: Pergamon.

Harris, S. L. (1986). Parents as teachers: A four to seven year follow up of parents of children with autism. *Child and Family Behavior Therapy, 8,* 39–47.

Hastings, R. (2003). Brief report: Behavioral adjustment of siblings of children with autism. *Journal of Autism and Developmental Disorders, 33,* 99–104.

Hersen, M., Bellack, A. S., & Harris, F. (1993). Staff training and consultation. In A. Bellack & M. Hersen (Eds.), *Handbook of behavior therapy in the psychiatric setting* (pp. 143–164). New York: Plenum Press.

Himle, M. B., Miltenberger, R. G., Flessner, C., & Gatheridge, B. (2004). Teaching safety skills to children to prevent gun play. *Journal of Applied Behavior Analysis, 37,* 1–9.

Himle, M. B., Miltenberger, R. G., Gatheridge, B. J., & Flessner, C. A. (2004). An evaluation of two procedures for training skills to prevent gun play in children. *Pediatrics, 113,* 70–7.

Holmes, N., & Carr, J. (1991). The pattern of care in families of adults with a mental handicap: A comparison between families of autistic adults and Down syndrome adults. *Journal of Autism and Developmental Disorders, 21,* 159–176.

Howlin, P. A. (1981). The results of a home-based language training programme with autistic children. *British Journal of Disorders of Communication, 16,* 73–88.

Ingham, P., & Greer, R. D. (1992). Changes in student and teacher responses in observed and generalized settings as a function of supervisor observations. *Journal of Applied Behavior Analysis, 25,* 153–164.

Iwata, B. A., Wallace, M. D., Kahng, S., Lindberg, J. S., Roscoe, E. M., Conners J., et al. (2000). Skill acquisition in the implementation of functional analysis methodology. *Journal of Applied Behavior Analysis, 33,* 181–194.

Iwata, B. A., Wong, S. E., Riordan, M. M., Dorsey, M. F., & Lau, M. M. (1982). Assessment and training of clinical interviewing skills: Analogue analysis and field replication. *Journal of Applied Behavior Analysis, 15,* 191–203.

Jahr, E. (1998). Current issues in staff training. *Research in Developmental Disabilities, 19,* 73–87.

Jarbrink, K., Fombonne, E., & Knapp, M. (2003). Measuring the parental, service and cost impacts of children with autistic spectrum disorders: A pilot study. *Journal of Autism and Developmental Disorders, 33,* 395–402.

Jocelyn, L. J., Casiro, O. G., Beattie, D., Bow, J., & Kneisz, J. (1998). Treatment of children with autism: A randomized controlled trial to evaluate a caregiver-based intervention program in community day-care centers. *Journal of Developmental and Behavioral Pediatrics, 19,* 326–334.

Jones, F. H., Fremouw, W., & Carples, S. (1977). Pyramid training of elementary school teachers to use a classroom management skills package. *Journal of Applied Behavior Analysis, 10,* 239–253.

Judge, S. L. (1997). Parental perceptions of help-giving practices and control appraisals in early intervention programs. *Topics in Early Childhood Special Education, 17,* 457–476.

Kazdin, A. E. (1982). *Single-case research designs.* New York: Oxford University Press.

Kazdin, A. E. (1984). *Behavior modification in applied settings.* Homewood, IL: Dorsey Press.

Kissel, R. C., Whitman, T. L., & Reid, D. H. (1983). An institutional staff training and self-management program for developing multiple self-care skills in severely/profoundly retarded individuals. *Journal of Applied Behavior Analysis, 16,* 395–415.

Koegel, R. L., Bimbela, A., & Schreibman, L. (1996). Collateral effects of parent training on family interactions. *Journal of Autism and Developmental Disorders, 26,* 347–359.

Koegel, R. L., Russo, D. C., & Rincover, A. (1977). Assessing and training teachers in the generalized use of behavior modification with autistic children. *Journal of Applied Behavior Analysis, 10,* 197–205.

Koegel, R. L., Schreibman, L., Britten, K. R., Burke, J. C., & O'Neill, R. E. (1982). A comparison of parent training to direct child treatment. In R. L. Koegel, A. Rincover, & A. L. Egel (Eds.), *Educating and understanding autistic children* (pp. 260–279). San Diego, CA: College Hill.

Koshes, R. J. (1997). Use of fluoxetine for obsessive compulsive behavior in adults with autism. *American Journal of Psychiatry, 154,* 578.

Krantz, P. J., MacDuff, M. T., & McClannahan, L. E. (1993). Programming participation in family activities for children with autism: Parents' use of photographic activity schedules. *Journal of Applied Behavior Analysis, 26,* 137–138.

Krauss, M. W., Gulley, S., Sciegaj, M., & Wells, N. (2003). Access to specialty medical care for children with mental retardation, autism, and other special health care needs. *Mental Retardation, 41,* 329–339.

Kuhn, S. A. C., Lerman, D. C., & Vorndran, C. M. (2003). Pyramidal training for families of children with problem behavior. *Journal of Applied Behavior Analysis, 36,* 77–88.

Laski, K. E., Charlop, M. H., & Schreibman, L. (1988). Training parents to use the natural language paradigm to increase their autistic child's speech. *Journal of Applied Behavior Analysis, 21,* 391–400.

Lavie, T., & Sturmey, P. (2002). Training staff to conduct a paired-stimulus preference assessment. *Journal of Applied Behavior Analysis, 35,* 209–211.

Lobato, D. J., & Kao, B. T. (2002). Integrated sibling–parent group intervention to improve sibling knowledge and adjustment to chronic illness and disability. *Journal of Pediatric Psychology, 27,* 711–716.

Lovaas, O. I. (1987). Behavioral treatment and normal educational and intellectual functioning in young autistic children. *Journal of Consulting and Clinical Psychology, 55,* 3–9.

Mandell, D. S., Listerud, J., Levy, S. E., & Pinto-Martin, J. A. (2002). Race differences in age at diagnosis among Medicaid-eligible children with autism. *Journal of the American Academy of Child and Adolescent Psychiatry, 41,* 1447–1453.

McClannahan, L. E., & Krantz, P. J. (1993). On systems analysis in autism intervention programs. *Journal of Applied Behavior Analysis, 26,* 589–596.

McDougle, C. J., Holmes, J. P., Carlson, D. C., Pelton, G. H., Cohen, D. J., & Price, L. H. (1998). A double-blind placebo-controlled study of risperidone in adults with autistic disorder and other pervasive developmental disorders. *Archives of General Psychiatry, 55,* 633–641.

McDougle, C. J., Kresch, L. E., Goodman, W. K., Naylor, S. T., Volkmar, F. R., Cohen, D. J., et al. (1995). A case-controlled study of repetitive thoughts and behavior in adults with autistic disorder and obsessive-compulsive disorder. *American Journal of Psychiatry, 152,* 772–777.

McDougle, C. J., Kresch, L. E., & Posey, D. J. (2000). Repetitive thoughts and behavior in pervasive developmental disorders: Treatment with serotonin reuptake inhibitors. *Journal of Autism and Developmental Disorders, 30,* 427–435.

McGimsey, J. F., Greene, B. F., & Lutzker, J. R. (1995). Competence in aspects of behavioral treatment and consultation: Implications for service delivery and graduate training. *Journal of Applied Behavior Analysis, 28,* 301–315.

Meichenbaum, D., & Turk, D. C. (1987). *Facilitating treatment adherence: A practitioner's guidebook.* New York: Plenum Press.

Meyer, D. J., & Vadasy, P. F. (1994). *Sibshops: Workshops for siblings of children with special needs.* Baltimore: Brookes.

Miltenberger, R., Flessner, C., Gatheridge, B., Johnson, B., Satterlund, M., & Egemo, K. (2004). Evaluation of behavioral skills training to prevent gun play in children. *Journal of Applied Behavior Analysis, 37,* 513–516.

Moes, D. R., & Frea, W. D. (2002). Contextualized behavioral support in early intervention for children with autism and their families. *Journal of Autism and Developmental Disorders, 32,* 519–533.

Moore, S. T. (2002). *Asperger syndrome and the elementary school experience.* Shawnee Mission, KS: Autism Asperger Publishing.

Morgan, S. B. (1988). The autistic child and family functioning: A developmental family-systems perspective. *Journal of Autism and Developmental Disorders, 18,* 263–280.

Mueller, M. M., Piazza, C. C., Moore, J. W., Kelley, M. E., Bethke, S. A., Pruett, A. E., et al. (2003). Training parents to implement pediatric feeding protocols. *Journal of Applied Behavior Analysis, 36,* 545–562.

National Research Council. (2001). *Educating children with autism.* Committee on educational interventions for children with autism. C. Lord & J. P. McGee (Eds.), Division of Behavioral and Social Sciences and Education. Washington, DC: National Academy Press.

Neef, N. A. (1995). Pyramidal parent training by peers. *Journal of Applied Behavior Analysis, 28,* 333–337.

New Jersey Department of Education. (2004). *Autism program quality indicators.* Trenton: New Jersey Department of Education.

New York State Department of Health Early Intervention Program. (1999). *Clinical practice guideline. Report of the recommendations. Autism/pervasive developmental disorders.* Albany: New York Department of Health.

Nixon, C. D., & Singer, G. S. (1993). Group cognitive-behavioral treatment for excessive parental blame and guilt. *American Journal on Mental Retardation, 97,* 665–672.

Noell, G. H., & Witt, J. C. (1999). When does consultation lead to effective implementation? Critical issues for research and practice. *Journal of Special Education, 33,* 29–35.

Noell, G. H., Witt, J. C., LaFleur, L. H., Mortenson, B. P., Ranier, D. D., & LeVelle, J. (2000). Increasing intervention implementation in general education following consultation: A comparison of two follow-up strategies. *Journal of Applied Behavior Analysis, 33,* 271–284.

Northup, J., Edwards S., Gulley, V., Fusilier, I., Swanson, V., & Dunaway, D. (1999). A brief assessment of methylphenidate effects in the classroom. *Proven Practice, 1,* 49–54.

Northup, J., Fusilier, I., Swanson, V., Roane, H., & Borrero, J. (1997). An evaluation of methylphenidate as a potential establishing operation for some common classroom reinforcers. *Journal of Applied Behavior Analysis, 30,* 615–625.

Northup, J., George, T., Jones, K., & Broussard, C. (1996). A comparison of reinforcer assessment methods: The utility of verbal and pictorial choice procedures. *Journal of Applied Behavior Analysis, 29,* 201–212.

Page, T. J., Iwata, B. A., & Reid, D. H. (1982). Pyramidal training: A large-scale application with institutional staff. *Journal of Applied Behavior Analysis, 15,* 335–351.

Parsons, M. B., & Reid, D. H. (1995). Training residential supervisors to provide feedback for maintaining staff teaching skills with people who have severe difficulties. *Journal of Applied Behavior Analysis, 28,* 317–322.

Parsons, M. B., Reid, D. H., & Green, C. W. (1993). Preparing direct service staff to teach people with severe disabilities: A comprehensive evaluation of effective and acceptable training program. *Behavioral Residential Treatment, 8,* 163–186.

Parsonson, B. S., Baer, A. M., & Baer, D. M. (1974). The application of generalized correct social contingencies: An evaluation of a training program. *Journal of Applied Behavior Analysis, 7,* 427–437.

Peterson, L., Homer, A., & Wonderlich, S. (1982). The integrity of independent variables in behavior analysis. *Journal of Applied Behavior Analysis, 15,* 477–492.

Pommer, D. A., & Streedbeck, D. (1974). Motivating staff performance in an operant learning program for children. *Journal of Applied Behavior Analysis, 7,* 217–221.

Powell, J., Edwards, A., Edwards, M., Pandit, B. S., Sungum-Paliwal, S. R., & White-house, B. S. (2000). Changes in the incidence of childhood autism and other autistic spectrum disorders in preschool children from two areas of West Midlands, U.K. *Developmental Medicine and Child Neurology, 42,* 624–628.

Prieto-Bayard, M., & Baker, B. L. (1986). Parent training for Spanish speaking families with a retarded child. *Journal of Community Psychology, 14,* 134–143.

Reid, D. H., & Green, C. W. (1990). Staff training. In J. L. Matson (Ed.), *Handbook of behavior modification with the mentally retarded* (pp. 71–90). New York: Plenum Press.

Reid, D. H., & Parsons, M. B. (1995). Comparing choice and questionnaire measures of the acceptability of a staff training procedure. *Journal of Applied Behavior Analysis, 28,* 95–96.

Reid, D. H., Rotholz, D. A., Parsons, M. B., Morris, L., Braswell, B. A., Green, C. W., et al. (2003). Training human service supervisors in aspects of positive behavior support. Evaluation of a state-wide, performance-based program. *Journal of Positive Behavior Interventions, 5,* 35–46.

Richman, G. S., Riordan, M. R., Reiss, M. L., Pyles, D. A. M., & Bailey, J. S. (1988). The effects of self-monitoring and supervisor feedback on staff performance in a residential setting. *Journal of Applied Behavior Analysis, 21,* 401–409.

Rivers, J. W., & Stoneman, Z. (2003). Sibling relationships when a child has autism: Marital stress and support coping. *Journal of Autism and Developmental Disorders, 33,* 383–394.

Rodrigue, J. R., Geffken, G. R., & Morgan, S. B. (1993). Perceived competence and behavioral adjustment of siblings of children with autism. *Journal of Autism and Developmental Disorders, 23,* 665–674.

Ruble, L. A., Helfinger, C. A., Renfrew, J. W., & Saunders, R. C. (2005). Access and service use by children with autism spectrum disorders in Medicaid managed care. *Journal of Autism and Developmental Disorders, 35,* 3–13.

Rumsey, J. M., Rapoport, J. L., & Sceery, W. R. (1985). Autistic children as adults: Psychiatric, social, and behavioral outcomes. *Journal of the American Academy of Child Psychiatry, 24,* 465–473.

Rutter, M., Bailey, A., Simonoff, E., & Pickles, A. (1997). Genetic influences and autism. In D. J. Cohen & F. R. Volkmar (Eds.), *Handbook of autism and pervasive developmental disorders* (2nd ed., pp. 370–387). New York: Wiley.

Sarokoff, R. A., & Sturmey, P. (2004). The effects of behavioral skills training on staff implementation of discrete-trial training. *Journal of Applied Behavior Analysis, 37,* 535–538.

Schepis, M. M., Reid, D. H., Ownbey, J., & Parsons, M. B. (2001). Training support staff to embed teaching within natural routines of young children with disabilities in an inclusive preschool. *Journal of Applied Behavior Analysis, 34,* 313–327.

Schreibman, L., O'Neill, R. E., & Koegel, R. L. (1983). Behavioral training for siblings of autistic children. *Journal of Applied Behavior Analysis, 16*, 129–138.

Scorgie, K., & Sobsey, D. (2000). Transformational outcomes associated with parenting children who have disabilities. *Mental Retardation, 38*, 195–206.

Selinske, J. E., Greer, R. D., & Lodhi, S. (1991) A functional analysis of comprehensive application of behavior analysis to schooling. *Journal of Applied Behavior Analysis, 24*, 107–117.

Shook, G. L., & Favell, J. E. (1996). Identifying qualified professionals in behavior analysis. In C. Maurice, G. Green, & S. C. Luce (Eds.), *Behavioral intervention for young children with autism* (pp. 221–229). Austin TX: PRO-ED.

Shore, B. A., Iwata, B. A., Vollmer, T. R., Lerman, D. C., & Zarcone, J. R. (1995). Pyramidal staff training in the extension of treatment for severe behavior disorders. *Journal of Applied Behavior Analysis, 28*, 323–332.

Singh, A. N., Matson, J. L., Cooper, C. L., Dixon, D., & Sturmey, P. (2005.) The use of risperidone among individuals with mental retardation: Clinically supported or not? *Research in Developmental Disabilities, 26*, 203–218.

Sivberg, B. (2002). Family system and coping behaviors. *Autism, 6*, 397–409.

Skinner, D. G., Bailey, D. B., Correa, V., & Rodriguez, P. (1999). Narrating self and disability: Latino mothers' construction of identities vis-à-vis their child with special needs. *Exceptional Children, 65*, 481–495.

Skinner, D. G., Correa, V., Skinner, M., & Bailey, D. B. (2001). Role of religion in the lives of Latino families of young children with developmental delays. *American Journal on Mental Retardation, 106*, 297–313.

Smith, T., Groen, A. D., & Wynn, J. W. (2000). Randomized trial of intensive early intervention for children with pervasive developmental disorder. *American Journal on Mental Retardation, 105*, 269–285.

Smith Myles, B., & Southwick, J. (1999). *Asperger Syndrome and difficult moments: Practical solutions for tantrums, rage, and meltdowns.* Shawnee Mission, KS: Autism Asperger Publishing.

Sofronoff, K., & Farbotko, M. (2002). The effectiveness of parent management training to increase self-efficacy in parents of children with Asperger disorder. *Autism, 6*, 271–286.

Steingard, R. J., Zimnitsky, B., DeMaso, D. R., Bauman, M. L., & Bucci, J. P. (1997). Sertraline treatment of transition-induced anxiety and agitation in children with autistic disorder. *Journal of Child and Adolescent Psychopharmacology, 7*, 9–15.

Stoneman, Z., Brody, G. H., Davis, C. H., Crapps, J. M., & Malone, D. M. (1991). Ascribed role relations between children with mental retardation and their younger siblings. *American Journal on Mental Retardation, 95*, 537–550.

Sturmey, P. (2005.) Secretin is an ineffective treatment for pervasive developmental disabilities: A review of 15 double-blind randomized controlled trials. *Research in Developmental Disabilities, 26*, 87–97.

Tsai, L. (1996). Brief report: Comorbid psychiatric disorders in autistic disorders. *Journal of Autism and Developmental Disorders, 26*, 159–164.

Tunali, B., & Power, T. G. (2002). Coping by redefinition: Cognitive appraisals in mothers of children with autism and children without autism. *Journal of Autism and Developmental Disorders, 32*, 25–34.

Van Houten, R., Axelrod, S., Bailey, J. S., Foxx, R. M., Iwata, B. A., & Lovaas, O. I. (1988). The right to effective behavioral treatment. *Journal of Applied Behavior Analysis, 21*, 381–384.

Volkmar, F. R., Klin, A., & Cohen, D. J. (1997). Diagnosis and classification of autism and related conditions: Consensus and issues. In D. J. Cohen & F. R. Volkmar (Eds.), *Handbook of autism and pervasive developmental disorders* (2nd ed., pp. 5–40). New York: Wiley.

Wallace, M. D., Doney, J. K., Mintz-Resudek, C. M., & Tarbox, R. S. F. (2004). Training educators to implement functional analyses. *Journal of Applied Behavior Analysis, 37*, 89–92.

Watson, L. S., & Uzzell, R. A. (1980). A program for teaching behavior modification skills to institutional staff. *Applied Research in Mental Retardation, 1*, 41–53.

Weiss, M. J. (2002). Hardiness and social support as predictors of stress in mothers of typical children, children with autism, and children with mental retardation. *Autism, 6*, 115–130.

Winnett, R. A., Kramer, K. D., Walker, W. B., Malone, S. W., & Lane, M. K. (1988). Modifying food purchases in supermarkets with modeling, feedback and goal-setting procedures. *Journal of Applied Behavior Analysis, 21*, 73–80.

Witt, J. C., Noell, G. H., LaFleur, L. H., & Mortenson, B. P. (1997). Teacher use of interventions in general education settings: Measurement and analysis of the independent variable. *Journal of Applied Behavior Analysis, 30*, 693–696.

Wolery, M. (1997). Encounters with general early education: Lessons being learned. *Journal of Behavioral Education, 7*, 91–98.

Wright, P. W. D., & Wright, P. D. (1999). *Wrightslaw: Special education law.* Hartfield, VA: Harbor House Law Press.

Zaharia, E. S., & Baumeister, A. A. (1979). Technician losses in public residential facilities. *American Journal of Mental Deficiency, 84*, 36–39.

Author Index

Wright, P. D., 252
Wright, P. W. D., 252
Wynn, J. W., 243

Yarbrough, S. C., 15
Yeargin-Allsopp, M., 7
Yeung-Courchesne, R., 6

Yoder, P., 174, 176
Young, A., 59, 113
Young, J. M., 59
Young, P. J., 92

Zager, D. B., 85
Zaharia, E. S., 242

Zanolli, K., 127, 128, 130, 133, 134, 138
Zarcone, J. R., 12, 193, 204, 209, 216, 221, 241
Zeiler, M., 212
Zhou, L., 70, 94
Zimnitsky, B., 248

SUBJECT INDEX

AAC. *See* Augmentative and alternative communication (AAC) systems
ABA. *See* Applied behavior analysis (ABA)
ABC recording, 199–201
ABLLS. *See Assessment of Basic Language and Learning Skills* (ABLLS)
Access to services, 250–252
Activity schedules. *See* Schedules
ADHD (Attention-Deficit/Hyperactivity Disorder), 250
Adult-mediated interventions for social behavior, 129–137, 143
African Americans, 250, 252
Aggression, 188
Analog analyses, 193
Anecdotal assessment, 203–204
Angelman syndrome, 166
Antecedent-based interventions for problem behaviors, 215–217
Antecedent-behavior-consequence (ABC) model, 199–201
Anticonvulsant medications, 248
Antidepressant medications, 248
Antihypertensive medications, 248
Antipsychotic medications, 8, 20–21, 247–248
Applied behavior analysis (ABA). *See also* Communication intervention; Readiness skills; Self-help skills; Social behavior
    basic principles and key elements of, 12, 39, 41–42
    behaviorism and, 9–11
    certification of behavior analysts, 252–253
    for children with autism generally, 11–16
    conclusion on, 71–72
    current issues and future directions of, 18–20

    current status of, 15–16
    definition of, 7, 31
    development of, 12–15
    for difficult problems generally, 16–18
    discrimination and generalization in, 42–56, 72–73
    environment as causal agent and, 34–35
    generalization strategies for, 13
    goal of, 34–35
    incidental teaching methods and, 14
    misconceptions about, 32–34
    origins of, 11–12
    practitioner recommendations on, 21, 72–74
    prompting procedures in, 56–64
    reinforcement in and reinforcers for, 41–42, 64–71
    as science of the individual, 36–39
    for social interaction, 17–18
    systems level approach to, 15
    training in, 18–19, 235–244
    for verbal behavior, 16–17
Arbitrary matching-to-sample, 47–48, 50, 51, 52, 72–73
ASD. *See* Autism Spectrum Disorders (ASD)
Asperger's Disorder, 4–5, 6, 115–116
Assessment
    ABC recording, 199–201
    anecdotal assessment, 203–204
    of communication skills, 154–157
    continuous recording, 201–203
    experimental (or functional) analysis, 192–197
    functional assessment, 192–206
    functional behavioral assessment, 192
    scatter plots, 197–199
    stimulus preference assessment (SPA), 67–71, 73–74, 137

CONTRIBUTORS

William H. Ahearn, PhD, BCBA serves as the director of research at the New England Center for Children and is a clinical assistant professor in Northeastern University's Master's Program in Applied Behavior Analysis. Dr. Ahearn's research interests include pediatric feeding disorders, behavioral economics, behavioral momentum, and translating basic learning principles into practical applications.

William V. Dube, PhD received his doctorate in experimental psychology from Northeastern University in 1987. He is a senior scientist at the University of Massachusetts Medical School (UMMS) Shriver Center and associate professor of psychiatry at UMMS. Dr. Dube's research interests include stimulus control, discrimination learning, and behavioral choice in individuals with developmental disabilities.

Adrienne Fitzer, MA is an advanced doctoral student in the Learning Processes Program, a subprogram of Psychology at the Graduate Center, City University of New York, and a Board Certified Behavior Analyst. She has worked with learners with autism and other developmental delays for ten years. Her research interest is in the applied use of stimulus equivalence technology with learners with varying disabilities, and she has coauthored several papers that have been published in the *Journal of the Experimental Analysis of Behavior* in the area of categorization and concept learning.

Richard B. Graff, MS, BCBA is a program director at The New England Center for Children. He currently serves on the editorial boards of the *Journal of Applied Behavior Analysis* and *Behavioral Interventions*. He also teaches in Northeastern University's Master's Program in Applied Behavior Analysis. His research interests include preference and reinforcer assessment and the effects of choice on behavior.

Sandra L. Harris, PhD is a Board of Governors Distinguished Service Professor of Clinical Psychology at the Graduate School of Applied and Professional Psychology and the Department of Psychology at Rutgers, The State University of New Jersey. She is executive director of the Douglass Developmental Disabilities Center, a Rutgers program for people with autism. Her most recent book, *Incentives for Change: Motivating People with Autism Spectrum Disorders to Learn and Gain Independence*, is coauthored with Lara Delmolino.

Giulio E. Lancioni, PhD received his PhD in Child Development and Psychology from the University of Kansas in 1978. He is professor in the Department of Psychology at the University of Bari, Italy. His research interests include development and evaluation of assistive technologies, social skills training, and strategies for examining and teaching choice and preference to individuals with severe or profound and multiple disabilities.

Robert H. LaRue, PhD is a research assistant professor at the Graduate School of Applied and Professional Psychology at Rutgers University. He is the Assistant Director of Training at the Douglass Developmental Disabilities Center (DDDC). He earned a dual doctorate in biological and school psychology from Louisiana State University. He has coauthored articles published in peer-reviewed journals and presented at national and international conferences. He currently supervises several doctoral students providing behavioral consultation at the DDDC.

Linda A. LeBlanc, PhD is an associate professor of psychology at Western Michigan University (WMU). She is the codirector of the WMU Center for Autism, a university-based outpatient clinic serving families of children with ASD. Her primary research interests in the area of autism and developmental disabilities are interventions for language and social skills and patterns of development of ritualistic behavior in children with autism. She has published many articles and book chapters on language and social skills interventions and has served on the editorial boards of several journals focusing on behavioral interventions for children with special needs.

Dorothea C. Lerman, PhD is an associate professor of psychology at the University of Houston, Clear Lake, where she is the coordinator of a graduate program in applied behavior analysis. Her primary research interests include the functional analysis and treatment of behavior disorders, early intervention, and teacher training. She has served as associate editor for two journals focusing on behavioral interventions and has published numerous articles in this area.

Rebecca MacDonald, PhD, BCBA serves as the Director of Intensive Instructional Preschool Program at the New England Center for Children. She is an adjunct professor in Northeastern University's Master's Program in Applied Behavior Analysis. Dr. MacDonald's research interests currently include assessing and teaching joint attention skills, teaching play and social reciprocity, and measuring clinical outcomes of early intensive behavior intervention.

David McAdam, PhD received his doctoral degree in Developmental and Child Psychology from the University of Kansas and is a Board Certified Behavior Analyst. Currently, he is a senior instructor in pediatrics at the University of Rochester School of Medicine. His current research interests include the stereotypic behaviors of persons with autism, preference assessment procedures, and the functional analysis of problem behavior.

Deborah Napolitano, PhD, BCBA is senior instructor in pediatrics at the University of Rochester Medical Center. She is a coinvestigator in a study funded by the National Institute on Child Health and Human Development on compulsive food seeking and food motivation in Prader-Willi syndrome. She also has coauthored several papers on medication evaluation and treatment in persons with developmental disabilities.

Mark F. O'Reilly, PhD obtained his PhD in special education at the University of Illinois. He is currently a professor for the Autism and Developmental Disabilities Program in the Department of Special Education at the University of Texas at Austin. His research interests include behavior analysis (especially examining how basic principles of behavior can be translated into applied settings), self-injury (particularly biobehavioral interactions), and social skills training (effectiveness of cognitive–behavioral models of intervention).

Ruth Anne Rehfeldt, PhD is an assistant professor in the Rehabilitation Services Program in the Rehabilitation Institute at Southern Illinois University. She also has academic responsibilities in the Behavior Analysis and Therapy program and Doctoral program within the Rehabilitation Institute. She is a Board Certified Behavior Analyst with more than 55 published articles and book chapters focused primarily on autism and other developmental disabilities. Her interests are largely concentrated on derived relational responding, stimulus equivalence, and verbal behavior in such populations. Dr. Rehfeldt is a member of Phi Kappa Phi Honor Society and has been awarded the Rehabilitation Institute's Teacher of the Year Award for 2001, 2002, and 2004. She is currently an editorial board member of both the *Journal of Applied Behavior Analysis* and *Journal of the Experimental Analysis of Behavior.*

Rocio Rosales is a graduate student in the Master's program for Behavior Analysis and Therapy at Southern Illinois University, Carbondale, and holds a BA in psychology from the University of Nevada, Reno (2001). She is a Board Certified Associate Behavior Analyst and has served children with autism in public schools, homes, and center-based settings. Her research interests include assessment and treatment for children with ASD, skill acquisition in adults with developmental disabilities, and verbal behavior. She is a member of the Outstanding Student Honor Society and the Golden Key National Honor Society and has been a recipient of a number of academic achievement awards.

Ralf W. Schlosser, PhD received his PhD in special education from Purdue University in 1994. He currently holds an appointment as an associate professor in the Department of Speech–Language Pathology and Audiology at Northeastern University in Boston. He teaches in the area of augmentative and alternative communication, evidence-based practice, and research design. Dr. Schlosser has published 37 peer-reviewed articles, nine book chapters, and two books related to augmentative and alternative communication.

Jeff Sigafoos, PhD received his PhD in educational psychology from the University of Minnesota in 1990. His most recent appointment is as professor of education and director of the Centre for Transforming Learning Communities within the School of Education at the University of Tasmania. He teaches in the area of developmental disabilities and conducts research on communication intervention, use of assistive technology, and assessment and treatment of challenging behavior. He has published more than 100 journal articles and four books describing educational and behavioral interventions for individuals with developmental disabilities.

Richard G. Smith, PhD is associate professor and chair of the Department of Behavior Analysis at the University of North Texas. His research interests include assessment and treatment of behavior disorders in persons with developmental disabilities, translational research on behavioral principles underlying intervention effects, and assessment of antecedent influences on behavior. Dr. Smith is currently serving as associate editor for the *Journal of Applied Behavior Analysis* and was the 1998 recipient of the B. F. Skinner New Researcher Award (American Psychological Association [APA]), as well as the 2002 Texas Association on Mental Retardation Distinguished Research Award.

Tristram Smith, PhD is an assistant professor of pediatrics at the University of Rochester Medical Center (URMC). He serves as the research director for the Multisite Young Autism Project, which is a federally funded study on early, intensive behavioral intervention based on the UCLA/Lovaas model for children with autism. He is also an investigator in a study in the Center for Studies to Advance Autism Research and Treatment at the University of Rochester. He has authored or coauthored a number of the most widely cited studies on treatment outcomes for individuals with ASD.

Claire St. Peter Pipkin is a doctoral student at the University of Florida. Her primary research interests include the assessment and treatment of maladaptive behavior in school settings, including treatment integrity failures, and the effects of history on current responding. She is also interested in translational research and the basic-to-applied continuum, especially the use of human operant preparations to inform applied work. She has been the recipient of the Sidney and Janet Bijou Fellowship, University of Florida Alumni Fellowship, and Adele Lewis Grant.

Peter Sturmey, PhD is a professor at Queens College, City University of New York and a faculty member in the Learning Processes and Neuropsychology Programs of the Graduate Center, City University of New York. He is also affiliated with the doctoral internship in psychology program at Louisiana State University and Pinecrest Developmental Center and is an honorary senior lecturer at the GKT Dental Institute, Kings College, London. He has published several books, including *Functional Analysis in Clinical Psychology*, more than 100 peer-reviewed papers, and more than 25 book chapters related to applied behavior analysis and developmental disabilities. He is on the editorial board of several journals, including *Research in Developmental Disabilities, Journal of Positive Behavioral Interventions, Journal of Applied Research in Intellectual Disabilities, International Journal of Consultation and Therapy, Journal of Intellectual Disabilities Research,* and *Research in Autism Spectrum Disorders.*

Valerie M. Volkert, MS is currently working on a doctoral degree in school psychology at Louisiana State University. Her current research interests include the treatment of behavior disorders, side effects of extinction, variables that influence interspersal procedures, and interventions for social behavior in children with autism.

Timothy R. Vollmer, PhD is an associate professor at the University of Florida. His primary research interest is applied behavior analysis, with an emphasis on developmental disabilities. His research spans the basic-to-applied spectrum with studies in an operant rat lab, an operant human lab, and school-based applications. Additionally, he is the primary investigator for an ongoing project in conjunction with the Florida Department of Children in Families, teaching parenting skills to foster parents. Dr. Vollmer is a past associate editor of the *Journal of Applied Behavior Analysis,* was the 1996 recipient of the B. F. Skinner New Researcher Award (APA), the 2004 Distinguished Contributions to Applied Behavior Analysis Award (APA), and the University of Florida Research Foundation Professorship.

Mary Jane Weiss, PhD is a research associate professor of clinical psychology at the Graduate School of Applied and Professional Psychology, Rutgers University. She is the director of the Division of Research and Training at the Douglass Developmental Disabilities Center at Rutgers. One of her most recent books, *Reaching out, Joining in: Teaching Social Skills to Young Children with Autism,* is co-authored with Sandra Harris.